DIFFERENTIAL EQUATION ANALYSIS IN BIOMEDICAL SCIENCE AND ENGINEERING

DIFFERENTIAL EQUATION ANALYSIS IN BIOMEDICAL SCIENCE AND ENGINEERING

ORDINARY DIFFERENTIAL EQUATION APPLICATIONS WITH R

William E. Schiesser
Department of Chemical Engineering
Lehigh University
Bethlehem, PA

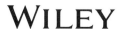

Copyright © 2014 by John Wiley & Sons, Inc. All rights reserved.

Published by John Wiley & Sons, Inc., Hoboken, New Jersey.
Published simultaneously in Canada.

For general information on our other products and services or for technical support, please contact our Customer Care Department within the United States at (800) 762-2974, outside the United States at (317) 572-3993 or fax (317) 572-4002.

Wiley also publishes its books in a variety of electronic formats. Some content that appears in print may not be available in electronic formats. For more information about Wiley products, visit our web site at www.wiley.com.

Library of Congress Cataloging-in-Publication Data:

Schiesser, W. E.
    Differential equation analysis in biomedical science and engineering : ordinary differential equation applications with R / William E. Schiesser, Department of Chemical Engineering, Lehigh University, Bethlehem, PA.
        pages cm
    Includes bibliographical references and index.
    ISBN 978-1-118-70548-3 (cloth)
    1. Biomedical engineering–Mathematics. 2. Biomathematics. 3. Bioreactors–Data processing. 4. Differential equations. I. Title.
    R857.M34O34 2013
    610.280285–dc23

                                                                        2013020440

Printed in the United States of America.
10 9 8 7 6 5 4 3 2 1

To John Backus and Leon Lapidus,
and their research groups

CONTENTS

■■■■■ PREFACE

This book focuses on the rapidly expanding development and use of computer-based mathematical models in the life sciences, designated here as biomedical science and engineering (BMSE). The mathematical models are stated as systems of ordinary differential equations (ODEs) and generally come from papers in the current research literature that typically include the following steps:

1. The model is presented as a system of ODEs that explain associated chemistry, physics, biology, and physiology.
2. A numerical solution to the model equations is presented, particularly a discussion of the important features of the solution.

What is missing in this two-step approach are the details of how the solution was computed, particularly the details of the numerical algorithms. Also, because of the limited length of a research paper, the computer code used to produce the numerical solution is not provided. Thus, for the reader to reproduce (confirm) the solution and extend it is virtually impossible with reasonable effort.

The intent of this book is to fill in the steps for selected example applications that will give the reader the knowledge to reproduce and possibly extend the numerical solutions with reasonable effort. Specifically, the numerical algorithms are discussed in some detail, with additional background references, so that the reader will have some understanding of how the calculations were performed, and a set of transportable routines in R^1 is provided so that the reader can execute to produce and extend the solutions.

Thus, the typical format of a chapter includes the following steps:

1. The model is presented as a system of ODEs with explanation of the associated chemistry, physics, biology, and physiology. The requirements of a well-posed set of equations such as the number of dependent variables, the number of ODEs, algebraic equations used to calculate intermediate variables, and the initial conditions for the ODEs are included (which is often not the case in research papers so that all of the details of the model are not included or known to the reader).

2. The features of the model that determine the selection of numerical algorithms are discussed; for example, how derivatives are approximated, whether the ODEs are nonstiff or stiff, and therefore, whether an explicit or implicit integration algorithm is used. The computational requirements of the particular selected algorithms are identified such as the solution of nonlinear equations, banded matrix processing, or sparse matrix processing.

3. The routines that are the programming of the ODEs and numerical algorithms are completely listed and then each section of code is explained, including referral to the mathematical model and the algorithms. Thus, all of the computational details for producing a numerical solution are in one place. Referring to another source for the software, possibly with little or no documentation, is thereby avoided.

4. A numerical solution to the model equations is presented, particularly a discussion of the important features of the solution.

---

[1] R is a quality open source scientific programming system that can be easily downloaded from the Internet (http://www.R-project.org/). In particular, R has (i) vector-matrix operations that facilitate the programming of linear algebra, (ii) a library of quality ODE integrators, and (iii) graphical utilities for the presentation of the numerical solutions. All of these features and utilities are demonstrated through the applications in this book.

5. The accuracy of the computed solution is inferred using established methods such as h and p refinement. Alternative algorithms and computational details are considered, particularly to extend the model and the numerical solution.

In this way, a complete picture of the model and its computer implementation is provided without having to try to fill in the details of the numerical analysis, algorithms, and computer programming (often a time-consuming procedure that leads to an incomplete and unsatisfactory result). The presentation is not heavily mathematical, for example, no theorems and proofs, but rather is in terms of detailed examples of BMSE applications.

End of the chapter problems have not been provided. Rather, the instructor can readily construct problems and assignments that will be in accordance with the interests and objectives of the instructor. This can be done in several ways by developing variations and extensions of the applications discussed in the chapters. For example,

1. Parameters in the model equations can be varied, and the effects on the computed solutions are observed and explained. Exploratory questions can be posed such as whether the changes in the solutions are as expected. In addition, the terms in the right- hand sides (RHSs) of the ODEs (without the derivatives in the independent variable) can be computed and displayed numerically and graphically to explain in detail why the parameter changes had the observed effect. The computation and display of ODE RHS terms is illustrated in selected chapters to serve as a guide.

2. Additional terms can be added to the ODE RHSs to model physical, chemical, and biological effects that might be significant in determining the characteristics of the problem system. These additional terms can be computed and displayed along with the original terms to observe which terms have a significant effect on the computed model solution.

3. One or more ODEs can be added to an existing model to include additional phenomena that are considered possibly relevant to the analysis and understanding of the problem system.

4. An entirely new model can be proposed and programmed for comparison with an existing model. The existing routines might serve as a starting point, for example, a template.

These suggested problem formats are in the order of increasing generality to encourage the reader to explore new directions, including the revision of an existing model and the creation of a new model. This process is facilitated through the availability of existing routines for a model that can first be executed and then modified. The trial-and-error development of a model can be explored, particularly if experimental data that can be used as the basis for model development are provided, starting from parameter estimation based on the comparison of experimentally measured data and computed solutions from an existing model up to the development of a new model to interpret the data.

The focus of this book is primarily on models expressed as systems of ODEs that generally result by neglecting spatial effects so that the dependent variables of ODE, for example, concentrations, are uniform in space. The independent variable of the ODE systems is, therefore, time in most applications.

The assumption of spatial uniformity is quite accurate for a spectrum of BMSE systems, for example, a mixed reactor as considered in Chapter 1. However, the assumption of spatial uniformity is not correct for BMSE systems that function according to the spatial distribution of their principal variables, such as corneal curvature discussed in the concluding Chapter 8. This chapter, therefore, serves as an introduction to models based on partial differential equations (PDEs) in which both space and time are the independent variables. The additional spatial variables require boundary conditions for a complete specification of the PDE model. These details are introduced in Chapter 8 and are considered in detail in a companion volume titled *Differential Equation Analysis in Biomedical Science and Engineering: Partial Differential Equation Applications with R.*

In summary, my intention is to provide a set of basic computational procedures for ODE/PDE models in the two volumes that readers can use with modest effort without becoming deeply involved in the details of the numerical methods for ODE/PDEs and computer programming. All of the R routines discussed in the two volumes are available from a software download site, booksupport.wiley.com, which requires the ISBN: 9781118705483 for the ODE volume or 9781118705186 for the PDE volume. I welcome comments and will be pleased to respond to questions to the extent possible by e-mail (wes1@lehigh.edu).

WILLIAM E. SCHIESSER

Bethlehem, PA
January 2014

## CHAPTER 1

Introduction to Ordinary Differential Equation Analysis: Bioreactor Dynamics

1.1 Introduction

Mathematical models formulated as systems of ordinary differential equations (ODEs) and partial differential equations (PDEs) have been reported for a spectrum of applications in biomedical science and engineering (BMSE). The intent of this research is to provide a quantitative understanding of the biological, chemical, and physical phenomena that determine the characteristics of BMSE systems and to provide a framework for the analysis and interpretation of experimental data observed in the study of BMSE systems.

In the subsequent discussion in this chapter, we consider the programming of a 7×7 (seven equations in seven unknowns) ODE system to illustrate the integration (solution) of ODE systems using R, a quality, open source, scientific programming system [10]. The intent is to provide the reader with a complete and thoroughly documented example of the numerical integration of an ODE system, including (i) the use of library ODE integrators, (ii) the programming of ODE integration algorithms, and (iii) graphical output of the numerical solutions. This example application can then serve as a prototype or template which the reader can modify and extend for an ODE model of interest.

Differential Equation Analysis in Biomedical Science and Engineering: Ordinary Differential Equation Applications with R, First Edition. William E. Schiesser.
© 2014 John Wiley & Sons, Inc. Published 2014 by John Wiley & Sons, Inc.

1.2   A 7 × 7 ODE System for a Bioreactor

The reaction system for the conversion of xylose to ethanol by fermentation is now formulated and coded (programmed) in R. The ODE model is discussed in detail in [1, pp 35–42]; this discussion is recommended as a starting point for the details of the chemical reactions, particularly the various intermediates, so that the discussion to follow can concentrate on the numerical algorithms and R programming.

The reaction system is given in Table 1.1.

TABLE 1.1   Summary of reactions.[a]

Reaction Number	Reaction Stoichiometry
1	xylose $\rightleftharpoons$ xylitol
2	xylitol $\rightleftharpoons$ xylulose
3	2 xylulose $\rightleftharpoons$ 3 acetaldehyde
4	acetaldehyde $\rightleftharpoons$ ethanol
5	acetaldehyde $\rightleftharpoons$ acetate
6	2 xylulose $\rightleftharpoons$ 3 glycerol

[a] From [1], Table 2.1, p 39.

The corresponding ODE system is [1, p 39]

$$\frac{d[\text{xylose}]}{dt} = -J_1 \tag{1.1a}$$

$$\frac{d[\text{xylitol}]}{dt} = J_1 - J_2 \tag{1.1b}$$

$$\frac{d[\text{xylulose}]}{dt} = J_2 - 2J_3 - 2J_6 \tag{1.1c}$$

$$\frac{d[\text{acetaldehyde}]}{dt} = 3J_3 - J_4 - J_5 \tag{1.1d}$$

$$\frac{d[\text{ethanol}]}{dt} = J_4 \tag{1.1e}$$

$$\frac{d[\text{acetate}]}{dt} = J_5 \tag{1.1f}$$

$$\frac{d[\text{glycerol}]}{dt} = 3J_6 \tag{1.1g}$$

The concentrations in eqs. (1.1), denoted as [ ], are expressed in total (intraplus extracellular) moles per unit cell dry weight.

J_1 to J_6 are the kinetic rates for the six reactions listed in Table 1.1. The multiplying constants are stoichiometric coefficients. For example, reaction 3 (with rate J_3) in Table 1.1 produces 3 mol of acetaldehyde for every 2 mol of xylulose consumed. Therefore, eq. (1.1c) for $d[\text{xylulose}]/dt$ has -2 multiplying J_3 and eq. (1.1d) for $d[\text{acetaldehyde}]/dt$ has $+3$ multiplying J_3.

The reaction rates, J_1 to J_6, are expressed through mass action kinetics.

$$J_1 = k_1[\text{xylose}] \tag{1.2a}$$

$$J_2 = k_2[\text{xylitol}] - k_{-2}[\text{xylulose}][\text{ethanol}] \tag{1.2b}$$

$$J_3 = k_3[\text{xylulose}] - k_{-3}[\text{acetaldehyde}][\text{ethanol}] \tag{1.2c}$$

$$J_4 = k_4[\text{acetaldehyde}] \tag{1.2d}$$

$$J_5 = k_5[\text{acetaldehyde}] \tag{1.2e}$$

$$J_6 = k_6[\text{xylulose}] \tag{1.2f}$$

Note in particular the product terms for the reverse reactions in eqs. (1.2b) and (1.2c), $-k_{-2}[\text{xylulose}][\text{ethanol}]$ and $-k_{-3}[\text{acetaldehyde}][\text{ethanol}]$, which are nonlinear and therefore make the associated ODEs nonlinear (with right-hand side (RHS) terms in eqs. (1.1) that include J_2 and J_3). This nonlinearity precludes the usual procedures for the analytical solution of ODEs based on the linear algebra, that is, a numerical procedure is required for the solution of eqs. (1.1).

k_1 to k_6, k_{-2}, k_{-3}, in eqs. (1.2) are kinetic constants (adjustable parameters) that are selected so that the model output matches experimental data in some manner, for example, a least squares sense. Two sets of numerical values are listed in Table 1.2

BP000 refers to a wild-type yeast strain, while BP10001 refers to an engineered yeast strain.

TABLE 1.2   Kinetic constants for two yeast strains.[a]

Parameter	Value (BP000)	Value (BP10001)	Units
k_1	7.67×10^{-3}	8.87×10^{-3}	h^{-1}
k_2	3.60	13.18	h^{-1}
k_3	0.065	0.129	h^{-1}
k_4	0.867	0.497	h^{-1}
k_5	0.045	0.027	h^{-1}
k_6	1.15×10^{-3}	0.545×10^{-3}	h^{-1}
k_{-2}	88.0	88.7	$gh^{-1} \, mol^{-1}$
k_{-3}	99.0	99.9	$gh^{-1} \, mol^{-1}$

[a]From [1], Table 2.2, p 41.

To complete the specification of the ODE system, each of eqs. (1.1) requires an initial condition (IC) (and only one IC because these equations are first order in t).

TABLE 1.3   Initial conditions (ICs) for eqs. (1.1).

Equation	IC (t=0)
(1.1a)	[xylose] = 0.10724
(1.1b)	[xylitol] = 0
(1.1c)	[xylulose] = 0
(1.1d)	[acetaldehyde] = 0
(1.1e)	[ethanol] = 0
(1.1f)	[acetate] = 0
(1.1g)	[glycerol] = 0

The 7×7 ODE system is now completely defined and we can proceed to programming the numerical solution.

1.3 In-Line ODE Routine

An ODE routine for eqs. (1.1) is listed in the following.

```
#
# Library of R ODE solvers
```

```
  library("deSolve")
#
# Parameter values for BP10001
  k1=8.87e-03;
  k2=13.18;
  k3=0.129;
  k4=0.497;
  k5=0.027;
  k6=0.545e-3;
  km2=87.7;
  km3=99.9;
#
# Initial condition
  yini=c(y1=0.10724,y2=0,y3=0,y4=0,y5=0,y6=0,y7=0)
  yini
  ncall=0;
#
# t interval
  nout=51
  times=seq(from=0,to=2000,by=40)
#
# ODE programming
  bioreactor_1=function(t,y,parms) {
  with(as.list(y),
    {
#
# Assign state variables:
  xylose       =y1;
  xylitol      =y2;
  xylulose     =y3;
  acetaldehyde=y4;
  ethanol      =y5;
  acetate      =y6;
  glycerol     =y7;
#
# Fluxes
  J1=k1*xylose;
  J2=k2*xylitol-km2*xylulose*ethanol;
  J3=k3*xylulose-km3*acetaldehyde*ethanol;
  J4=k4*acetaldehyde;
  J5=k5*acetaldehyde;
```

```
  J6=k6*xylulose;
#
# Time derivatives
  f1=-J1;
  f2=J1-J2;
  f3=J2-2*J3-2*J6;
  f4=3*J3-J4-J5;
  f5=J4;
  f6=J5;
  f7=3*J6;
#
# Calls to bioreactor_1
  ncall <<- ncall+1
#
# Return derivative vector
  list(c(f1,f2,f3,f4,f5,f6,f7))
  })
}
#
# ODE integration
  out=ode(y=yini,times=times,func=bioreactor_1,parms=NULL)
#
# ODE numerical solution
  for(it in 1:nout){
   if(it==1){
   cat(sprintf(
   "\n        t      y1      y2      y3      y4      y5
     y6       y7"))}
   cat(sprintf("\n %8.0f%8.4f%8.4f%8.4f%8.4f%8.4f%8.4f
     %8.4f",
   out[it,1],out[it,2],out[it,3],out[it,4],
   out[it,5],out[it,6],out[it,7],out[it,8]))
   }
#
# Calls to bioreactor_1
  cat(sprintf("\n ncall = %5d\n\n",ncall))
#
# Set of 7 plots
  plot(out)
```

Listing 1.1: ODE routine.

We can note the following details about Listing 1.1.

- The R library of ODE numerical integrators, deSolve, is specified. The contents of this library will be discussed subsequently through examples.

```
#
# Library of R ODE solvers
  library("deSolve")
```

- The parameters from Table 1.2 for the engineered yeast strain BP10001 are defined numerically.

```
#
# Parameter values for BP10001
  k1=8.87e-03;
  k2=13.18;
  k3=0.129;
  k4=0.497;
  k5=0.027;
  k6=0.545e-3;
  km2=87.7;
  km3=99.9;
```

- The ICs of Table 1.3 are defined numerically through the use of the R vector utility c (which defines a vector, in this case yini). This statement illustrates a feature of R that requires careful attention, that is, there are reserved names such as c that should not be used in other ways such as the definition of a variable with the name c.

```
#
# Initial condition
  yini=c(y1=0.10724,y2=0,y3=0,y4=0,y5=0,y6=0,y7=0)
  yini
  ncall=0;
```

Also, the naming of the variables is open for choice (except for reserved names). Here, we select something easy to program, that is, $y1$ to $y7$ but programming in terms of problem-oriented variables is illustrated subsequently. Also, the elements in the

IC vector `yini` are displayed by listing the name of the vector on a separate line. This is an obvious but important step to ensure that the ICs are correct as a starting point for the solution. Finally, the number of calls to the ODE function, `bioreactor_1`, is initialized.

- The values of t (in eqs. (1.1)) at which the solution is to be displayed are defined as the vector `times`. In this case, the R function `seq` is used to define the sequence of 51 values $t = 0, 40, \ldots, 2000$.

```
#
# t interval
  nout=51
  times=seq(from=0,to=2000,by=40)
```

To give good resolution (smoothness) of the plots of the solutions, 51 was selected (discussed subsequently).

- Eqs. (1.1) are programmed in a function `bioreactor_1`.

```
#
# ODE programming
  bioreactor_1=function(t,y,parms) {
  with(as.list(y),
    {
```

We can note the following details about function `bioreactor_1`.

— The function is defined with three input arguments, `t,y,parms`. Also, a left brace, `{`, is used to start the function that is matched with a right brace, `}`, at the end of the function.

— The input argument `y` is a list (rather than a numerical vector) specified with `with(as.list(y)`, (this statement is optional and is not used in subsequent ODE routines). The second `{` starts the `with` statement.

— The seven dependent variables, `y1` to `y7`, are placed in problem-oriented variables, `xylose` to `glycerol`, to facilitate the programming of eqs. (1.1).

```
#
# Assign state variables:
  xylose      =y1;
  xylitol     =y2;
  xylulose    =y3;
  acetaldehyde=y4;
  ethanol     =y5;
  acetate     =y6;
  glycerol    =y7;
```

— The fluxes of eqs. (1.2) are programmed.

```
#
# Compute fluxes
  J1=k1*xylose;
  J2=k2*xylitol-km2*xylulose*ethanol;
  J3=k3*xylulose-km3*acetaldehyde*ethanol;
  J4=k4*acetaldehyde;
  J5=k5*acetaldehyde;
  J6=k6*xylulose;
```

— The ODEs of eqs. (1.1) are programmed, with the left-hand side (LHS) derivatives placed in the variables f1 to f7. For example, $d[\text{xylose}]/dt \rightarrow$ f1.

```
#
# Time derivatives
  f1=-J1;
  f2=J1-J2;
  f3=J2-2*J3-2*J6;
  f4=3*J3-J4-J5;
  f5=J4;
  f6=J5;
  f7=3*J6;
```

— The number of calls to bioreactor_1 is incremented and returned to the calling program with <<-.

```
#
# Calls to bioreactor_1
  ncall <<- ncall+1
```

This use of <<- illustrates a basic property of R, that is, numerical values set in a subordinate routine are not shared with higher level routines without explicit programming such as <<-.

— The vector of derivatives is returned from bioreactor_1 as a list.

```
#
# Return derivative vector
  list(c(f1,f2,f3,f4,f5,f6,f7))
  })
}
```

Note the use of the R vector utility c. The }) ends the with statement and the second } concludes the function bioreactor_1. In other words, the derivative vector is returned from bioreactor_1 as a list. This is a requirement of the ODE integrators in the library deSolve. This completes the programming of bioreactor_1. We should note that this function is part of the program of Listing 1.1. That is, this function is in-line and is defined (programmed) before it is called (used). An alternative would be to formulate bioreactor_1 as a separate function; this is done in the next example.

• Eqs. (1.1) are integrated numerically by a call to the R library integrator ode (which is part of deSolve).

```
#
# ODE integration
  out=ode(y=yini,times=times,func=bioreactor_1,
    parms=NULL)
```

We can note the following details about this call to ode.

— The inputs to ode are (i) yini, the IC vector; (ii) times, the vector of output values of t; and (iii) bioreactor_1 to define the RHSs of eqs. (1.1). These inputs define the ODE system of eqs. (1.1) as expected.

— The fourth input argument, parms, can be used to provide a vector of parameters. In the present case, it is unused. However, a vector of parameters, k1 to km3, was defined previously for use in bioreactor_1. This sharing of the parameters with bioreactor_1 illustrates a basic property of R: Numerical values set in a higher level routine are shared with subordinate routines (e.g., functions) without any special designation for this sharing to occur.

— ode has as a default the ODE integrator lsoda [10]. The a in the name lsoda stands for "automatic," meaning that lsoda automatically switches between a stiff option and a nonstiff option as the numerical integration of the ODE system proceeds. The significance of stiffness will be discussed in the following and in subsequent chapters. Here we mention only that this is a sophisticated feature intended to relieve the analyst of having to specify a stiff or nonstiff integrator. lsoda also has a selection of options that can be specified when it is called via ode such as error tolerances for the ODE integration. Experimentation with these options (rather than the use of the defaults) may improve the performance of ode. In the present case, only the defaults are used.

— The numerical solution of the ODE system is returned from ode as a 2D array, in this case out. The first index of this solution array is for the output values of the independent variable (t). The second index is for the numerical solution of the ODEs. For example, out in the present case has the dimensions out[51,1+7] corresponding to (i) the 51 output values $t = 0, 40, \ldots, 2000$ (defined previously) and (ii) the seven dependent variables of eqs. (1.1) plus the one independent variable t. For example, out[1,1] is the value $t = 0$ and out[51,1] is the value $t = 2000$. out[1,2] is (from eq. (1.1a) and Table 1.3) [xylose]($t = 0$) = 0.10724 and out[51,2] is [xylose]($t = 2000$). out[1,8] is (from eq. (1.1g) and Table 1.3) [glycerol]($t = 0$) = 0 and out[51,8] is [glycerol]($t = 2000$). An understanding of the arrangement of the output array is essential for subsequent numerical and graphical (plotted) display of the solution.

— ode receives the number of output values of the solution from the length of the vector of output values of the independent variable. For example, times has 51 elements ($t = 0, 40, \ldots, 2000$) that define the first dimension of the output array as 51 (in out[51,1+7]).

— ode receives the number of ODEs to be integrated from the length of the IC vector. For example, yini has seven elements that define the second dimension of the output array as out[51,1+7] (with the one added to include t).

• The numerical solution is displayed at the nout $=51$ output values of t through a for loop. For it=1 ($t = 0$), a heading for the numerical solution is displayed.

```
#
# ODE numerical solution
  for(it in 1:nout){
  if(it==1){
  cat(sprintf(
  "\n          t        y1       y2       y3       y4
      y5        y6        y7"))}
  cat(sprintf("\n %8.0f%8.4f%8.4f%8.4f%8.4f%8.4f%8.4f
     %8.4f",
  out[it,1],out[it,2],out[it,3],out[it,4],
  out[it,5],out[it,6],out[it,7],out[it,8]))
  }
```

Note the use of the $51 \times (1 + 7)$ values in out. Also, the combination of the R utilities cat and sprintf provides formatting that is used in other languages (e.g., C, C++, Matlab).

• The number of calls to bioreactor_1 is displayed at the end of the solution to give an indication of the computational effort required to compute the solution.

```
#
# Calls to bioreactor_1
  cat(sprintf("\n ncall = %5d\n\n",ncall))
```

- Finally, the solutions of eqs. (1.1) are plotted with the R utility plot.

```
#
# Set of 7 plots
  plot(out)
```

A complete plot is produced with just this abbreviated use of out. plot has a variety of options to format the graphical output that will be considered in subsequent applications.

1.4   Numerical and Graphical Outputs

Abbreviated numerical output from Listing 1.1 is given in Table 1.4. We can note the following details about this output.

TABLE 1.4   Abbreviated numerical output from Listing 1.1.

t	y1	y2	y3	y4	y5	y6	y7
0	0.1072	0.0000	0.0000	0.0000	0.0000	0.0000	0.0000
40	0.0752	0.0020	0.0153	0.0009	0.0195	0.0011	0.0006
80	0.0527	0.0053	0.0221	0.0008	0.0361	0.0020	0.0018
120	0.0370	0.0081	0.0245	0.0006	0.0497	0.0027	0.0034
160	0.0259	0.0101	0.0248	0.0005	0.0608	0.0033	0.0050
200	0.0182	0.0112	0.0239	0.0004	0.0702	0.0038	0.0066
	.					.	
	.					.	
	.					.	

Output for t = 240 to 1760 removed

t	y1	y2	y3	y4	y5	y6	y7
	.					.	
	.					.	
	.					.	
1800	0.0000	0.0004	0.0004	0.0000	0.1303	0.0071	0.0222
1840	0.0000	0.0003	0.0004	0.0000	0.1304	0.0071	0.0223
1880	0.0000	0.0003	0.0004	0.0000	0.1305	0.0071	0.0223
1920	0.0000	0.0003	0.0003	0.0000	0.1306	0.0071	0.0223
1960	0.0000	0.0003	0.0003	0.0000	0.1306	0.0071	0.0223
2000	0.0000	0.0002	0.0003	0.0000	0.1307	0.0071	0.0223

ncall =   427

- The ICs (at $t = 0$) correspond to the values in Table 1.3. While this may seem to be an obvious fact, it is a worthwhile check to ensure that the solution has the correct starting values.
- The solutions approach steady-state conditions as $t \to 2000$. Note in particular that y1 (for xylose from eq. (1.1a)) approaches zero as the the reactant that drives the system is nearly consumed. Also, y5 (for ethanol from eq. (1.1e)) approaches 0.1307 indicating a significant production of ethanol, the product of primary interest (e.g., possibly to be used as a fuel). y7 (for glycerol from eq. (1.1g)) approaches 0.0223 and might represent a contaminant that would have to be subsequently reduced by a separation process; this is rather typical of reaction systems, that is, they usually produce undesirable by-products.
- The computational effort is quite modest, ncall = 427 (the reason for calling this "modest" is explained subsequently).

The graphical output is given in Fig. 1.1. We can note the following about Fig. 1.1.

- The plotting utility plot provides automatic scaling of each of the seven dependent variables. Also, the default of plot is the solid lines connecting the values in Table 1.4; alternative options provide discrete points, or points connected by lines.
- The initial ($t = 0$) values reflect the ICs of Table 1.3 and the final values ($t \to 2000$) reflect the values of Table 1.4.
- The solutions have their largest derivatives at the beginning which is typical of ODE systems (the LHSs of eqs. (1.2) is largest initially).
- The plots are smooth with 51 points.

A fundamental question remains concerning the accuracy of the solution in Table 1.4. As an exact (i.e., analytical, mathematical, closed form) solution is not available for eqs. (1.1) (primarily because they are nonlinear as discussed previously), we cannot directly determine the accuracy of the numerical solution by comparison with an

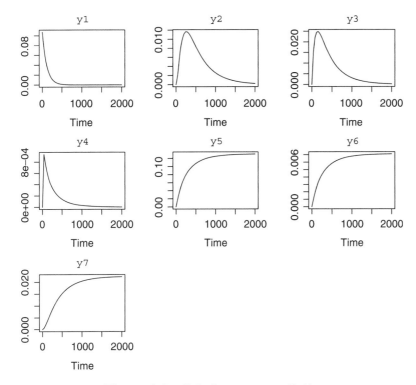

Figure 1.1 Solutions to eqs. (1.1).

exact solution (and if such a solution was available, there would really be no need to compute a numerical solution).

We therefore must use a method of accuracy evaluation that is built on the numerical approach. For example, we could change the specified error tolerances for lsoda (via the call to ode) and compare the solutions as the error tolerances are changed. Or we could use other ODE integrators (other than lsoda) and compare the solutions from different integrators (this approach is discussed in a subsequent example). In any case, some form of error analysis is an essential part of any numerical procedure to give reasonable confidence that the numerical solution has acceptable accuracy.

Finally, with the operational code of Listing 1.1, we can now perform studies (experiments) that will contribute to an understanding of the problem system (which is usually the ultimate objective in developing a mathematical model) on the computer. For example, the effect of changing the model parameters, termed the *parameter sensitivity*, can be carried out by observing the changes in the solutions as parameters are varied. As an example, the BP000 parameters of Table 1.2 can be used in place of the BP10001 parameters (in Listing 1.1) to investigate the effect of using an engineered yeast strain (BP10001) in place of a wild-type yeast strain (BP000). Ideally, an increase in ethanol production would be observed (the final value of y5 in Table 1.4 would increase), indicating that the engineered yeast strain can improve the efficiency of ethanol production.

This type of parameter sensitivity analysis presupposes available values of the model parameters that reflect the performance of the problem system, and these parameters might have to be measured experimentally, for example, by comparing the model solution with laboratory data, and/or estimated using available theory. A good example of the comparison of the ethanol model solution with experimental data is given in [1] for BP000 (Fig. 2.7) and BP10001 (Fig. 2.8).

1.5 Separate ODE Routine

Variations of the coding in Listing 1.1 will now be considered. The intent is to produce a more flexible modular format and to enhance the graphical output. The main program now is in Listing 1.2 (in place of Listing 1.1)

```
#
# Library of R ODE solvers
  library("deSolve")
#
# ODE routine
  setwd("c:/R/bme_ode/chap1")
  source("bioreactor_2.R")
#
# Parameter values for BP10001
  k1=8.87e-03;
  k2=13.18;
  k3=0.129;
  k4=0.497;
```

```
  k5=0.027;
  k6=0.545e-3;
  km2=87.7;
  km3=99.9;
#
# Initial condition
  yini=c(0.10724,0,0,0,0,0,0)
  ncall=0;
#
# t interval
  nout=51
  times=seq(from=0,to=2000,by=40)
#
# ODE integration
  out=ode(y=yini,times=times,func=bioreactor_2,parms=NULL)
#
# ODE numerical solution
  for(it in 1:nout){
   if(it==1){
   cat(sprintf(
   "\n          t       y1       y2       y3       y4       y5
      y6       y7"))}
   cat(sprintf("\n %8.0f%8.4f%8.4f%8.4f%8.4f%8.4f%8.4f
      %8.4f",
   out[it,1],out[it,2],out[it,3],out[it,4],
   out[it,5],out[it,6],out[it,7],out[it,8]))
   }
#
# Calls to bioreactor_2
  cat(sprintf("\n ncall = %5d\n\n",ncall))
#
# Single plot
  par(mfrow=c(1,1))
#
# y1
  plot(out[,1],out[,2],type="l",xlab="t",ylab="y1(t),...,
     y7(t)",
   xlim=c(0,2000),ylim=c(0,0.14),lty=1, main="y1(t),...,
      y7(t) vs t",
   lwd=2)
#
```

```
# y2
  lines(out[,1],out[,3],type="l",lty=2,lwd=2)
#
# y3
  lines(out[,1],out[,4],type="l",lty=3,lwd=2)
#
# y4
  lines(out[,1],out[,5],type="l",lty=4,lwd=2)
#
# y5
  lines(out[,1],out[,6],type="l",lty=5,lwd=2)
#
# y6
  lines(out[,1],out[,7],type="l",lty=6,lwd=2)
#
# y7
  lines(out[,1],out[,8],type="l",lty=7,lwd=2)
```

Listing 1.2: Main program with separate ODE routine.

We can note the following details about Listing 1.2.

- `library("deSolve")` is used again (as in Listing 1.1) in order to access the ODE integrator `ode`. In addition, the separate ODE routine `bioreactor_2` is accessed through the `setwd` and `source` R utilities.

```
#
# Library of R ODE solvers
  library("deSolve")
#
# ODE routine
  setwd("c:/R/bme_ode/chap1")
  source("bioreactor_2.R")
```

To explain the use of `setwd` and `source`:

— `setwd`, set woking directory, is used to go to a directory (folder) where the R routines are located. Note in particular the use of the forward slash / rather than the usual backslash \.

— `source` identifies a particular file within the directory identified by the `setwd`; in this case, the ODE routine `bioreactor_2` is called by `ode`.

— These two statements could be combined as

```
source("c:/R/bme_ode/chap1/bioreactor_2.R")
```

If the R application uses a series of files from the same directory, using the `setwd` is usually simpler; a series of `source` statements can then be used access the required files.

• The sections of Listing 1.2 for setting the parameters, IC and t interval, are the same as in Listing 1.1 and are therefore not discussed here. The call to `ode` uses the ODE routine `bioreactor_2` (Listing 1.3) rather than `bioreactor_1` (Listing 1.1).

```
#
# ODE integration
  out=ode(y=yini,times=times,func=bioreactor_2,
      parms=NULL)
```

Again, the ODE solution is returned in 2D array `out` for subsequent display. `bioreactor_2` is in a separate routine rather than placed in-line as in Listing 1.1, which makes the coding more modular and easier to follow.

• The display of the numerical solution is the same as in Listing 1.1 so this code is not discussed here.

• The number of calls to `bioreactor_3` (returned from `bioreactor_2` at the end of the solution, i.e., at $t = 2000$) is displayed.

```
#
# Calls to bioreactor_2
  cat(sprintf("\n ncall = %5d\n\n",ncall))
```

• The graphical output is extended to produce a single plot with the seven ODE solution curves.

```
#
# Single plot
```

```
   par(mfrow=c(1,1))
#
# y1
   plot(out[,1],out[,2],type="l",xlab="t",ylab="y1(t),
      ...,y7(t)",
     xlim=c(0,2000),ylim=c(0,0.14),lty=1, main="y1(t),
         ...,y7(t) vs t",
     lwd=2)
#
# y2
   lines(out[,1],out[,3],type="l",lty=2,lwd=2)
#
# y3
   lines(out[,1],out[,4],type="l",lty=3,lwd=2)
#
# y4
   lines(out[,1],out[,5],type="l",lty=4,lwd=2)
#
# y5
   lines(out[,1],out[,6],type="l",lty=5,lwd=2)
#
# y6
   lines(out[,1],out[,7],type="l",lty=6,lwd=2)
#
# y7
   lines(out[,1],out[,8],type="l",lty=7,lwd=2)
```

To explain this coding,

— A 1×1 array of plots is specified, that is, a single plot;

```
#
# Single plot
   par(mfrow=c(1,1))
```

— plot is used with a series of parameters for $y_1(t)$.

```
#
# y1
   plot(out[,1],out[,2],type="l",xlab="t",ylab="y1
      (t),...,y7(t)",
```

```
xlim=c(0,2000),ylim=c(0,0.14),lty=1, main="y1
   (t),...,y7(t) vs t",
lwd=2)
```

These parameters are:

out[,1],out[,2] plotted to give a solution curve for eq. (1.1a) of y_1 versus t;

type="l" designates a line type of the solution curve (rather than a point type);

xlab="t" specifies the label t on the abcissa (horizontal) axis;

ylab="y1(t),...,y7(t)" specifies the label on the ordinate (vertical) axis;

xlim=c(0,2000) scales the horizontal axis for $0 \le t \le 2000$;

ylim=c(0,0.14) scales the vertical axis to include the range of values from y_1 to y_7;

lty=1 sets the type of line for the first solution as reflected in Fig. 1.2;

main="y1(t),...,y7(t) vs t" specifies a main label or title for the plot as reflected in Fig. 1.2;

lwd=2 sets the line width for the first solution as reflected in Fig. 1.2.

- $y_2(t)$ is included as a second solution with the R utility lines by plotting out[,1],out[,3]. The parameters are the same as for the previous call to plot except lty=2, which specifies a second type of line as reflected in Fig. 1.2.

```
#
# y2
  lines(out[,1],out[,3],type="l",lty=2,lwd=2)
```

- $y_3(t)$ to $y_7(t)$ are plotted in the same way with lines. For example, $y_7(t)$ is plotted as

```
#
# y7
```

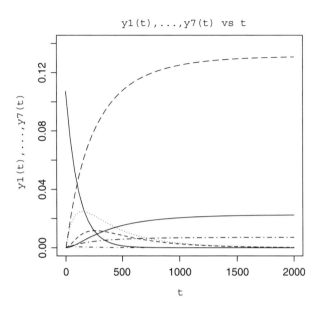

Figure 1.2   Solutions to eqs. (1.1) using a separate ODE routine.

```
lines(out[,1],out[,8],type="l",lty=7,lwd=2)
```

with a line type specified as lty=7, which specifies a seventh type of line as reflected in Fig. 1.2.

bioreactor_2 in Listing 1.3 is a separate routine called by ode.

```
bioreactor_2=function(t,y,parms) {
#
# Assign state variables:
  xylose      =y[1];
  xylitol     =y[2];
  xyluLose    =y[3];
  acetaldehyde=y[4];
  ethanol     =y[5];
  acetate     =y[6];
  glycerol    =y[7];
#
# Compute fluxes
  J1=k1*xylose;
  J2=k2*xylitol-km2*xyluLose*ethanol;
```

```
  J3=k3*xylulose-km3*acetaldehyde*ethanol;
  J4=k4*acetaldehyde;
  J5=k5*acetaldehyde;
  J6=k6*xylulose;
#
# Time derivatives
  f1=-J1;
  f2=J1-J2;
  f3=J2-2*J3-2*J6;
  f4=3*J3-J4-J5;
  f5=J4;
  f6=J5;
  f7=3*J6;
#
# Calls to bioreactor_2
  ncall <<- ncall+1
#
# Return derivative vector
  return(list(c(f1,f2,f3,f4,f5,f6,f7)))
}
```

Listing 1.3: ODE routine `bioreactor_2`.

`bioreactor_2` is the same as `bioreactor_1` of Listing 1.1 except for the following details.

- The function is defined as in Listing 1.1, but the statement specifying y as a list (`with(as.list(y))`) is not used.

  ```
  bioreactor_2=function(t,y,parms) {
  ```

- The dependent variables constitute a vector ($y[1],...,y[7]$) rather than a list of scalars ($y1,...,y7$) as in Listing 1.1. In other words, the input argument of `bioreactor_2`, y, is a vector and not a list.

- At the end, the calls to `bioreactor_3` is incremented and returned to the main program of Listing 1.2 with `<<-`.

  ```
  #
  # Calls to bioreactor_2
    ncall <<- ncall+1
  ```

- Finally, the derivatives `f1` to `f7` are placed in a vector with c that is returned from `bioreactor_2` (to `lsoda` in `ode`) as a list (as required by the ODE integrators in `deSolve`).

```
#
# Return derivative vector
  return(list(c(f1,f2,f3,f4,f5,f6,f7)))
}
```

The right-hand bracket } concludes `bioreactor_2`.

The numerical output from Listing 1.2 is identical to that of Listing 1.1 as expected because the only difference in the coding is the use of the separate ODE routine `bioreactor_2`. The graphical output is given in Fig. 1.2. Note the composite plot of Fig 1.2 rather than the separate plots of Fig 1.1.

This concludes the example with a separate ODE routine. The intent is primarily to demonstrate the use of subordinate functions to modularize the code (rather than having it all in one routine such as in Listing 1.1). This modularization becomes increasingly useful as the complexity of the application increases because it can be used to organize the code into small, more easily manageable sections.

1.6   Alternative Forms of ODE Coding

We now consider variations of the coding in the preceding Listings 1.1–1.3. The intention is primarily to introduce alternatives that can be useful, particularly as the number of ODEs increases (beyond the 7 of eqs. (1.1)).

In the following example, the main program is the same as in Listing 1.2 except for the use of `bioreactor_3` in place of `bioreactor_2`.

```
#
# ODE integration
  out=ode(y=yini,times=times,func=bioreactor_3,parms=NULL)
```

`bioreactor_3` is similar to `bioreactor_2` in Listing 1.3, except that the fluxes and the derivatives are programmed as vectors (Listing 1.4).

```
bioreactor_3=function(t,y,parms) {
#
# Assign state variables:
  xylose      =y[1];
  xylitol     =y[2];
  xylulose    =y[3];
  acetaldehyde=y[4];
  ethanol     =y[5];
  acetate     =y[6];
  glycerol    =y[7];
#
# Compute fluxes
  J=rep(0,n)
  J[1]=k1*xylose;
  J[2]=k2*xylitol-km2*xylulose*ethanol;
  J[3]=k3*xylulose-km3*acetaldehyde*ethanol;
  J[4]=k4*acetaldehyde;
  J[5]=k5*acetaldehyde;
  J[6]=k6*xylulose;
#
# Time derivatives
  f=rep(0,n)
  f[1]=-J[1];
  f[2]=J[1]-J[2];
  f[3]=J[2]-2*J[3]-2*J[6];
  f[4]=3*J[3]-J[4]-J[5];
  f[5]=J[4];
  f[6]=J[5];
  f[7]=3*J[6];
#
# Calls to bioreactor_3
  ncall <<- ncall+1
#
# Return derivative vector
  return(list(c(f)))
}
```

Listing 1.4: ODE routine with vectors to facilitate the ODE programming.

We can note the following details about `bioreactor_3`.

- The sizes of the vectors for the fluxes and derivatives are declared using the R utility `rep` before the vectors are used.

```
#
# Compute fluxes
  J=rep(0,n)
      .
      .
      .
#
# Time derivatives
  f=rep(0,n)
```

This is in contrast with some other programming languages that dynamically allocate memory as arrays are defined (first used). Thus, we might say that the `rep` "preallocates" the vectors J and f. In this case, initial values of the n elements of J and f are set to zero, then reset with the subsequent programming.

- The derivative vector f is returned from `bioreactor_3` (to `lsoda` in `ode`) as a list (as required by the ODE integrators in `deSolve`).

```
#
# Return derivative vector
  return(list(c(f)))
}
```

The intent of this example is to demonstrate how vectors can be used in programming ODEs, which can be particularly useful as the number of ODEs increases. As expected, the numerical and graphical outputs are the same as in the preceding discussion.

1.7   ODE Integrator Selection

As mentioned previously, the R utility `ode` is based (as a default) on the `lsoda` ODE integrator which has the distinguishing feature of switching between stiff and nonstiff algorithms.[1] Another variation that is quite important for stiff ODE systems is the use of sparse matrix algorithms to conserve storage (memory) and enhance computational efficiency.

Here, we will not consider sparse matrix methods other than to point out that they have been implemented in an ODE integrator lsodes where the final "s" in this name designates sparse. lsodes is part of the deSolve library of ODE integrators and can be readily accessed. To illustrate how this is done, the previous main program in Listing 1.2 can be modified with the statements for the ODE integration.

```
#
# ODE integration
# out=   ode(y=yini,times=times,func=bioreactor_4,
   parms=NULL,method="lsodes")
  out=lsodes(y=yini,times=times,func=bioreactor_4,
    parms=NULL)
```

Listing 1.5: Modification of Listing 1.2 to call ODE integrator lsodes.

We can note the following details about this code.

- In the call to ode (inactive or commented), lsodes is called as method="lsodes". This form of argument can be applied to an extensive set of ODE integrators in ode, both stiff and nonstiff.
- In the second line (without ode), lsodes is called explicitly.

As expected, both forms give the same numerical output as in Table 1.4. Also, they are based on the default options for lsodes. A variety of options are available, particularly pertaining to sparse matrix ODE integration that might be very effective as the number of ODEs increases. The details of these options are given in the R

---

[1]The concepts of stiffness and explicit integration are discussed in detail in [6]; Appendix C, [8].

documentation for `lsodes` and in [10]. The ODE routine called by `lsodes`, `bioreactor_4`, is the same as `bioreactor_3` in Listing 1.4 (the number was changed just to keep each case of the programming distinct and self-contained).

1.8 Euler Method

We have so far numerically integrated eqs. (1.1) by using a library integrator in `deSolve`. The integrators that are available in this way are of high quality and well established. However, we do not have access to the source code of these integrators and therefore the programmed details of the numerical integration are not available explicitly. We, therefore, now consider the programing of some classic ODE integration algorithms mainly to demonstrate how systems of ODEs can be integrated numerically. In other words, the discussion of numerical ODE integration to follow is intended to be introductory and instructional, and thereby give some insight into the computation performed by library integrators such as those in `deSolve`.[2]

The Taylor series is the starting point for most numerical integrators. We illustrate this approach starting with the most basic of all ODE integrators, the Euler method. A single ODE with an IC is considered in the following development.

$$\frac{dy}{dt} = f(y, t); \; y(t = t_0) = y_0 \qquad \text{(1.3a),(1.3b)}$$

where the derivative function $f(y, t)$ and the IC y_0 at t_0 are specified for a particular ODE problem.

The solution of eq. (1.3a) is expressed as a Taylor series at point i

$$y_{i+1} = y_i + \frac{dy_i}{dt} h + \frac{d^2 y_i}{dt^2} \frac{h^2}{2!} + \cdots$$

where $h = t_{i+1} - t_i$. We can truncate this series after the linear term in h

$$y_{i+1} \approx y_i + \frac{dy_i}{dt} h \qquad \text{(1.4)}$$

[2]Numerical methods for initial-value ODEs are discussed in [2–5 and 9].

and use this approximation to step along the solution from y_0 to y_1 (with $i = 0$), then from y_1 to y_2 (with $i = 1$), etc., for a specified integration step h. This is the famous Euler method, the most basic of all ODE numerical integration methods. Note that eq. (1.4) requires only dy_i/dt, which is available from eq. (1.3a). The starting value for this stepping procedure, y_0, is available from eq. (1.3b).

Eq. (1.4) is implemented in the following variation of Listing 1.2 (Listing 1.6a) in which the ODE integration via ode is replaced with in-line coding of eq. (1.4).

```
#
# ODE routine
  setwd("c:/R/bme_ode/chap1")
  source("bioreactor_5.R")
#
# Parameter values for BP10001
  k1=8.87e-03;
  k2=13.18;
  k3=0.129;
  k4=0.497;
  k5=0.027;
  k6=0.545e-3;
  km2=87.7;
  km3=99.9;
#
# Initial condition
  n=7;nout=51;t=0;ncall=0;
  y=c(0.10724,0,0,0,0,0,0)
  cat(sprintf(
  "\n         t       y1       y2       y3       y4       y5
     y6       y7"))
  cat(sprintf("\n %8.0f%8.4f%8.4f%8.4f%8.4f%8.4f%8.4f
     %8.4f",
  t,y[1],y[2],y[3],y[4],y[5],y[6],y[7]))
#
# Arrays for output
  out=matrix(0,nrow=nout,ncol=(n+1))
  out[1,-1]=y
  out[1,1]=t
#
```

```
# Parameters for t integration
# nt=400;h=0.10  # unstable
  nt=800;h=0.05  # stable
#
# Euler integration
  for(i1 in 2:nout){
#
#   nt Euler steps
    for(i2 in 1:nt){
      yt=bioreactor_5(t,y);
      y=y+yt*h; t=t+h;
    }
#
#   Solution after nt Euler steps
    cat(sprintf("\n %8.0f%8.4f%8.4f%8.4f%8.4f%8.4f%8.4f
      %8.4f",
    t,y[1],y[2],y[3],y[4],y[5],y[6],y[7]))
    out[i1,-1]=y
    out[i1,1]=t
  }
#
# Calls to bioreactor_5
  cat(sprintf("\n ncall = %5d\n\n",ncall))
#
# Single plot
  par(mfrow=c(1,1))
#
# y1
  plot(out[,1],out[,2],type="l",xlab="t",ylab="y1(t),...,
    y7(t)",
    xlim=c(0,2000),ylim=c(0,0.14),lty=1, main="y1(t),...,
      y7(t) vs t",
    lwd=2)
#
# y2
  lines(out[,1],out[,3],type="l",lty=2,lwd=2)
#
# y3
  lines(out[,1],out[,4],type="l",lty=3,lwd=2)
#
# y4
```

```
  lines(out[,1],out[,5],type="l",lty=4,lwd=2)
#
# y5
  lines(out[,1],out[,6],type="l",lty=5,lwd=2)
#
# y6
  lines(out[,1],out[,7],type="l",lty=6,lwd=2)
#
# y7
  lines(out[,1],out[,8],type="l",lty=7,lwd=2)
```

Listing 1.6a: Main program with in-line explicit Euler method.

We can note the following details about Listing 1.6a.

- reactor_5.R is the ODE routine (rather than reactor_3.R, reactor_4.R). The differences in reactor_5.R are considered subsequently.

  ```
  #
  # ODE routine
    setwd("c:/R/bme_ode/chap1")
    source("bioreactor_5.R")
  ```

- The section for setting the parameters k1 to km3 is the same as in Listings 1.1 and 1.2 and is therefore not repeated here.
- The IC is placed in vector c, then displayed with a heading.

  ```
  #
  # Initial condition
    n=7;nout=51;t=0;ncall=0;
    y=c(0.10724,0,0,0,0,0,0)
    cat(sprintf(
    "\n          t      y1      y2      y3      y4      y5
       y6       y7"))
    cat(sprintf("\n %8.0f%8.4f%8.4f%8.4f%8.4f%8.4f%8.4f
       %8.4f",
    t,y[1],y[2],y[3],y[4],y[5],y[6],y[7]))
  ```

Note in particular the number of ODEs, n=7, and the number of output points nout=51.

- An array out is defined for the numerical solution that has the same format as out in Listings 1.1 and 1.2.

```
#
# Arrays for output
  out=matrix(0,nrow=nout,ncol=(n+1))
  out[1,-1]=y
  out[1,1]=t
```

To further explain this programming,

— out is defined as a 2D array with the R utility matrix. outs has nout ($=51$) rows for the output points in t set previously and $(n+1) = 7 + 1$ columns for the seven dependent variables of eqs. (1.1) and the independent variable t.

```
  out=matrix(0,nrow=nout,ncol=(n+1))
```

— The first index of out is 1 corresponding to $t = 0$.
— The second index (subscript) of out indicates all values except 1, that is, -1. In this case, there are seven values corresponding to the ICs for y set previously.

```
  out[1,-1]=y
```

— The initial value of $t (= 0)$ is placed in out with the second subscript set to 1.

```
  out[1,1]=t
```

- The integration step h in eq. (1.4) is set numerically. This is typically done by some trial and error. For example, because $0 \le t \le 2000$, $h = 0.1$ corresponds to $(2000)/(0.1) = 20,000$ Euler steps. However, when this value is used, the solution is unstable as will be demonstrated subsequently. With $h = 0.05$, the solution is stable (and as we will observe, also accurate). In other words, h generally has to be selected so that the numerical solution is stable and accurate.

```
#
# Parameters for t integration
```

```
# nt=400;h=0.10  # unstable
  nt=800;h=0.05  # stable
```

Once h is defined, the number of Euler steps, nt, to span the output interval of 40 is nt $= 40/0.05 = 800$. In other words, 800 Euler steps according to eq. (1.4) are completed for each output at $t = 40, 80, \ldots, 2000$. This is in contrast with the variable step integrators in ode which adjust h to achieve a prescribed accuracy of the numerical solution and therefore may take many fewer steps than 800 for each output interval 40. For example, lsoda required ncall = 427 (Table 1.4) calls to the ODE integrator, whereas the Euler integrator of Listing 1.6a requires 2000/0.05 $= 40,000$ calls to the ODE routine, bioreactor_5. This larger number (40,000 rather than 427) is a manifestation of stiffness of eqs. (1.1). In other words, the Euler method requires 40,000 steps to main stability of the numerical solution rather than accuracy. Thus, the effectiveness of the stiff integrator of lsoda for this example (eqs. (1.1)) is clear.

- The Euler integration proceeds with two for loops.

```
#
# Euler integration
  for(i1 in 2:nout){
#
#    nt Euler steps
    for(i2 in 1:nt){
      yt=bioreactor_5(t,y);
      y=y+yt*h; t=t+h;
    }
```

The first loop with index i1 steps through the 50 output points $t = 40, 80, \ldots, 2000$ (after $t = 0$). The second loop with index i2 steps through the 800 Euler steps for each output (so that there are a total of $50 \times 800 = 40,000$ Euler steps for the complete solution to $t = 2000$). Within this second loop, the derivative vector dy_i/dt in eq. (1.4) is computed by a call to the ODE routine bioreactor_5 (yt has seven elements but the vector facility of R is used so that subscripting is not required). Then, the solution is advanced from i to $i + 1$ according to eq. (1.4). Also, t is advanced by the integration step h, that is, $t_{i+1} = t_i + h$.

- After each pass of the loop in i1, the solution is put into array out for subsequent plotting.

```
#
#    Solution after nt Euler steps
     cat(sprintf("\n %8.0f%8.4f%8.4f%8.4f%8.4f%8.4f
        %8.4f%8.4f",
     t,y[1],y[2],y[3],y[4],y[5],y[6],y[7]))
     out[i1,-1]=y
     out[i1,1]=t
   }
```

Note the use of index i1 when writing out. The final } completes the loop in i1.

- Since array out is used in the same way as in Listings 1.1, 1.2, and 1.5 (with ode and lsodes), the plotting used previously can be used again (listed above but not here).

bioreactor_5 called by the main program in Listing 1.6a is in Listing 1.6b. It is the same as bioreactor_3 and bioreactor_4 except for the final line that returns the derivative vector f.

```
bioreactor_5=function(t,y,parms) {
    .                        .
    .                        .
  (same as bioreactor_3, bioreactor_4)
    .                        .
    .                        .
#
# Return derivative vector
  return(c(f))
}
```

Listing 1.6b: bioreactor_5.R called in Listing 1.6a.

The difference in the return statements

```
From Listing 1.4
```

```
return(list(c(f))
```

```
From Listing 1.6b
return(c(f))
```

is small but important.

For Listing 1.4, `return(list(c(f))` returns the derivative vector f as a list that is required by the integrators in deSolve, for example, ode, lsodes. For Listing 1.6b, `return(c(f))` returns the derivative vector f as a numerical vector, which is required in the programming of the Euler method in Listing 1.6a. In particular, the arithmetic multiplication * used in y=y+yt*h must operate on two numerical objects, in this case yt and h. If yt is a list rather than a numerical vector, the multiplication * will not function (an error message results). While this may seem like a minor detail, the distinction between a list and a numerical object must be taken into consideration.

Abbreviated numerical output from Listings 1.6a and 1.6b is in Table 1.5.

This output is identical to the output in Table 1.4 to four figures, for example, at $t = 2000$,

```
Table 1.4

  2000  0.0000  0.0002  0.0003  0.0000  0.1307  0.0071
        0.0223

  ncall =    427

Table 1.5

  2000  0.0000  0.0002  0.0003  0.0000  0.1307  0.0071
        0.0223

  ncall = 40000
```

Thus, we conclude that the Euler method reproduces the output from ode and lsodes for eqs. (1.1), which can be considered a check on the numerical solutions. However, an essential difference in the programming was the need to provide an integration

TABLE 1.5 Numerical output from Listings 1.6a and 1.6b, $h = 0.05$.

t	y1	y2	y3	y4	y5	y6	y7
0	0.1072	0.0000	0.0000	0.0000	0.0000	0.0000	0.0000
40	0.0752	0.0020	0.0153	0.0009	0.0195	0.0011	0.0006
80	0.0527	0.0053	0.0221	0.0008	0.0361	0.0020	0.0018
120	0.0370	0.0081	0.0246	0.0006	0.0497	0.0027	0.0034
160	0.0259	0.0101	0.0248	0.0005	0.0609	0.0033	0.0050
200	0.0182	0.0112	0.0239	0.0004	0.0702	0.0038	0.0066
240	0.0128	0.0116	0.0224	0.0004	0.0780	0.0042	0.0081

.
.
.

Output for t = 280 to 1720 removed

.
.
.

1760	0.0000	0.0004	0.0005	0.0000	0.1303	0.0071	0.0222
1800	0.0000	0.0004	0.0004	0.0000	0.1303	0.0071	0.0222
1840	0.0000	0.0003	0.0004	0.0000	0.1304	0.0071	0.0222
1880	0.0000	0.0003	0.0004	0.0000	0.1305	0.0071	0.0223
1920	0.0000	0.0003	0.0003	0.0000	0.1306	0.0071	0.0223
1960	0.0000	0.0003	0.0003	0.0000	0.1306	0.0071	0.0223
2000	0.0000	0.0002	0.0003	0.0000	0.1307	0.0071	0.0223

ncall = 40000

step (h in eq. (1.4)) for the Euler method, whereas ode and lsodes automatically adjusted the step in accordance with the default error tolerances for ode (lsoda) and lsodes. We next consider some additional consequences of using eq. (1.4).

1.9 Accuracy and Stability Constraints

We return to the important detail in Listing 1.6a pertaining to the value of the integration step h and the stability of the numerical solution.

```
#
# Parameters for t integration
# nt=400;h=0.10  # unstable
  nt=800;h=0.05  # stable
```

This limit on the value of h reflects the stability limit of the explicit Euler method in eq. (1.4) where explicit refers to the direct (explicit) calculation of y_{i+1} from y_i. This calculation is straightforward but also has a limit on h for the calculation to remain stable (as demonstrated by the transition from $h = 0.05$ to $h = 0.10$).

To further investigate this limit with some basic ideas from linear algebra [7, Appendix 2], we consider a $n \times n$ linear, constant coefficient ODE system for which there will be an associated set of n eigenvalues. The ODE system will be stable (have a stable solution) if and only if (iff) all of the eigenvalues are in the left half of the complex plane, that is, iff the real parts of the eigenvalues are nonpositive. However, even with a stable ODE system, the numerical solution from an explicit algorithm such as the Euler method of eq. (1.4) can be unstable unless the integration step h is restricted. For the explicit Euler method, this stability limit is [4, p 230]

$$|\lambda h| \le c \tag{1.5}$$

with $c = 2$ for each eigenvalue λ; if the eigenvalue is complex, then $|\ |$ denotes a modulus (absolute value).

Eq. (1.5) indicates that the maximum step h for a stable solution is set by the eigenvalue with the largest modulus, λ_{max}. However, the timescale for the ODE system, for example, $0 \le t \le 2000$ of eqs. (1.1), is determined by the eigenvalue with the smallest modulus, λ_{min}. Thus, the ratio

$$SR = \frac{\lambda_{max}}{\lambda_{min}} \tag{1.6}$$

termed the *stiffness ratio* (SR), is an indicator of the number of steps required to compute a complete solution to an ODE system with an explicit integrator such as eq. (1.4). As a qualitative guideline, the following Table 1.6 provides approximate ranges of values of SR.

TABLE 1.6   Qualitative degree of stiffness.

SR	Stiffness
<100	nonstiff
$100 \leq SR \leq 1000$	moderately stiff
>1000	stiff

The effect of an increase in SR in Table 1.6 can be interpreted as increased stiffness with the spread (spectrum, spectral radius) of the ODE eigenvalues, that is, for a stiff ODE system, $|\lambda_{max}| >> |\lambda_{min}|$. The requirement of using $h = 0.05$ (and not $h = 0.1$) with $(2000)(20) = 40,000$ Euler steps for a complete solution (in Listing 1.6a) suggests eqs. (1.1) are effectively stiff.

However, there is one additional complication. The preceding discussion of the SR based on eigenvalues presupposes a linear constant coefficient ODE system. But eqs. (1.1) are nonlinear, so the use of the concept of eigenvalues is not straightforward. We will just conclude that if an ODE systems requires a large number of integration steps for a complete numerical solution, the ODE system is effectively stiff and therefore requires a stiff integrator to produce a solution with a modest number of steps.

Then we have to consider what is a stiff integrator. The general answer is that it is implicit rather than explicit. For example, rather than use the explicit Euler method of eq. (1.4), we can use the implicit form

$$y_{i+1} \approx y_i + \frac{dy_{i+1}}{dt}h \qquad (1.7)$$

The only difference between eqs. (1.4) and (1.7) is the point along the solution at which the derivative dy/dt is evaluated (i for eq. (1.4) and $i+1$ for eq. (1.7)). While this may seem like a minor point, it is important for at least two reasons.

- The constant c in eq. (1.5) is ∞. In other words, the implicit Euler method is unconditionally stable and, therefore, there is no stability restriction placed on h (the only restriction is from accuracy).

- Since y_{i+1} appears on both the sides of eq. (1.7), it is implicit in the solution at the next point along the solution. For systems of ODEs, this means that the solution of a system of simultaneous algebraic equations is required to move from point i to point $i + 1$ along the solution. If the ODEs are nonlinear, a system of nonlinear algebraic equations must be solved numerically which can be a formidable requirement (depending on the number of ODEs and the form of their nonlinearities). Generally a variant of Newton's method is used to solve the nonlinear algebraic system.

This discussion indicates that the stability limit of explicit methods can be circumvented by using an implicit method, but this increased stability comes at the cost of substantially increased computational complexity.

Two other points should be mentioned.

- Because implicit (stiff) integrators require rather substantial computation, they should be used only if the ODE system is actually stiff. In other words, a nonstiff (explicit) integrator should be tried first, and if it requires a small step (as in Listing 1.6a) to maintain stability, a stiff (implicit) integrator should be considered.
- Nonlinearity in an ODE system does not necessarily mean that the ODEs are stiff (a common misconception is to equate nonlinearity and stiffness).

These two points indicate that the choice of a stiff versus a nonstiff ODE integrator may not be straightforward and clear cut. To assist with this requirement, lsoda, the default integrator of ode switches automatically between stiff and nonstiff options as the solution proceeds; the "a" denotes the automatic switching, which is based on the eigenvalue analysis. The details of lsoda are rather complicated, but the final result is a well-established quality integrator that can be used, for example, in ode without becoming involved in the details.

To conclude this discussion of the Euler method, if the integration is done with $h = 0.10$ rather than $h = 0.05$, the output from Listing 1.6a (abbreviated) is given in Table 1.7.

TABLE 1.7   Numerical output from Listings 1.6a and 1.6b, $h = 0.10$.

t	y1	y2	y3	y4	y5	y6	y7
0	0.1072	0.0000	0.0000	0.0000	0.0000	0.0000	0.0000
40	0.0752	0.0020	0.0153	0.0009	0.0195	0.0011	0.0006
80	0.0527	0.0053	0.0221	0.0008	0.0361	0.0020	0.0018
120	0.0370	0.0081	0.0246	0.0006	0.0497	0.0027	0.0034
160	0.0259	0.0101	0.0248	0.0005	0.0609	0.0033	0.0050
200	0.0182	94287.4828	-211142.0815	175269.8277		11.5836	0.6293
							-0.0091
240	0.0127	NaN	NaN	NaN	NaN	NaN	NaN
280	0.0089	NaN	NaN	NaN	NaN	NaN	NaN
320	0.0063	NaN	NaN	NaN	NaN	NaN	NaN
360	0.0044	NaN	NaN	NaN	NaN	NaN	NaN
400	0.0031	NaN	NaN	NaN	NaN	NaN	NaN
.						.	
.						.	
.						.	
	Output from t = 440 to 1760 deleted						
.						.	
.						.	
.						.	
1800	0.0000	NaN	NaN	NaN	NaN	NaN	NaN
1840	0.0000	NaN	NaN	NaN	NaN	NaN	NaN
1880	0.0000	NaN	NaN	NaN	NaN	NaN	NaN
1920	0.0000	NaN	NaN	NaN	NaN	NaN	NaN
1960	0.0000	NaN	NaN	NaN	NaN	NaN	NaN
2000	0.0000	NaN	NaN	NaN	NaN	NaN	NaN

ncall = 20000

We can note the following details about this output.

- The solutions starts at the same ICs ($t = 0$) as in Table 1.5.

- At $t = 200$, the numbers (not the correct numerical solution) suddenly change, reflecting an instability in the calculations.
- For the remaining values of t, NaN (not a number) indicates the calculations have failed.
- The number of calls to bioreactor_5 is 20,000, as expected (because the integration h is doubled from 0.05 to 0.01). But clearly, the doubling has violated the stability criterion (1.5).

In summary, lsoda performed 427 derivative evaluations while the explicit Euler integrator performed $(2000)(20) = 40,000$, a difference of nearly two orders of magnitude (a factor of 10^2). This example clearly indicates the effectiveness of a stiff integrator (in lsoda). However, we again indicate that a nonstiff integrator should be tried first in case the ODE system is not stiff (and therefore the increased computations for each step of a stiff integrator are not required).

The integration step for explicit integrators may be constrained by accuracy and/or stability. In the case of eqs. (1.1), h is constrained by stability as reflected in Listing 1.6a and apparently not by accuracy (recall the agreement of the solutions in Tables 1.4 and 1.5). However, the explicit Euler method of eq. (1.4) can be constrained by accuracy because it is only first-order correct $(O(h))$. Therefore, the explicit integrators we discuss next are worth considering for a new nonstiff ODE problem application because they are of higher order than the first-order explicit Euler method of eq. (1.4). However, higher order explicit methods do not have improved stability. For example, c in eq. (1.5) generally does not exceed 3 even for higher order explicit methods.

As a point of notation, $O(h)$ used above denotes "of first order in h" or "first-order correct" and is intended to indicate the error resulting from the truncated Taylor series. For example, the Taylor series is truncated after the h term to give the Euler method. This can be stated alternatively, the truncation error is

$$\text{error} = O(h) = c_t h$$

where c_t is taken as a constant (generally it will vary along the solution). To demonstrate that the Euler method is first order, the reader might compute the numerical solution of an ODE with an exact solution (eqs. (1.1) does not have a known exact solution), then use the exact error (as the absolute value of the difference between the Euler solution and the exact solution at a particular t) for a series of h values in a plot of the exact error versus h. This plot, for sufficiently small h, will be a straight line with slope 1. For an nth order method with $O(h^n)$, a plot in log-log format will be a line with slope n since

$$\text{error} = O(h^n) = c_t h^n$$

or

$$\log(\text{error}) = n\log(h) + \log(c_t)$$

This type of graphical error analysis is usually done with the model problem (a special case of eq. (1.3))

$$\frac{dy}{dt} = \lambda y; \ y(0) = y_0$$

and the exact solution

$$y(t) = y_0 e^{\lambda t}$$

Note that for the eigenvalue $\lambda \leq 0$, the exact solution is stable. Therefore, this test problem can also be used to test the Euler stability criterion of eq. (1.5) (with $c = 2$) by using a value of h greater than $2/|\lambda|$. The calculations for this accuracy and stability analysis can be carried out with a straightforward modification of Listings 1.6a and 1.6b (routines for this purpose are provided with the software download for this book).

If the ODE system is stiff and therefore the integration step of an explicit method is constrained by stability, this constraint can usually be circumvented by using an implicit method such as the implicit Euler method of eq. (1.7); but the implicit Euler method of eq. (1.7) is only first order so that a higher order implicit method is generally used to give both good accuracy and stability, for example, the stiff integrator in `lsoda`. Implicit methods have the cost of additional calculations for the solution of systems of nonlinear algebraic equations, but the additional calculations are worthwhile for stiff systems (recall again the improvement of two orders of magnitude between the explicit Euler method of eq. (1.4) and the higher order implicit method of `lsoda`).

1.10 Modified Euler Method as a Runge–Kutta Method

The preceding discussion of the explicit Euler method of eq. (1.4) indicated the limited first-order accuracy (the error is $O(h)$) resulting from the truncation of the Taylor series after the h term. We now consider how this order can be increased, basically by using additional terms in the Taylor series.

$$y_{i+1} = y_i + \frac{dy_i}{dt}h + \frac{d^2y_i}{dt^2}\frac{h^2}{2!} + \cdots \tag{1.8}$$

For example, we might consider including the h^2 term. To do this, we have to use the second derivative d^2y_i/dt^2 which is generally unavailable because the ODE, eq. (1.3a), provides only the first derivative. One possibility would be to repeatedly differentiate the derivative function (RHS of eq. (1.3a)) to obtain the higher order derivatives that are required as more terms are included in the Taylor series. But this quickly becomes impractical if we are considering an ODE system. In other words, we need to have a procedure for including the higher order terms in the Taylor series without having to differentiate the ODEs. We now consider how this can be done with the Runge–Kutta method.

If the second derivative is approximated as the finite difference of the first derivative,

$$\frac{d^2y_i}{dt^2} \approx \frac{dy_{i+1}/dt - dy_i/dt}{h} \tag{1.9}$$

then substitution of eq. (1.9) in eq. (1.8) with truncation after the h^2 term gives

$$y_{i+1} = y_i + \frac{dy_i}{dt}h + \frac{\frac{dy_{i+1}}{dt} - \frac{dy_i}{dt}}{h}\frac{h^2}{2!}$$

$$= y_i + \frac{\frac{dy_{i+1}}{dt} + \frac{dy_i}{dt}}{2}h \tag{1.10}$$

Eq. (1.10) indicates that the derivatives at the base point i and the advanced point $i + 1$ are averaged in stepping along the solution (from y_i to y_{i+1}). The derivative y_{i+1}/dt can be computed by substituting y_{i+1} from eq. (1.4) in the ODE, eq. (1.3a). This leads to an algorithm with the following steps:

- Starting at the base point y_i, t_i, the ODE, eq. (1.3a), is used to calculate dy_i/dt

$$\frac{dy_i}{dt} = f(y_i, t_i) \tag{1.11a}$$

- Eq. (1.4) is used to calculate y_{i+1} (with $t_{i+1} = t_i + h$) from the result of eq. (1.11a).

$$y_{i+1} = y_i + \frac{dy_i}{dt}h \tag{1.11b}$$

- The ODE, eq. (1.3a), is used to calculate dy_{i+1}/dt from the result of eq. (1.11b).

$$\frac{dy_{i+1}}{dt} = f(y_{i+1}, t_i + h) \tag{1.11c}$$

- Eq. (1.10) is used to calculate an improved y_{i+1} from the results of eqs. (11.1a) and (1.11c).

$$y_{i+1} = y_i + \frac{\frac{dy_{i+1}}{dt} + \frac{dy_i}{dt}}{2}h \tag{1.11d}$$

Eqs. (1.11) are the modified Euler method (also termed the *extended Euler method* or *Heun's method*). Also, if we consider y_{i+1} from eq. (1.11b) to be a predicted value, and y_{i+1} from eq. (1.11d) to be a corrected value, eqs. (1.11) can be considered as a predictor–corrector scheme. An important point to note is that eqs. (1.11) do not require differentiating the ODE, eq. (1.3a) (only the ODE is used), but the final result of eq. (1.11d) is second-order correct (the error is $O(h^2)$). The cost of this improved accuracy ($O(h)$ of the Euler method, eq. (1.4), improved to $O(h^2)$ of the modified Euler method, eqs. (1.11)), is an increase of one derivative evaluation in eq. (1.4) to two derivatives evaluation in eqs. (1.11). Usually, the increased accuracy is well worth the additional calculational effort (additional derivative evaluations from the ODE).

In other words, we have achieved higher order accuracy without differentiating the ODE by evaluating the derivative from the ODE at selected points along the solution. In the case of the modified Euler method, the selected points for derivative evaluation are (y_i, t_i) and (y_{i+1}, t_{i+1}) as reflected in eq. (1.11d). This idea of multiple evaluation of the ODE derivative function along selected points of the numerical solution to produce higher order methods is the basis of the Runge–Kutta method.[3] Therefore, we restate eqs. (1.11) in the Runge–Kutta format so that we can then logically extend them to higher order methods stated in the Runge–Kutta format.

$$k_1 = f(y_i, t_i)h \qquad\qquad (1.12a)$$

$$y_{i+1} = y_i + k_1 \qquad\qquad (1.12b)$$

$$k_2 = f(y_{i+1}, t_{i+1})h = f(y_i + k_1, t_i + h)h \qquad\qquad (1.12c)$$

$$y_{i+1} = y_i + \frac{k_1 + k_2}{2}h \qquad\qquad (1.12d)$$

Note that the derivatives (multiplied by h) are given the names k_1, k_2 by convention.

We now consider the programming of eqs. (1.11) and (1.12) (two cases). A main program with these equations is in Listing 1.7.

```
#
# ODE routine
  setwd("c:/R/bme_ode/chap1")
```

---

[3]The Runge–Kutta methods are discussed in [2] and [3].

```
  source("bioreactor_6.R")
#
# Select modified Euler format
#
# ncase = 1: Taylor series format
#
# ncase = 2: Runge Kutta format
  ncase=1;
#
# Parameter values for BP10001
  k1=8.87e-03;
  k2=13.18;
  k3=0.129;
  k4=0.497;
  k5=0.027;
  k6=0.545e-3;
  km2=87.7;
  km3=99.9;
#
# Initial condition
  n=7;nout=51;t=0;ncall=0;
  y=c(0.10724,0,0,0,0,0,0)
  cat(sprintf(
  "\n          t        y1       y2       y3       y4       y5
     y6       y7"))
  cat(sprintf("\n %8.0f%8.4f%8.4f%8.4f%8.4f%8.4f%8.4f
     %8.4f",
  t,y[1],y[2],y[3],y[4],y[5],y[6],y[7]))
#
# Arrays for output
  out=matrix(0,nrow=nout,ncol=(n+1))
  out[1,-1]=y
  out[1,1]=t
#
# Parameters for t integration
# nt=400;h=0.10  # unstable
  nt=800;h=0.05  # stable
#
# Modified Euler integration
  for(i1 in 2:nout){
#
```

```
#   nt modified Euler steps
    for(i2 in 1:nt){
    if(ncase==1){
      yb=y
      ytb=bioreactor_6(t,y)
      y=yb+ytb*h; t=t+h
      yt=bioreactor_6(t,y)
      y=yb+(ytb+yt)/2*h
    }
    if(ncase==2){
      yb=y
      rk1=bioreactor_6(t,y)*h
      y=yb+rk1; t=t+h
      rk2=bioreactor_6(t,y)*h
      y=yb+(rk1+rk2)/2
    }
    }
#
#   Solution after nt modified Euler steps
    cat(sprintf("\n %8.0f%8.4f%8.4f%8.4f%8.4f%8.4f%8.4f
       %8.4f",
    t,y[1],y[2],y[3],y[4],y[5],y[6],y[7]))
    out[i1,-1]=y
    out[i1,1]=t
  }
#
# Calls to bioreactor_6
  cat(sprintf("\n ncall = %5d\n\n",ncall))
#
# Single plot
  par(mfrow=c(1,1))
#
# y1
  plot(out[,1],out[,2],type="l",xlab="t",ylab="y1(t),...,
     y7(t)",
    xlim=c(0,2000),ylim=c(0,0.14),lty=1, main="y1(t),...,
       y7(t) vs t",
    lwd=2)
#
# y2
  lines(out[,1],out[,3],type="l",lty=2,lwd=2)
```

```
#
# y3
  lines(out[,1],out[,4],type="l",lty=3,lwd=2)
#
# y4
  lines(out[,1],out[,5],type="l",lty=4,lwd=2)
#
# y5
  lines(out[,1],out[,6],type="l",lty=5,lwd=2)
#
# y6
  lines(out[,1],out[,7],type="l",lty=6,lwd=2)
#
# y7
  lines(out[,1],out[,8],type="l",lty=7,lwd=2)
```

Listing 1.7: Main program with the in-line modified Euler method.

Listing 1.7 is similar to Listing 1.6a for the Euler method but it is included here because of some of the following significant differences.

- The ODE routine is bioreactor_6, which is the same as bioreactor_5 of Listing 1.6b

```
#
# ODE routine
  setwd("c:/R/bme_ode/chap1")
  source("bioreactor_6.R")
#
# Select modified Euler format
#
# ncase = 1: Taylor series format
#
# ncase = 2: Runge Kutta format
  ncase=1;
```

ncase has the values 1 for eqs. (1.11) or 2 for eqs. (1.12).
- The parameters for BP1001 of Listing 1.6a are used again.

- The ICs of Listing 1.6a are used again. Note in particular that the counter ncall is initialized.

```
#
# Initial condition
  n=7;nout=51;t=0;ncall=0;
  y=c(0.10724,0,0,0,0,0,0)
  cat(sprintf(
  "\n          t        y1        y2        y3        y4        y5
     y6        y7"))
  cat(sprintf("\n %8.0f%8.4f%8.4f%8.4f%8.4f%8.4f%8.4f
     %8.4f",
  t,y[1],y[2],y[3],y[4],y[5],y[6],y[7]))
```

- The array out for the solution again has the same format as produced by the integrators in deSolve.

```
#
# Arrays for output
  out=matrix(0,nrow=nout,ncol=(n+1))
  out[1,-1]=y
  out[1,1]=t
#
# Parameters for t integration
# nt=400;h=0.10   # unstable
  nt=800;h=0.05   # stable
```

The integration step is $h = 0.05$, which is stable (the value of c in eq. (1.5) is again 2 for the modified Euler method [4, p 230, Fig. 6.2]).

- The programming of eqs. (1.11) (ncase = 1) is similar to the programming of the Euler method of Listing 1.6a.

```
#
# Modified Euler integration
  for(i1 in 2:nout){
#
#   nt modified Euler steps
    for(i2 in 1:nt){
    if(ncase==1){
```

```
        yb=y
        ytb=bioreactor_6(t,y)
        y=yb+ytb*h;  t=t+h
        yt=bioreactor_6(t,y)
        y=yb+(ytb+yt)/2*h
      }
```

The correspondence of the coding with eqs. (1.11) (for ncase=1) is clear. Note that two calls to the ODE routine, bioreactor_6, are used to achieve the second-order accuracy of the modified Euler method as explained previously.

• The programming of eqs. (1.12) (ncase=2) is straightforward. k_1 and k_2 in eqs. (1.12) are programmed as rk1 and rk2 to avoid a conflict with the kinetic rate constants k1,k2 defined previously.

```
    if(ncase==2){
        yb=y
        rk1=bioreactor_6(t,y)*h
        y=yb+rk1;  t=t+h
        rk2=bioreactor_6(t,y)*h
        y=yb+(rk1+rk2)/2
      }
    }
```

• The numerical and graphical displays of the solutions are the same as in Listing 1.6a. Note also the display of the counter ncall.

```
    #
    # Calls to bioreactor_6
      cat(sprintf("\n ncall = %5d\n\n",ncall))
```

ODE routine bioreactor_6 is not listed here because it is the same as in Listing 1.6b.

The output from these routines is the same as in Tables 1.4 and 1.5, except the number of calls to bioreactor_6 is 80000 as expected (twice the calls for the Euler method because of two derivative evaluations in each integration step according to eqs. (1.12)).

The comparison of the output from the Euler method and the modified Euler method suggests a way to evaluate the accuracy of the numerical solution, that is, compare the numerical solutions computed by two different methods. This idea is used in the following reprogramming of the numerical integration in Listing 1.7.

```
#
# ODE routine
  setwd("c:/R/bme_ode/chap1")
  source("bioreactor_7.R")
#
# Select modified Euler format
#
# ncase = 1: RK format
#
# ncase = 2: RK format with explicit error estimate
  ncase=2;
#
# Parameter values for BP10001
  k1=8.87e-03;
  k2=13.18;
  k3=0.129;
  k4=0.497;
  k5=0.027;
  k6=0.545e-3;
  km2=87.7;
  km3=99.9;
#
# Initial condition
  n=7;nout=51;t=0;ncall=0;
  y=c(0.10724,0,0,0,0,0,0)
  cat(sprintf(
  "\n           t       y1       y2       y3       y4       y5
     y6       y7"))
  if(ncase==2){
  ee=c(0,0,0,0,0,0,0)
    cat(sprintf(
  "\n                   e1       e2       e3       e4       e5
     e6       e7"))}
  cat(sprintf("\n %8.0f%8.4f%8.4f%8.4f%8.4f%8.4f%8.4f
     %8.4f",
```

```
  t,y[1],y[2],y[3],y[4],y[5],y[6],y[7]))
  if(ncase==2){
    cat(sprintf("\n             %8.4f%8.4f%8.4f%8.4f%8.4f%8.4f
      %8.4f\n",
    ee[1],ee[2],ee[3],ee[4],ee[5],ee[6],ee[7]))}
#
# Arrays for output
  out=matrix(0,nrow=nout,ncol=(n+1))
  out[1,-1]=y
  out[1,1]=t
#
# Parameters for t integration
# nt=400;h=0.10  # unstable
  nt=800;h=0.05  # stable
#
# Modified Euler integration
  for(i1 in 2:nout){
#
#   nt modified Euler steps
    for(i2 in 1:nt){
    if(ncase==1){
       yb=y
       rk1=bioreactor_7(t,y)*h
       y=yb+rk1; t=t+h
       rk2=bioreactor_7(t,y)*h
       y=yb+(rk1+rk2)/2
    }
    if(ncase==2){
       yb=y
       rk1=bioreactor_7(t,y)*h
       y1=yb+rk1; t=t+h
       rk2=bioreactor_7(t,y1)*h
       y=yb+(rk1+rk2)/2
       ee=y-y1
    }
    }
#
#   Solution after nt modified Euler steps
    cat(sprintf("\n %8.0f%8.4f%8.4f%8.4f%8.4f%8.4f%8.4f
      %8.4f",
    t,y[1],y[2],y[3],y[4],y[5],y[6],y[7]))
```

```
      if(ncase==2){
        cat(sprintf("\n                %8.4f%8.4f%8.4f%8.4f%8.4f
            %8.4f%8.4f\n",
          ee[1],ee[2],ee[3],ee[4],ee[5],ee[6],ee[7]))}
      out[i1,-1]=y
      out[i1,1]=t
    }
#
# Calls to bioreactor_7
  cat(sprintf("\n ncall = %5d\n\n",ncall))
#
# Single plot
  par(mfrow=c(1,1))
#
# y1
  plot(out[,1],out[,2],type="l",xlab="t",ylab="y1(t),...,
      y7(t)",
    xlim=c(0,2000),ylim=c(0,0.14),lty=1, main="y1(t),...,
        y7(t) vs t",
    lwd=2)
#
# y2
  lines(out[,1],out[,3],type="l",lty=2,lwd=2)
#
# y3
  lines(out[,1],out[,4],type="l",lty=3,lwd=2)
#
# y4
  lines(out[,1],out[,5],type="l",lty=4,lwd=2)
#
# y5
  lines(out[,1],out[,6],type="l",lty=5,lwd=2)
#
# y6
  lines(out[,1],out[,7],type="l",lty=6,lwd=2)
#
# y7
  lines(out[,1],out[,8],type="l",lty=7,lwd=2)
```

Listing 1.8: Comparison of the solutions of eqs. (1.1) from the Euler and the modified Euler methods.

We can note the following details about Listing 1.8.

- The ODE routine is `bioreactor_7` and is the same as Listing 1.6b. Also, two cases are programmed. ncase=1 is the same as the integration in Listing 1.7. ncase=2 gives an estimate of the solution error by comparing the solutions from the Euler method (eq. (1.4)) and the modified Euler method (eqs. (1.11)).

```
#
# ODE routine
  setwd("c:/R/bme_ode/chap1")
  source("bioreactor_7.R")
#
# Select modified Euler format
#
# ncase = 1: RK format
#
# ncase = 2: RK format with explicit error estimate
  ncase=2;
```

- The programming of the parameters for eqs. (1.1) is the same as in Listing 1.7.
- The ICs of Listing 1.7 are now extended to include the estimated integration error ee. The initial values (at $t = 0$) of the error are zero (ee=c(0,0,0,0,0,0,0)) because the numerical solutions for the Euler and modified Euler methods are the same (they have the same IC, y=c(0.10724,0,0,0,0,0,0)).

```
#
# Initial condition
  n=7;nout=51;t=0;ncall=0;
  y=c(0.10724,0,0,0,0,0,0)
  cat(sprintf(
  "\n        t       y1       y2       y3       y4       y5
     y6       y7"))
  if(ncase==2){
  ee=c(0,0,0,0,0,0,0)
    cat(sprintf(
  "\n                 e1       e2       e3       e4       e5
```

```
      e6        e7"))}
  cat(sprintf("\n %8.0f%8.4f%8.4f%8.4f%8.4f%8.4f%8.4f
     %8.4f",
  t,y[1],y[2],y[3],y[4],y[5],y[6],y[7]))
  if(ncase==2){
    cat(sprintf("\n                %8.4f%8.4f%8.4f%8.4f%8.4f
       %8.4f%8.4f\n",
     ee[1],ee[2],ee[3],ee[4],ee[5],ee[6],ee[7]))}
```

Output with a heading and the ICs is included. Also, the initial values of the estimated error, ee, are displayed.

- The output array, out, and the parameters for the t integration are the same as in Listing 1.7.
- The two cases for the ODE integration are programmed as

```
#
# Modified Euler integration
  for(i1 in 2:nout){
#
#   nt modified Euler steps
    for(i2 in 1:nt){
    if(ncase==1){
      yb=y
      rk1=bioreactor_7(t,y)*h
      y=yb+rk1; t=t+h
      rk2=bioreactor_7(t,y)*h
      y=yb+(rk1+rk2)/2
    }
    if(ncase==2){
      yb=y
      rk1=bioreactor_7(t,y)*h
      y1=yb+rk1; t=t+h
      rk2=bioreactor_7(t,y1)*h
      y=yb+(rk1+rk2)/2
      ee=y-y1
    }
    }
```

The ODE routine is bioreactor_7 and is the same as Listing 1.6b. For ncase=1, the programming is the same as in Listing 1.7.

For ncase=2, the error ee is estimated as the difference between the Euler solution, y1, and the modified Euler solution, y, that is, ee=y-y1. Note that the R vector facility is used because y1, y, ee are vectors with seven elements. The final left } concludes the for loop in i2.

- The solution and estimated errors are displayed after nt modified Euler steps (performed in the for loop with index i2).

```
#
#    Solution after nt modified Euler steps
     cat(sprintf("\n %8.0f%8.4f%8.4f%8.4f%8.4f%8.4f
        %8.4f%8.4f",
     t,y[1],y[2],y[3],y[4],y[5],y[6],y[7]))
     if(ncase==2){
       cat(sprintf("\n           %8.4f%8.4f%8.4f%8.4f
          %8.4f%8.4f%8.4f\n",
       ee[1],ee[2],ee[3],ee[4],ee[5],ee[6],ee[7]))}
     out[i1,-1]=y
     out[i1,1]=t
   }
```

The final left } concludes the for in i1.

- The number of calls to the ODE routine bioreactor_7, ncall, and the plotting are the same as in Listing 1.7.

Abbreviated output from Listing 1.8 is given in Table 1.8.

We can note the following details about this output.

- The ICs ($t = 0$) are confirmed for the solution and the estimated error.
- The estimated errors throughout the solution are zero to four figures as expected, because the Euler solution from Listing 1.6a and the modified Euler solution from Listings 1.9 and 1.10 agree to at least four figures.
- The number of calls to bioreactor_7 remains at (2) (40000)=80000 from Listing 1.7 as expected.

As a concluding point, we were able to estimate the error in the numerical solution (ncase=2) without any additional computation (beyond ncase=1).

TABLE 1.8   Abbreviated numerical output from Listing 1.8.

t	y1	y2	y3	y4	y5	y6	y7
	e1	e2	e3	e4	e5	e6	e7
0	0.1072	0.0000	0.0000	0.0000	0.0000	0.0000	0.0000
	0.0000	0.0000	0.0000	0.0000	0.0000	0.0000	0.0000
40	0.0752	0.0020	0.0153	0.0009	0.0195	0.0011	0.0006
	0.0000	0.0000	-0.0000	0.0000	-0.0000	-0.0000	0.0000

Output from t = 80 to 1920 removed

1960	0.0000	0.0003	0.0003	0.0000	0.1306	0.0071	0.0223
	0.0000	0.0000	-0.0000	0.0000	-0.0000	-0.0000	0.0000
2000	0.0000	0.0002	0.0002	0.0000	0.1307	0.0071	0.0223
	0.0000	0.0000	-0.0000	0.0000	-0.0000	-0.0000	0.0000

ncall = 80000

To conclude this section, we can note that eqs. (1.12) are a particular second-order Runge–Kutta method from a group generally defined by the selection of some arbitrary constants. However, the Euler method of eq. (1.4) is the only (unique) first-order Runge–Kutta method.

1.11   Modified Euler Method as an Embedded Method

Since the Euler and the modified Euler solutions in the preceding section are the same, this suggests that the numerical solution has been confirmed (at least to four figures) by agreement of the solutions from algorithms of two different orders. Also, as the first Runge–Kutta derivative, k_1, is the same for both the methods, this suggests that the first-order (Euler) method is embedded in the second-order (modified Euler) method. The idea that two embedded algorithms can be used as the basis for estimating the errors in a numerical solution (e.g., as programmed in Listing 1.8 for `ncase=2`) is now considered. Eqs. (1.12) can be written in an alternate form that provides an explicit estimate of the error, ε.

$$k_1 = f(y_i, t_i)h \tag{1.13a}$$

$$y_{i+1}^p = y_i + k_1 \tag{1.13b}$$

$$k_2 = f(y_{i+1}^p, t_{i+1})h = f(y_i + k_1, t_i + h)h \tag{1.13c}$$

$$\varepsilon_{i+1} = \frac{k_2 - k_1}{2} \tag{1.13d}$$

$$y_{i+1}^c = y_{i+1}^p + \varepsilon_{i+1} \tag{1.13e}$$

where the superscripts p and c indicate a predicted value and a corrected value, respectively. Note that

$$y_{i+1}^c = y_i + k_1 + \frac{k_2 - k_1}{2} = y_i + \frac{k_1 + k_2}{2} \tag{1.13f}$$

which is just the modified Euler method.

We can note the following properties of eqs. (1.13).

- Eq. (1.13a) gives the first Runge–Kutta derivative, k_1.
- Eq. (1.13b) is the Euler method (eq. (1.4)), a first-order method based on k_1, that gives the predicted value y_{i+1}^p.
- Eq. (1.13c) gives the second Runge–Kutta derivative, k_2, from the predicted value y_{i+1}^p
- Eq. (1.13d) is an explicit estimate of the solution error, ε, computed from k_1 and k_2.
- Eq. (1.13e) gives a corrected value of the solution, y_{i+1}^c, by adding the estimated error to the predicted value as a correction.
- Eq. (1.13f) confirms that the corrected value is the same as that for the second-order modified Euler method. Thus, we can consider the result of eq. (1.13e) as a first-order method embedded in a second-order method. The key to this idea of an embedded pair is the same Runge–Kutta derivative k_1 for both methods.

The implementation (programming) of eqs. (1.13) is a straightforward modification of the `ncase=2` programming in Listing 1.8.

```
#
# Modified Euler integration
  for(i1 in 2:nout){
#
#    nt modified Euler steps
    for(i2 in 1:nt){
    if(ncase==1){
      yb=y
      rk1=bioreactor_8(t,y)*h
      y1=yb+rk1; t=t+h
      rk2=bioreactor_8(t,y1)*h
      y=yb+(rk1+rk2)/2
      ee=y-y1
    }
    if(ncase==2){
      yb=y
      rk1=bioreactor_8(t,y)*h
      y1=yb+rk1; t=t+h
      rk2=bioreactor_8(t,y1)*h
      ee=(rk2-rk1)/2
      y=y1+ee
    }
    }
```

Listing 1.9: Programming of the Euler and modified Euler methods as an embedded pair.

The ODE routine is `bioreactor_8` and is the same as Listing 1.6b. Eqs. (1.13) is programmed as `ncase=2`. The correspondence of the programming and eqs. (1.13) is clear. Note that the estimated error `ee` computed according to eq. (1.13d), `ee=(rk2-rk1)/2`, is added as a correction, `y=y1+ee`, according to eq. (1.13e). The final left `}` concludes the `for` loop in `i2`.

The explicit error estimate ε_{i+1} can be used to adjust the integration step h according to a specified error tolerance. If ε_{i+1} is above the specified tolerance, h can be reduced and the step from i to $i + 1$ is repeated. This reduction in h can be repeated until the estimated error is less than the specified error tolerance, at which point h can be considered small enough to achieve the required accuracy in the numerical solution (from the Euler method of eq. (1.13b)). The estimated error can then be added as a correction to the (predicted) solution at $i + 1$ (eq. (1.13e)) to produce an improved (corrected) value that is the starting value for the next step along the solution, from $i + 1$ to $i + 2$.

Note that this procedure of using the estimated error to adjust the integration step requires only the ODE (eq. (1.3a)) and not an exact solution of the ODE. However, we should keep in mind that eq. (1.13d) provides an estimate of the error and not the exact error (that would generally require the exact solution). The details of adjusting the integration step h is not considered here. However, step size adjustment to meet a specified error tolerance is used in most quality library integrators such as lsoda (in the R utility ode) and lsodes.

We can now apply these basic ideas to higher order Runge–Kutta methods, including the use of an estimated error computed from an embedded Runge–Kutta pair. In conclusion, this development and implementation (programming) of higher order Runge–Kutta methods is based on the fundamental idea that these methods fit the underlying Taylor series of the ODE solution to any number of terms without having to differentiate the ODE (they require only the first derivative in $\dfrac{dy}{dt} = f(y, t)$ of eq. (1.3a) at selected points along the solution).

1.12 Classic Fourth-Order Runge–Kutta Method as an Embedded Method

The classic fourth-order Runge–Kutta method, which was reported more than 100 years ago, is

$$k_1 = f(y_i, t_i)h \tag{1.14a}$$

$$k_2 = f(y_i + k_1/2, t_i + h/2)h \tag{1.14b}$$

$$k_3 = f(y_i + k_2/2, t_i + h/2)h \tag{1.14c}$$

$$k_4 = f(y_i + k_3, t_i + h)h \tag{1.14d}$$

$$y_{4,i+1} = y_i + (1/6)(k_1 + 2k_2 + 2k_3 + k_4); \quad t_{i+1} = t_i + h$$

$$(1.14e)$$

Eqs. (1.14) fit the Taylor series up to and including the fourth-order derivative term, $\dfrac{d^4y}{dt^4}\dfrac{h^4}{4!}$, that is, the resulting numerical solution is $O(h^4)$. This higher order is achieved by evaluating the Runge–Kutta derivatives k_1, k_2, k_3, and k_4 at the points $t_i, t_i + h/2, t_i + h/2$, and $t_i + h$, respectively.

The second-order Runge–Kutta method can be used in combination with eqs. (1.14).

$$k_1 = f(y_i, t_i)h \tag{1.15a}$$

$$k_2 = f(y_i + k_1/2, t_i + h/2)h \tag{1.15b}$$

$$y_{2,i+1} = y_i + k_2; \quad t_{i+1} = t_i + h \tag{1.15c}$$

which is the midpoint method. As the name suggests, k_2 is computed at the midpoint between i and $i + 1$, that is, at $t_i + h/2$.

The second-order midpoint Runge–Kutta method of eqs. (1.15) has the same k_1 and k_2 as the classic fourth-order Runge–Kutta method (compare eqs. (1.14a) and (1.15a), eqs. (1.14b) and (1.15b)), and therefore, this second-order method is embedded in the fourth-order method. An error estimate for this second-order method can be obtained by subtracting the second-order solution $y_{2,i+1}$ (eq. (1.15c)) from the fourth-order solution $y_{4,i+1}$ (eq. (1.14e)).

$$\epsilon_{i+1} = y_{4,i+1} - y_{2,i+1} = y_i + (1/6)(k_1 + 2k_2 + 2k_3 + k_4) - (y_i + k_2)$$
$$= (1/6)(k_1 - 4k_2 + 2k_3 + k_4) \tag{1.16}$$

Note how the k_1 and k_2 terms combine in arriving at eq. (1.16) because they are the same for both algorithms. As this error estimate was achieved by subtracting the second-order solution from the fourth order solution, it actually represents two terms in the Taylor series, $\dfrac{d^3y}{dt^3}\dfrac{h^3}{3!}$ and $\dfrac{d^4y}{dt^4}\dfrac{h^4}{4!}$, that is, ϵ_i from eq. (1.16) is a two-term error estimate, and therefore, we might expect that it will be more accurate than the one-term error estimate of eq. (1.13d). Experience has indicated this is the case.

The following are the principal conclusions from this discussion of embedded methods:

- The Runge–Kutta derivatives generally can be computed once for both the lower order and the higher order methods of an embedded pair. In other words, the common Runge–Kutta derivatives are the basis for embedded pairs.
- Correction of the lower order solution using the estimated error (the difference between the higher and lower order solutions) gives a substantially improved lower order solution. In other words, the higher order solution is used as the base point for the next step along the solution.
- The estimated error could be used to adjust the integration step h according to a prescribed error tolerance.

Listing 1.9 is an extension of Listing 1.8 for eqs. (1.14) and (1.15).

```
#
# ODE routine
  setwd("c:/R/bme_ode/chap1")
  source("bioreactor_9.R")
#
# Select classical fourth order Runge Kutta method
#
# ncase = 1: RKC4
#
# ncase = 2: RKC4 with embedded second order midpoint
#            method and error estimate
  ncase=2;
#
# Parameter values for BP10001
  k1=8.87e-03;
  k2=13.18;
  k3=0.129;
  k4=0.497;
  k5=0.027;
  k6=0.545e-3;
  km2=87.7;
  km3=99.9;
#
```

```
# Initial condition
  n=7;nout=51;t=0;ncall=0;
  y=c(0.10724,0,0,0,0,0,0)
  cat(sprintf(
  "\n          t       y1      y2      y3      y4      y5
     y6       y7"))
  if(ncase==2){
  ee=c(0,0,0,0,0,0,0)
    cat(sprintf(
  "\n              e1      e2      e3      e4      e5
     e6       e7"))}
  cat(sprintf("\n %8.0f%8.4f%8.4f%8.4f%8.4f%8.4f%8.4f
     %8.4f",
  t,y[1],y[2],y[3],y[4],y[5],y[6],y[7]))
  if(ncase==2){
    cat(sprintf("\n          %8.4f%8.4f%8.4f%8.4f%8.4f%8.4f
       %8.4f\n",
    ee[1],ee[2],ee[3],ee[4],ee[5],ee[6],ee[7]))}
#
# Arrays for output
  out=matrix(0,nrow=nout,ncol=(n+1))
  out[1,-1]=y
  out[1,1]=t
#
# Parameters for t integration
# nt=400;h=0.10   # unstable
  nt=800;h=0.05   # stable
#
# rkc4 integration
  for(i1 in 2:nout){
#
#   nt rkc4 steps
    for(i2 in 1:nt){
    if(ncase==1){
      yb=y; tb=t
      rk1=bioreactor_9(tb,yb)*h
      y=yb+0.5*rk1; t=tb+0.5*h
      rk2=bioreactor_9(t,y)*h
      y=yb+0.5*rk2; t=tb+0.5*h
      rk3=bioreactor_9(t,y)*h
      y=yb+rk3; t=tb+h
```

```
      rk4=bioreactor_9(t,y)*h
      y=yb+(1/6)*(rk1+2*rk2+2*rk3+rk4)
    }
    if(ncase==2){
      yb=y; tb=t
      rk1=bioreactor_9(tb,yb)*h
      y=yb+0.5*rk1; t=tb+0.5*h
      rk2=bioreactor_9(t,y)*h
      y2=yb+rk2
      y=yb+0.5*rk2; t=tb+0.5*h
      rk3=bioreactor_9(t,y)*h
      y=yb+rk3; t=tb+h
      rk4=bioreactor_9(t,y)*h
      y=yb+(1/6)*(rk1+2*rk2+2*rk3+rk4)
      ee=y-y2
    }
    }
#
#    Solution after nt rkc4 steps
    cat(sprintf("\n %8.0f%8.4f%8.4f%8.4f%8.4f%8.4f%8.4f
      %8.4f",
    t,y[1],y[2],y[3],y[4],y[5],y[6],y[7]))
    if(ncase==2){
      cat(sprintf("\n            %8.4f%8.4f%8.4f%8.4f%8.4f
        %8.4f%8.4f\n",
      ee[1],ee[2],ee[3],ee[4],ee[5],ee[6],ee[7]))}
    out[i1,-1]=y
    out[i1,1]=t
  }
#
# Calls to bioreactor_9
  cat(sprintf("\n ncall = %5d\n\n",ncall))
#
# Single plot
  par(mfrow=c(1,1))
#
# y1
  plot(out[,1],out[,2],type="l",xlab="t",ylab="y1(t),...,
    y7(t)",
    xlim=c(0,2000),ylim=c(0,0.14),lty=1, main="y1(t),...,
      y7(t) vs t",
```

```
  lwd=2)
#
# y2
  lines(out[,1],out[,3],type="l",lty=2,lwd=2)
#
# y3
  lines(out[,1],out[,4],type="l",lty=3,lwd=2)
#
# y4
  lines(out[,1],out[,5],type="l",lty=4,lwd=2)
#
# y5
  lines(out[,1],out[,6],type="l",lty=5,lwd=2)
#
# y6
  lines(out[,1],out[,7],type="l",lty=6,lwd=2)
#
# y7
  lines(out[,1],out[,8],type="l",lty=7,lwd=2)
```

Listing 1.10: The classic fourth-order Runge–Kutta with the embedded midpoint method.

We can note the following details about Listing 1.10.

- The ODE routine is bioreactor_9 and is the same as Listing
  1.6b. Also, two cases are programmed. ncase=1 is for eqs. (1.14).
  ncase=2 is for a combination of eqs. (1.14) and (1.15), including
  the estimated error.

```
#
# ODE routine
  setwd("c:/R/bme_ode/chap1")
  source("bioreactor_9.R")
#
# Select classical fourth order Runge Kutta method
#
# ncase = 1: RKC4
#
# ncase = 2: RKC4 with embedded second order midpoint
```

```
#                    method and error estimate
  ncase=2;
```

- The programming of the parameters for eqs. (1.1) is the same as in Listing 1.8.
- The ICs and the output array out of Listing 1.8 are repeated.
- The two cases for the ODE integration are programmed as

```
#
# Parameters for t integration
# nt=400;h=0.10  # unstable
  nt=800;h=0.05  # stable
#
# rkc4 integration
  for(i1 in 2:nout){
#
#   nt rkc4 steps
    for(i2 in 1:nt){
    if(ncase==1){
      yb=y; tb=t
      rk1=bioreactor_9(tb,yb)*h
      y=yb+0.5*rk1; t=tb+0.5*h
      rk2=bioreactor_9(t,y)*h
      y=yb+0.5*rk2; t=tb+0.5*h
      rk3=bioreactor_9(t,y)*h
      y=yb+rk3; t=tb+h
      rk4=bioreactor_9(t,y)*h
      y=yb+(1/6)*(rk1+2*rk2+2*rk3+rk4)
    }
    if(ncase==2){
      yb=y; tb=t
      rk1=bioreactor_9(tb,yb)*h
      y=yb+0.5*rk1; t=tb+0.5*h
      rk2=bioreactor_9(t,y)*h
      y2=yb+rk2
      y=yb+0.5*rk2; t=tb+0.5*h
      rk3=bioreactor_9(t,y)*h
      y=yb+rk3; t=tb+h
      rk4=bioreactor_9(t,y)*h
      y=yb+(1/6)*(rk1+2*rk2+2*rk3+rk4)
```

```
    ee=y-y2
}
}
```

The ODE routine is `bioreactor_9` and is the same as Listing 1.6b. For `ncase=1`, the programming is for eqs. (1.14). For `ncase=2`, the error `ee` is estimated as the difference between the fourth-order Runge–Kutta and the second-order midpoint method of eqs. (1.15) (`ee=y-y2`).

- The solution and estimated errors are displayed after `nt` steps (performed in the `for` loop with index `i2`). The final left `}` concludes the `for` loop in `i2`.

- The number of calls to the ODE routine `bioreactor_9` is `ncall=160000` as expected (four derivative evaluations for each Euler step, with 40,000 Euler steps). The numerical and graphical outputs are the same as for Listings 1.10 and 1.11 (including Table 1.6).

Eqs. (1.16) can easily be programmed as a variant of the `ncase=2` code.

```
ee=(1/6)*(rk1-4*rk2+2*rk3+k4)
y=y2+ee
```

Note also that the integration step is again $h = 0.05$. We might expect that the higher order method of eqs. (1.14) would permit a larger step. This is true with respect to accuracy, but it is not true with respect to stability. In fact, the constant c in eq. (1.5) for the fourth-order method of eqs. (1.14) is only 2.785. In other words, the calculation of four derivatives in eqs. (1.14) extended the stability limit of the Euler and modified Euler methods only slightly from $c = 2$ to $c = 2.785$; of course, the advantage of doing the additional derivative calculations is the increase in accuracy from $O(h^2)$ (modified Euler method) to $O(h^4)$ (the fourth-order method of eqs. (1.14)). But the numerical integration of eqs. (1.1) (which are stiff) is limited by stability to a step of $h = 0.05$ (and not limited by accuracy because all of the preceding numerical solutions were similar to four figures);

in other words, we might say the integration step of $h = 0.05$ was excessively small with regard to accuracy.

1.13 RKF45 Method

To conclude the discussion of ODE numerical integration with explicit Runge–Kutta methods, we consider a widely used embedded pair usually designated as RKF45 [5, p 84].

$$k_1 = f(y_i, t_i)h \qquad\qquad (1.17a)$$

$$k_2 = f(y_i + k_1/4, t_i + h/4)h \qquad\qquad (1.17b)$$

$$k_3 = f(y_i + (3/32)k_1 + (9/32)k_2, t_i + (3/8)h)h \qquad\qquad (1.17c)$$

$$k_4 = f(y_i + (1932/2197)k_1 - (7200/2197)k_2 + (7296/2197)k_3, t_i$$
$$+ (12/13)h)h \qquad\qquad (1.17d)$$

$$k_5 = f(y_i + (439/216)k_1 - 8k_2 + (3680/513)k_3$$
$$- (845/4104)k_4, t_i + h)h \qquad\qquad (1.17e)$$

$$k_6 = f(y_i - (8/27)k_1 + 2k_2 - (3544/2565)k_3 + (1859/4104)k_4$$
$$- (11/40)k_5, t_i + (1/2)h)h \qquad\qquad (1.17f)$$

An $O(h^4)$ method is then

$$y_{4,i+1} = y_i + (25/216)k_1 + (1408/2565)k_3$$
$$+ (2197/4104)k_4 - (1/5)k_5 \qquad\qquad (1.17g)$$

and an $O(h^5)$ method is (with the same ks)

$$y_{5,i+1} = y_i + (16/315)k_1 + (6656/12825)k_3 + (28561/56430)k_4$$
$$- (9/50)k_5 + (2/55)k_6 \qquad\qquad (1.17h)$$

An error estimate can then be obtained by subtracting eq. (1.17g) from eq. (1.17h).

$$\epsilon_{i+1} = y_{i+1,5} - y_{i+1,4} \qquad\qquad (1.17i)$$

Note that six derivative evaluations are required (k_1 through k_6), even though the final result from eq. (1.17h) is only $O(h^5)$ (the number of derivative evaluations will, in general, be equal to or greater than the order of the method).

The formulas of eqs. (1.17g) and (1.17h) match the Taylor series up to and including the terms $\dfrac{d^4 y_i}{dt^4} \dfrac{h^4}{4!}$ and $\dfrac{d^5 y_i}{dt^5} \dfrac{h^5}{5!}$, respectively.

Eqs. (1.17) is implemented in Listing 1.11.

```
#
# ODE routine
  setwd("c:/R/bme_ode/chap1")
  source("bioreactor_10.R")
#
# Select rkf45 format
#
# ncase = 1: No error estimation
#
# ncase = 2: With error estimation
  ncase=2;
#
# Parameter values for BP10001
  k1=8.87e-03;
  k2=13.18;
  k3=0.129;
  k4=0.497;
  k5=0.027;
  k6=0.545e-3;
  km2=87.7;
  km3=99.9;
#
# Initial condition
  n=7;nout=51;t=0;ncall=0;
  y=c(0.10724,0,0,0,0,0,0)
  cat(sprintf(
  "\n        t       y1      y2      y3      y4      y5
     y6       y7"))
  if(ncase==2){
  ee=c(0,0,0,0,0,0,0)
    cat(sprintf(
  "\n                e1      e2      e3      e4      e5
     e6       e7"))}
```

```
  cat(sprintf("\n %8.0f%8.4f%8.4f%8.4f%8.4f%8.4f%8.4f
     %8.4f",
  t,y[1],y[2],y[3],y[4],y[5],y[6],y[7]))
  if(ncase==2){
    cat(sprintf("\n            %8.4f%8.4f%8.4f%8.4f%8.4f%8.4f
       %8.4f\n",
    ee[1],ee[2],ee[3],ee[4],ee[5],ee[6],ee[7]))}
#
# Arrays for output
  out=matrix(0,nrow=nout,ncol=(n+1))
  out[1,-1]=y
  out[1,1]=t
#
# Parameters for t integration
# nt=400;h=0.10  # unstable
  nt=800;h=0.05  # stable
#
# rkf45 integration
  for(i1 in 2:nout){
#
#    nt rkf45 steps
    for(i2 in 1:nt){
    if(ncase==1){
      yb=y; tb=t;
      rk1=bioreactor_10(tb,yb)*h
      y=yb+0.25*rk1;
      t=tb+0.25*h;
      rk2=bioreactor_10(t,y)*h
      y=yb+(3/32)*rk1+(9/32)*rk2;
      t=tb+(3/8)*h;
      rk3=bioreactor_10(t,y)*h
      y=yb+(1932/2197)*rk1-(7200/2197)*rk2+(7296/2197)
         *rk3;
      t=tb+(12/13)*h;
      rk4=bioreactor_10(t,y)*h
      y=yb+(439/216)*rk1-8*rk2 +(3680/513)*rk3 -(845/4104)
         *rk4;
      t=tb+h;
      rk5=bioreactor_10(t,y)*h
      y=yb-(8/27)*rk1+2*rk2-(3544/2565)*rk3+(1859/4104)
         *rk4-(11/40)*rk5;
```

```
      t=tb+0.5*h;
      rk6=bioreactor_10(t,y)*h
      y=yb+(16/135)*rk1+(6656/12825)*rk3+(28561/56430)
         *rk4-(9/50)*rk5+
            (2/55)*rk6;
      t=tb+h;
    }
    if(ncase==2){
      yb=y; tb=t;
      rk1=bioreactor_10(tb,yb)*h
      y=yb+0.25*rk1;
      t=tb+0.25*h;
      rk2=bioreactor_10(t,y)*h
      y=yb+(3/32)*rk1+(9/32)*rk2;
      t=tb+(3/8)*h;
      rk3=bioreactor_10(t,y)*h
      y=yb+(1932/2197)*rk1-(7200/2197)*rk2+(7296/2197)
         *rk3;
      t=tb+(12/13)*h;
      rk4=bioreactor_10(t,y)*h
      y=yb+(439/216)*rk1-8*rk2 +(3680/513)*rk3 -(845/4104)
         *rk4;
      t=tb+h;
      rk5=bioreactor_10(t,y)*h
      y=yb-(8/27)*rk1+2*rk2-(3544/2565)*rk3+(1859/4104)
         *rk4-(11/40)*rk5;
      t=tb+0.5*h;
      rk6=bioreactor_10(t,y)*h
#
#     Fourth order step
      y4=yb+(25/216)*rk1+(1408/2565)*rk3  +(2197/4104)
         *rk4-( 1/5)*rk5;
#
#     Fifth order step
      y=yb+(16/135)*rk1+(6656/12825)*rk3+(28561/56430)
         *rk4-(9/50)*rk5+
            (2/55)*rk6;
      t=tb+h;
#
#     Truncation error estimate
      ee=y-y4
```

```
      }
    }
#
#    Solution after nt rkf45 steps
    cat(sprintf("\n %8.0f%8.4f%8.4f%8.4f%8.4f%8.4f%8.4f
       %8.4f",
    t,y[1],y[2],y[3],y[4],y[5],y[6],y[7]))
    if(ncase==2){
      cat(sprintf("\n            %8.4f%8.4f%8.4f%8.4f%8.4f
         %8.4f%8.4f\n",
      ee[1],ee[2],ee[3],ee[4],ee[5],ee[6],ee[7]))}
    out[i1,-1]=y
    out[i1,1]=t
  }
#
# Calls to bioreactor_10
  cat(sprintf("\n ncall = %5d\n\n",ncall))
#
# Single plot
  par(mfrow=c(1,1))
#
# y1
  plot(out[,1],out[,2],type="l",xlab="t",ylab="y1(t),...,
    y7(t)",
    xlim=c(0,2000),ylim=c(0,0.14),lty=1, main="y1(t),...,
      y7(t) vs t",
    lwd=2)
#
# y2
  lines(out[,1],out[,3],type="l",lty=2,lwd=2)
#
# y3
  lines(out[,1],out[,4],type="l",lty=3,lwd=2)
#
# y4
  lines(out[,1],out[,5],type="l",lty=4,lwd=2)
#
# y5
  lines(out[,1],out[,6],type="l",lty=5,lwd=2)
#
# y6
```

```
  lines(out[,1],out[,7],type="l",lty=6,lwd=2)
#
# y7
  lines(out[,1],out[,8],type="l",lty=7,lwd=2)
```

Listing 1.11: Implementation of the RKF45 method.

We can note the following details of Listing 1.11.

- The ODE routine is `bioreactor_10`, the same as Listing 1.6b.
  Also, two cases are programmed. `ncase=1` is for just the fifth-
  order method of eqs. (1.17). `ncase=2` is for a combination of the
  fourth- and fifth-order methods with an estimated error.

```
  #
  # ODE routine
    setwd("c:/R/bme_ode/chap1")
    source("bioreactor_10.R")
  #
  # Select rkf45 format
  #
  # ncase = 1: No error estimation
  #
  # ncase = 2: With error estimation
    ncase=2
```

- The programming of the parameters for eqs. (1.1) is the same as
  in Listing 1.10.
- The ICs, the output array `out`, and the integration parameters of
  Listing 1.10 are repeated.
- The two cases for the ODE integration are programmed as

```
  #
  # rkf45 integration
    for(i1 in 2:nout){
  #
  #    nt rkf45 steps
      for(i2 in 1:nt){
      if(ncase==1){
        yb=y; tb=t;
```

```
        rk1=bioreactor_10(tb,yb)*h
        y=yb+0.25*rk1;
        t=tb+0.25*h;
        rk2=bioreactor_10(t,y)*h
        y=yb+(3/32)*rk1+(9/32)*rk2;
        t=tb+(3/8)*h;
        rk3=bioreactor_10(t,y)*h
        y=yb+(1932/2197)*rk1-(7200/2197)*rk2+(7296/2197)
          *rk3;
        t=tb+(12/13)*h;
        rk4=bioreactor_10(t,y)*h
        y=yb+(439/216)*rk1-8*rk2 +(3680/513)*rk3
          -(845/4104)*rk4;
        t=tb+h;
        rk5=bioreactor_10(t,y)*h
        y=yb-(8/27)*rk1+2*rk2-(3544/2565)*rk3
          +(1859/4104)*rk4-(11/40)*rk5;
        t=tb+0.5*h;
        rk6=bioreactor_10(t,y)*h
        y=yb+(16/135)*rk1+(6656/12825)*rk3+(28561/56430)
          *rk4-(9/50)*rk5+
            (2/55)*rk6;
        t=tb+h;
      }
      if(ncase==2){
        yb=y; tb=t;
        rk1=bioreactor_10(tb,yb)*h
        y=yb+0.25*rk1;
        t=tb+0.25*h;
        rk2=bioreactor_10(t,y)*h
        y=yb+(3/32)*rk1+(9/32)*rk2;
        t=tb+(3/8)*h;
        rk3=bioreactor_10(t,y)*h
        y=yb+(1932/2197)*rk1-(7200/2197)*rk2+(7296/2197)
          *rk3;
        t=tb+(12/13)*h;
        rk4=bioreactor_10(t,y)*h
        y=yb+(439/216)*rk1-8*rk2 +(3680/513)*rk3-(845/
          4104)*rk4;
        t=tb+h;
        rk5=bioreactor_10(t,y)*h
```

```
            y=yb-(8/27)*rk1+2*rk2-(3544/2565)*rk3+(1859/
                4104)*rk4-(11/40)*rk5;
            t=tb+0.5*h;
            rk6=bioreactor_10(t,y)*h
#
#           Fourth order step
            y4=yb+(25/216)*rk1+(1408/2565)*rk3  +(2197/4104)
                *rk4-(1/5)*rk5;
#
#           Fifth order step
            y=yb+(16/135)*rk1+(6656/12825)*rk3+(28561/56430)
                *rk4-(9/50)*rk5+
                  (2/55)*rk6;
            t=tb+h;
#
#           Truncation error estimate
            ee=y-y4
          }
        }
```

For ncase=1, the programming is for the fifth-order method of eqs. (1.16) (eq. (1.17g) is not used). For ncase=2, the error ee is estimated as the difference between the fourth-order method (y4 from eq. (1.17g)) and the fifth- order method (y from eq. (1.17h)), that is, ee=y-y4.

- The solution and estimated errors are displayed after nt steps (performed in the for loop with index i2). The final left } concludes the for loop in i2.
- The number of calls to the ODE routine bioreactor_10 is ncall=240000. The numerical and graphical outputs are the same as for Listing 1.10. The value of ncall is from six derivative evaluations, (6)(40000)=240000.

The name RKF45 reflects the Runge–Kutta–Fehlberg method based on a fourth-order method embedded in a fifth-order method.

This concludes the discussion of the numerical integration of eqs. (1.1). The intent was to provide an introduction to the ODE integration in terms of some selected explicit Runge–Kutta methods, that is, the Euler, the modified Euler, the classic fourth order, and the RKF45 methods. An important point to note is the large number of derivative evaluations required to maintain stability, for example, `ncall=240000` for RKF45. In comparison, `lsoda` of `ode` required only 427 derivative evaluations (see Listing 1.7b and the related discussion). Thus, the automatic switching between stiff and nonstiff methods in `lsoda` was very effective.

Generally, an implicit integrator should be used for stiff ODEs. To this end, we consider some low order, fixed step implicit integrators in Appendix A1. However, for nonstiff ODEs, the explicit Runge–Kutta methods discussed previously can be very effective in computing an accurate ODE solution and should therefore be considered. For example, in Chapter 2, a nonstiff ODE model is considered for which explicit algorithms give an accurate solution with fewer derivative evaluations than `lsoda` in `ode`. In addition, explicit methods require fewer calculations at each point along the solution.

These integrators can be programmed as separate, stand-alone routines which would simplify the programming (make it more modular); examples of the use of a separate integrator routine are given in Chapter 2. Also, explicit Runge–Kutta library integrators such as RKF45 are included in `deSolve`. These library integrators have automatic step adjustment in accordance with a user-specified error tolerance (but the source code is not available as in the preceding listings).

References

[1] Beard, D.A. (2012), *Biosimulation: Simulation of Living Systems*, Cambridge University Press, Cambridge, UK.

[2] Butcher, J.W. (2003), *Numerical Methods for Ordinary Differential Equations*, John Wiley & Sons, Inc., Hoboken, NJ.

[3] Butcher, J.W., *Runge–Kutta Methods*, Scholarpedia, vol. 2, no. 9, 2007, p 3147; available at: http://www.scholarpedia.org/article/Runge-Kutta_methods.

[4] Deuflhard, P., and F. Bornemann (2002), *Scientific Computing with Ordinary Differential Equations*, Springer-Verlag, New York.

[5] Iserles, A. (1996), *A First Course in the Numerical Analysis of Differential Equations*, Cambridge University Press, Cambridge, UK.

[6] Lee, H.J., and W.E. Schiesser (2004), *Ordinary and Partial Differential Equation Routines, in C, C++, Fortran, Java, Maple and Matlab*, CRC Press, Boca Raton, FL.

[7] Schiesser, W.E. (2013), *Partial Differential Equation Analysis in Biomedical Engineering*, Cambridge University Press, Cambridge, UK.

[8] Shampine, L.F., and S. Thompson (2007a), Stiff systems, Scholarpedia, vol. 2, no. 3, p 2855; available at: `http://www.scholarpedia.org/article/Stiff_systems`.

[9] Shampine, L.F., and S. Thompson (2007b), *Initial value problems*, Scholarpedia, vol. 2, no. 3, p 2861; available at: `http://www.scholarpedia.org/article/Initial_value_problems`.

[10] Soetaert, K., J. Cash, and F. Mazzia (2012), *Solving Differential Equations in R*, Springer-Verlag, Heidelberg, Germany.

## CHAPTER 2

Diabetes Glucose Tolerance Test

2.1 Introduction

This case study has a two-fold purpose:

1. Application of the ODE numerical methods of Chapter 1 to a model for a diabetes glucose tolerance test [3].
2. Consideration of features of the model and its numerical solutions that illustrate some basic properties of the ODE models.

2.2 Mathematical Model

This chapter is based on the pioneering and highly informative mathematical model of the glucose tolerance test for diabetes presented by Randall ([3], p 69) and authors referenced therein. Although this model consists of just two ordinary ODEs in time, it provides a clear and basic introduction to the physiological response from changes in glucose level, particularly through variations in the insulin level. The two ODEs for the glucose and insulin levels, $G(t)$ and $I(t)$, respectively, are next represented in words followed by mathematical symbols.

Differential Equation Analysis in Biomedical Science and Engineering: Ordinary Differential Equation Applications with R, First Edition. William E. Schiesser.
© 2014 John Wiley & Sons, Inc. Published 2014 by John Wiley & Sons, Inc.

2.2.1   Glucose Balance

A mass balance on the glucose in the extracellular fluid can be stated as follows:

$$\begin{array}{l} \text{rate of change} \\ \text{of glucose} \end{array} = \begin{array}{l} \text{liver} \\ \text{production} \end{array} + \begin{array}{l} \text{glucose} \\ \text{infusion} \end{array} - \begin{array}{l} \text{insulin} \\ \text{control} \end{array}$$

$$- \begin{array}{l} \text{first order} \\ \text{metabolism} \end{array} - \begin{array}{l} \text{renal} \\ \text{removal} \end{array} \qquad (2.1a)$$

If eq. (2.1a) is applied to 100 ml of the extracellular fluid, a two-part ODE follows.

$$C_g \frac{dG}{dt} = Q + I_n - G_g IG - D_d G; \ G < G_k \qquad (2.1b)$$

$$C_g \frac{dG}{dt} = Q + I_n - G_g IG - D_d G - M_u(G - G_k); \ G \geq G_k \quad (2.1c)$$

We can then make a term-by-term comparison between eq. (2.1a) and eqs. (2.1b) and (2.1c).

Eq. (2.1a)	Eqs. (2.1b) and (2.1c)	Comments
rate of change of glucose	$C_g dG/dt$	$dG/dt < 0$, $G(t)$ decreasing with t $dG/dt > 0$, $G(t)$ increasing with t
liver production	Q	prescribed positive constant
glucose infusion	I_n	positive function of t
insulin control	$-G_g IG$	nonlinear from $I(t)G(t)$
first-order metabolism	$-D_d G$	decrease in $G(t)$ with $D_d > 0$
renal removal	$-M_u(G - G_k)$	negative function for $G \geq G_k$ zero function for $G < G_k$

$$\qquad (2.1d)$$

Numerical values and units for the model parameters for eqs. (2.1a), (2.1b), and (2.1c) are as follows:

G: extracellular glucose (mg glucose/100 ml extracellular fluid)

t: time (h)

C_g: glucose capacitance $= E_x/100$ (number of 100 ml extracellular volumes)

E_x: total extracellular space (ml)

Q: liver release of glucose (mg glucose/h)

I_n: glucose infusion, 0 or Q_t

Q_t: glucose infusion rate (mg glucose/h)

I: extracellular insulin (mg insulin/100 ml extracellular fluid)

G_g: controlled glucose loss

$$\left(\frac{\text{mg glucose}}{\text{h}}\right)\left(\frac{1}{\text{mg insulin/100 ml extracellular fluid}}\right)$$
$$\left(\frac{1}{\text{mg glucose/100 ml extracellular fluid}}\right)$$

D_d: first order glucose loss

$$\left(\frac{\text{mg glucose}}{\text{h}}\right)\left(\frac{1}{\text{mg glucose/100 ml extracellular fluid}}\right)$$

G_k: renal threshold (mg glucose/100 extracellular fluid)

M_u: renal loss rate

$$\left(\frac{\text{mg glucose}}{\text{h}}\right)\left(\frac{1}{\text{mg glucose/100 ml extracellular fluid}}\right)$$

We can note some interesting and important features of eqs. (2.1b) and (2.1c).

- The dependent variable $G(t)$ is the glucose concentration in units of mg glucose/100 ml of the extracellular fluid; these units are designated subsequently as mGml.

- These ODEs are nonlinear; for example, the term $G_g IG$ is a product of G with a second dependent variable, I, the insulin concentration. Therefore, an analytical solution to the ODE system is probably precluded and a numerical solution is required.

- The ODEs also have a variable coefficient in the sense that the term $M_u(G - G_k)$ is switched on to account for renal loss (kidney removal) of glucose. In addition, the glucose infusion, I_n, is an explicit function of the independent variable, t.

- Each term in eqs. (2.1b) and (2.1c) has the unit mg glucose/hr:

Q: mg glucose/hr

I_n: mg glucose/hr

$G_g IG$:

$$\left(\frac{\text{mg glucose}}{\text{hr}} \right) \left(\frac{1}{\text{mg insulin/100 ml extracellular fluid}} \right)$$

$$\left(\frac{1}{\text{mg glucose/100 ml extracellular fluid}} \right)$$

$$\left(\frac{\text{mg insulin}}{100 \text{ ml extracellular fluid}} \right) \left(\frac{\text{mg glucose}}{100 \text{ ml extracellular fluid}} \right)$$

$$= \text{mg glucose/hr}$$

$D_d G$:

$$\left(\frac{\text{mg glucose}}{\text{hr}} \right) \left(\frac{1}{\text{mg glucose/100 ml extracellular fluid}} \right)$$

$$\left(\frac{\text{mg glucose}}{100 \text{ ml extracellular fluid}} \right)$$

$$= \text{mg glucose/hr}$$

$M_u (G - G_k)$:

$$\left(\frac{\text{mg glucose}}{\text{hr}} \right) \left(\frac{1}{\text{mg glucose/100 ml extracellular fluid}} \right)$$

$$\left(\frac{\text{mg glucose}}{100 \text{ ml extracellular fluid}} \right)$$

$$= \text{mg glucose/hr}$$

$C_g \dfrac{dG}{dt}$:

(number of 100 ml extracellular volumes)

$$\left(\frac{\text{mg glucose}}{100 \text{ ml extracellular fluid}} \frac{1}{\text{hr}} \right)$$

$$= \text{mg glucose/hr}$$

The sign of the derivative $\dfrac{dG}{dt}$ is an important consideration because it determines if the glucose $G(t)$ is increasing with t $\left(\dfrac{dG}{dt} > 0\right)$, which might indicate that diabetes is a significant problem, that is, a condition of *hyperglycemia*; or decreasing with t $\left(\dfrac{dG}{dt} < 0\right)$, which might indicate that diabetes is not a problem or under control; or possibly a condition of excessively low glucose, that is, a condition of *hypoglycemia*.

- As all of the constants and variables are in hours, the timescale for the solution of eqs. (2.1b) and (2.1c) will also be in hours; this follows particularly from the derivative $C_g\dfrac{dG}{dt}$ which has the time units of h^{-1}. For the subsequent calculations, this timescale is taken as $0 \le t \le 12$ h, that is, $G(t), I(t)$ will be calculated for 12 hr.

In summary, this check for the consistency of units throughout eqs. (2.1b) and (2.1c) is essential to ensure that the solution $G(t)$ is correct. Also, these units provide additional insight into the physical/chemical significance of each term.

For example, the coefficient G_g in the nonlinear term G_gIG is particularly noteworthy because it is a direct indicator of the effect of insulin (I) on glucose level. If G_g is lower than normal, this could be interpreted as a condition for which insulin is less effective in determining glucose level than normal, that is, a resistance to insulin or Type II diabetes.

We now go through a similar analysis for the insulin mass balance, which leads to a second ODE for $I(t)$ that is used in eqs. (2.1b) and (2.1c); that is, the two ODE are *simultaneous* or *coupled*.

2.2.2 Insulin Balance

The insulin mass balance can be stated in words as

$$\begin{array}{ccc} \text{rate of change} \\ \text{of insulin} \end{array} = - \begin{array}{c} \text{first-order insulin} \\ \text{reduction} \end{array} + \begin{array}{c} \text{pancreas insulin} \\ \text{release rate} \end{array} \quad (2.2a)$$

If eq. (2.2a) is applied to 100 of the extracellular fluid, a two-part ODE results.

$$C_i \frac{dI}{dt} = -A_a I, \ G < G_0 \tag{2.2b}$$

$$C_i \frac{dI}{dt} = -A_a I + B_b(G - G_0), \ G \geq G_0 \tag{2.2c}$$

We can then make a term-by-term comparison between eq. (1.2a) and eqs. (1.2b) and (1.2c).

Eq. (2.2a)	Eqs. (2.2b), (2.2c)	Comments
rate of change of insulin	$C_{id} I / dt$	$dI/dt < 0$, $I(t)$ decreasing with t $dI/dt > 0$, $I(t)$ increasing with t
first-order insulin reduction	$-A_a I$	decrease in $I(t)$ for $A_a > 0$
pancreas insulin release rate	$B_b(G - G_0)$	positive function for $G \geq G_0$ zero function for $G < 0$

$$\tag{2.2d}$$

Numerical values and units for the model parameters for eqs. (2.2a), (2.2b), and (2.2c) are as follows:

I: extracellular insulin (mg insulin/100 ml extracellular fluid)

C_i: insulin capacitance $= E_x/100$ (number of 100 ml extracellular volumes)

A_a: first-order insulin reduction rate

$$\left(\frac{\text{mg insulin}}{\text{h}} \right) \left(\frac{1}{\text{mg insulin/100 ml extracellular fluid}} \right)$$

G_0: pancreas threshold (mg glucose/100 extracellular fluid)

B_b: pancreas insulin release rate

$$\left(\frac{\text{mg insulin}}{\text{h}} \right) \left(\frac{1}{\text{mg glucose/100 ml extracellular fluid}} \right)$$

We can note some interesting and important features of eqs. (2.2b) and (2.2c).

- The dependent variable $I(t)$ is the insulin concentration in units of mg insulin/100 ml of the extracellular fluid; these units are designated subsequently as mIml.
- The ODEs also have a variable coefficient in the sense that the term $B_b(G - G_0)$ is switched on to account for insulin production by the pancreas.
- Each term in eqs. (2.1b) and (2.1c) has the unit mg insulin/hr:

$A_a I$:

$$\left(\frac{\text{mg insulin}}{\text{hr}}\right)\left(\frac{1}{\text{mg insulin/100 ml extracellular fluid}}\right)$$

$$\left(\frac{\text{mg insulin}}{100 \text{ ml extracellular fluid}}\right)$$

$$= \text{mg insulin/hr}$$

$B_b(G - G_0)$:

$$\left(\frac{\text{mg insulin}}{\text{hr}}\right)\left(\frac{1}{\text{mg glucose/100 ml extracellular fluid}}\right)$$

$$\left(\frac{\text{mg glucose}}{100 \text{ ml extracellular fluid}}\right)$$

$$= \text{mg insulin/hr}$$

$C_i \dfrac{dI}{dt}$:

$$\text{(number of 100 ml extracellular volumes)}$$

$$\left(\frac{\text{mg insulin}}{100 \text{ ml extracellular fluid}}\frac{1}{\text{hr}}\right)$$

$$= \text{mg insulin/hr}$$

The sign of the derivative $\dfrac{dI}{dt}$ is an important consideration because it determines if the insulin $I(t)$ is increasing with t $\left(\dfrac{dI}{dt} > 0\right)$, which might indicate that diabetes is not a significant problem, or decreasing with t $\left(\dfrac{dI}{dt} < 0\right)$, which might indicate that diabetes is a problem.

- Since all of the constants and variables are in hours, the timescale for the solution of eqs. (2.2b) and (2.2c) will also be in hours as required to be consistent with the simultaneous solution of eqs. (2.1b) and (2.1c).

In summary, this check for the consistency of units throughout eqs. (2.2b) and (2.2c) is essential to ensure that the solution $I(t)$ is correct. Also, these units provide additional insight into the physical/chemical significance of each term.

For example, the coefficient B_b in the term $B_b(G - G_0)$ is noteworthy because it is a direct indicator of pancreatic insulin production. If B_b is lower than normal, this could be interpreted as a condition of below normal insulin production, that is, Type I diabetes. Variations in B_b are studied in the subsequent computer analysis.

Eqs. (2.1) and (2.2) constitute the mathematical model for the glucose tolerance test. We now consider a computer solution of these equations.

2.3   Computer Analysis of the Mathematical Model

Eqs. (2.1) and (2.2) constitute a 2×2 ODE system (two equations in two unknowns). These equations are *not stiff*, and therefore, an *explicit integrator* can be used for their solution.[1] In other words, the derivatives $\dfrac{dG}{dt}, \dfrac{dI}{dt}$ of eqs. (2.1) and (2.2) produce solutions $G(t), I(t)$ on approximately the same timescale (one dependent variable does not move at a much higher rate than the other). This is a somewhat loose description of a nonstiff ODE problem.

2.3.1   ODE Integration by lsoda

We start the discussion of the numerical solution of eqs. (2.1) and (2.2) with the library integrator lsoda in the R utility ode.[2]

---

[1]The concepts of stiffness and explicit integration are discussed in detail in [2], Appendix C, and [4].

[2]Numerical methods for initial-value ODEs are discussed in Chapter 1.

A main program with a call to ode is listed next. A discussion of this main program then follows the listing.

```
#
# Glucose Tolerance Test
#
# The glucose tolerance test is used clinically to
# evaluate the ability of the pancreas to release insulin
# in response to a large dose of glucose given either
# orally or intravenously.  The normal pancreas releases
# enough insulin to lower the plasma glucose within a few
# hours, sometimes to the point of hyperglycemia.  The
# deficiency of insulin release, characteristic of Type 1
# diabetes, also termed juvenile-onset diabetes, prolongs
# the fall of glucose for many hours (1).
#
# (1)  Randall, James E., Microcomputers and Physiological
# Simulation, Addison-Wesley Publishing Company, Inc.,
# Reading, MA, 1980, p69.
#
# The following differential equations can be used to
# compute the glucose and insulin levels as a function
# of time:
#
#    Cg*dG/dt = Q + In - (Gg*I*G) - Dd*G, G < Gk        (1)
#
#    Cg*dG/dt = Q + In - (Gg*I*G) - Dd*G - Mu*(G - Gk),
#       G >= Gk (2)
#
#    Ci*dI/dt = -Aa*I, G < GO                           (3)
#
#    Ci*dI/dt = -Aa*I + Bb*(G - GO), G >= GO            (4)
#
# where
#
#    Symbol         Parameters/Variables      Normal Values
#
#     Ex      extracellular space                15000 ml
#
#     Cg      glucose capacitance = Ex/100       150 ml
#
```

```
#      Ci      insulin capacitance = Ex/100       150 ml
#
#      Q       liver release of glucose          8400 mG/hr
#
#      Gt      glucose infusion rate            80000 mG/hr
#
#      In      glucose infusion, Gt or 0
#
#      Dd      first-order glucose loss     24.7 mG/hr/mGml
#
#      Gg      controlled glucose loss 13.9 mG/hr/mGml/mIml
#
#      Gk      renal threshold                   250 mGml
#
#      Mu      renal loss rate               72 mG/hr/mGml
#
#      G0      pancreas threshold                51 mGml
#
#      Bb      insulin release rate        14.3 mI/hr/mGml
#
#      Aa      first-order insulin rate      76 mI/hr/mGml
#
#      G       extracellular glucose         81 mGml (t = 0)
#
#      I       extracellular insulin        5.7 mIml (t = 0)
#
#      t       time                                   hr
#
# The mass and concentration units are:
#
#      mG      milligrams of glucose
#
#      mI      milligrams of insulin
#
#      mGml    milligrams of glucose/100 ml extracellular
#                  fluid
#
#      mIml    milligrams of insulin/100 ml extracellular
```

```
#                  fluid
#
#       ml      milliliter = cubic centimeter = 0.001 liter
#
# The glucose infusion function, In, is given by:
#
#              In = Gt, 0 <= t < 0.5
#
#              In = 0, 0.5 <= t <= 12
#
# Equations (1) to (4) are integrated for four cases:
#
#    (1)  (ncase = 1)
#
#         normal pancreatic sensitivity (Bb = 14.3)
#         (without glucose infusion, Gt = 0)
#
#    (2)  (ncase = 2)
#
#         normal pancreatic sensitivity (Bb = 14.3)
#         (with glucose infusion)
#
#    (3)  (ncase = 3)
#
#         reduced pancreatic sensitivity (Bb = 0.2(14.3))
#         (with glucose infusion)
#
#    (4)  (ncase = 4)
#
#         elevated pancreatic sensitivity (Bb = 2.0(14.3))
#         (with glucose infusion)
#
# Library of R ODE solvers
  library("deSolve")
#
# ODE routine
  setwd("c:/R/bme_ode/chap2")
  source("glucose_1.R")
```

```
#
# Vectors, matrices for the graphical output
  nout=49
  Gplot=matrix(0,nrow=nout,ncol=4)
  Iplot=matrix(0,nrow=nout,ncol=4)
  tplot=rep(0,nout)
#
# Step through four cases
  for(ncase in 1:4){
#
# Select the case parameters
  if(ncase==1){Bb=14.3;          Gt=0}
  if(ncase==2){Bb=14.3;       Gt=80000}
  if(ncase==3){Bb=0.2*14.3; Gt=80000}
  if(ncase==4){Bb=2.0*14.3; Gt=80000}
#
# Model parameters
  Ex=15000; Cg=150; Ci=150; Q=8400; Dd=24.7;
   Gg=13.9; Gk=250;  Mu=72;  G0=51;    Aa=76;
#
# Initialize counter for calls to glucose_1
  ncall=0
#
# Initial condition
  yini=c(81.14,5.671)
  yini
#
# t interval
  times=seq(from=0,to=12,by=12/(nout-1))
#
# ODE integration
  out=ode(y=yini,times=times,func=glucose_1,parms=NULL)
#
# ODE numerical solution
  for(it in 1:nout){
    if(it==1){
    cat(sprintf(
    "\n ncase = %2d \n\n          t        In        G
```

```
      I",ncase))}
#
#   Glucose infusion function
    t=times[it]
    if((t>=0)&(t<=0.51)){In=Gt}
    if( t>0.51)              {In=0 }
    cat(sprintf("\n %8.2f%8.0f%8.2f%8.3f",
                out[it,1],In,out[it,2],out[it,3]))
  }
#
# Store solution for plotting
  Gplot[,ncase]=out[,2]
  Iplot[,ncase]=out[,3]
  if(ncase==1)tplot=out[,1]
#
# Calls to glucose_1
  cat(sprintf("\n\n ncall = %5d\n\n",ncall))
#
# Next case
}
#
# Single plot for G
  par(mfrow=c(1,1))
#
# G, ncase = 1
  plot(tplot,Gplot[,1],xlab="t (hr)",
  ylab="G(t) (mg glucose/100 ml) vs t",
  xlim=c(0,12),ylim=c(0,300),type="b",lty=1,pch="1",lwd=2,
  main="Extracellular glucose, G(t), ncase = 1,2,3,4")
#
# G, ncase = 2
  lines(tplot,Gplot[,2],type="b",lty=1,pch="2",lwd=2)
#
# G, ncase = 3
  lines(tplot,Gplot[,3],type="b",lty=1,pch="3",lwd=2)
#
# G, ncase = 4
  lines(tplot,Gplot[,4],type="b",lty=1,pch="4",lwd=2)
```

```
#
# Single plot for I
  par(mfrow=c(1,1))
#
# I, ncase = 1
  plot(tplot,Iplot[,1],xlab="t (hr)",
  ylab="I(t) (mg insulin/100 ml) vs t",
  xlim=c(0,12),ylim=c(0,25),type="b",lty=1,pch="1",
     lwd=2,
  main="Extracellular insulin, I(t), ncase = 1,2,3,4")
#
# I, ncase = 2
  lines(tplot,Iplot[,2],type="b",lty=1,pch="2",lwd=2)
#
# I, ncase = 3
  lines(tplot,Iplot[,3],type="b",lty=1,pch="3",lwd=2)
#
# I, ncase = 4
  lines(tplot,Iplot[,4],type="b",lty=1,pch="4",lwd=2)
```

Listing 2.1 Main program for the numerical integration of eqs. (2.1) and (2.2).

We can note the following points about Listing 2.1.

- A block of comments documents the model of eqs. (2.1) and (2.2) (they are not repeated here to conserve space). In particular, four cases are explained, for ncase = 1 to ncase = 4, in which the pancreas sensitivity parameter B_b is varied. The details of these four cases are discussed in the comments and subsequently.

- The R library of the ODE integrators, deSolve, is accessed for the solution of eqs. (2.1) and (2.2).

```
#
# Library of R ODE solvers
  library("deSolve")
```

- The ODE routine `glucose_1` with the programming of eqs. (2.1) and (2.2) is accessed through `setwd` (set working directory) and `source` (to specify the file name).

```
#
# ODE routine
  setwd("c:/R/bme_ode/chap2")
  source("glucose_1.R")
```

- Two 2D matrices for plotting $G(t)$ from eq. (2.1) and $I(t)$ from eq. (2.2) are declared (preallocated) with the `matrix` utility for `nout=49` values of t and `ncol=4` cases (described previously in the comments).

```
#
# Vectors, matrices for the graphical output
  nout=49
  Gplot=matrix(0,nrow=nout,ncol=4)
  Iplot=matrix(0,nrow=nout,ncol=4)
  tplot=rep(0,nout)
```

The vector for `nout=49` values of t is also declared with the `rep` utility. Forty-nine output values were selected to give (i) three points for the glucose infusion function ($t = 0, 0.25, 0.5$) in the output and (ii) enough points for the plots without crowding.

- Four cases are programmed with a `for`. For each case, the model parameters `Bb`, `Gt` are defined numerically.

```
#
# Step through four cases
  for(ncase in 1:4){
#
# Select the case parameters
  if(ncase==1){Bb=14.3;              Gt=0}
  if(ncase==2){Bb=14.3;        Gt=80000}
  if(ncase==3){Bb=0.2*14.3; Gt=80000}
  if(ncase==4){Bb=2.0*14.3; Gt=80000}
```

Note in particular that for ncase = 1, Gt=0 so that no glucose infusion takes place. This corresponds to the normal condition without a glucose tolerance test. ncase = 2,3,4 then corresponds to the response to a glucose infusion of Gt=80000 (mg glucose) for three different values of the pancreas sensitivity parameter B_b.

- The remaining parameters in eqs. (2.1) and (2.2) are defined numerically.

```
#
# Model parameters
  Ex=15000; Cg=150; Ci=150; Q=8400; Dd=24.7;
  Gg=13.9; Gk=250;  Mu=72;  G0=51;   Aa=76;
```

These parameter values are available to the subordinate ODE routine glucose_1 (discussed subsequently).

- The counter for the number of calls to glucose_1 is initialized.

```
#
# Initialize counter for calls to glucose_1
  ncall=0
```

- The ICs for eqs. (2.1) and (2.2) are specified to start the solution.

```
#
# Initial condition
  yini=c(81.14,5.671)
  yini
```

Note the use of the R utility c to place the two ICs in a vector, yini, that is, G(t=0)=81.14, I(t=0)=5.671. The use of the name yini on a separate line displays the two numerical values for confirmation.

- The interval in t is defined as $0 \le t \le 12$ with the 49 values $t = 0, 12/(49 - 1) = 0.25, 0.50, \ldots, 12$ placed in the vector times (using the R utility seq).

```
#
# t interval
  times=seq(from=0,to=12,by=12/(nout-1))
```

- The ODE solution is computed by a call to ode that is available in deSolve.

```
#
# ODE integration
  out=ode(y=yini,times=times,func=glucose_1,
    parms=NULL)
```

Note the use of the IC vector yini and the output values of t in times as the input arguments y and times to ode. Also, the ODE routine glucose_1 with the programming of eqs. (2.1) and (2.2) is an input to ode through the argument func. In other words, y,times,func are reserved names. The numerical solution is returned from ode as a 2D array, out. The argument parms is unused.

- The numerical ODE solution in out is displayed for the nout=49 values of t with a for in it. For it=1 corresponding to $t = 0$, a heading for the solution is displayed.

```
#
# ODE numerical solution
  for(it in 1:nout){
    if(it==1){
    cat(sprintf(
    "\n ncase = %2d \n\n          t      In      G
      I",ncase))}
#
#    Glucose infusion function
    t=times[it]
    if((t>=0)&(t<=0.51)){In=Gt}
    if( t>0.51)           {In=0 }
    cat(sprintf("\n %8.2f%8.0f%8.2f%8.3f",
                out[it,1],In,out[it,2],out[it,3]))
  }
```

The infusion function In is computed to be included in the numerical output. if((t>=0)&(t<=0.51))In=Gt is used in place of if((t>=0)&(t<=0.5))In=Gt to avoid the test of equality t=0.5, which is unreliable in floating point arithmetic.

out[it,1] has the 49 values of t. out[it,2], out[it,3] have the 49 values of $G(t)$ and $I(t)$, respectively.

- The solution is placed in two 2D arrays for plotting. Note the use of , to include all (49) values of the first subscript. The second subscript is for each of the four solutions (set by the previous for(ncase in 1:4)).

```
#
# Store solution for plotting
  Gplot[,ncase]=out[,2]
  Iplot[,ncase]=out[,3]
  if(ncase==1)tplot=out[,1]
```

- The number of calls to glucose_1 is displayed.

```
#
# Calls to glucose_1
  cat(sprintf("\n ncall = %5d\n\n",ncall))
#
# Next case
}
```

The concluding } terminates the for in ncase.

- A composite plot with the four solutions for $G(t)$ is produced. For the first solution (ncase=1 with Gplot[,1] vs tplot), the plotting is similar to that in Listing 1.2 and therefore the details (input arguments to plot) are not repeated here.

```
#
# Single plot for G
  par(mfrow=c(1,1))
#
# G, ncase = 1
  plot(tplot,Gplot[,1],xlab="t (hr)",
  ylab="G(t) (mg glucose/100 ml) vs t",
  xlim=c(0,12),ylim=c(0,300),type="b",lty=1,pch="1",
    lwd=2,
  main="Extracellular glucose, G(t), ncase = 1,2,3,4")
```

pch="1" specifies the character 1 for the plot points in the first solution.

- The solutions for ncase=2,3,4 follow from the lines utility. The plot characters are 2,3,4.
- A similar set of statements provides the composite plot for $I(t)$.

The ODE routine, glucose_1, called by ode is in Listing 2.2.

```
glucose_1=function(t,y,parms) {
#
# Assign state variables
  G=y[1];
  I=y[2];
#
# Glucose infusion function
  if((t>=0)&(t<=0.51)){In=Gt}
  if( t>0.51)            {In=0 }
#
# ODEs
#
# Glucose equations
  if(G< Gk){dGdt=(1/Cg)*(Q+In-(Gg*I*G)-Dd*G)}
  if(G>=Gk){dGdt=(1/Cg)*(Q+In-(Gg*I*G)-Dd*G-Mu*(G-Gk))}
#
# Insulin equations
  if(G< G0){dIdt=(1/Ci)*(-Aa*I)}
  if(G>=G0){dIdt=(1/Ci)*(-Aa*I+Bb*(G-G0))}
#
# Calls to glucose_1
  ncall <<- ncall+1
#
# Return derivative vector
  return(list(c(dGdt,dIdt)))
}
```

Listing 2.2 ODE routine glucose_1 for the eqs. (2.1) and (2.2).

We can note the following details about glucose_1.

- The function is defined.

```
    glucose_1=function(t,y,parms) {
```

- The dependent variable vector y is expressed as two problem-oriented variables G, I to facilitate the programming of eqs. (2.1) and (2.2).

```
#
# Assign state variables
  G=y[1];
  I=y[2];
```

Note that y is an input vector (RHS argument) to glucose_1. It has two elements as specified by the number of ICs in the main program of Listing 2.1.

- The glucose infusion function In is defined at a particular value of the independent variable t (an input or RHS arguments to glucose_1).

```
#
# Glucose infusion function
  if((t>=0)&(t<=0.51)){In=Gt}
  if( t>0.51)          {In=0 }
```

In equals Gt for $0 \leq t \leq 0.5$ h and zero thereafter.

- Eqs. (2.1b) and (2.1c) are programmed in a straightforward manner, including the switch based on Gk to add the term -Mu*(G-Gk).

```
#
# Glucose equations
  if(G< Gk){dGdt=(1/Cg)*(Q+In-(Gg*I*G)-Dd*G)}
  if(G>=Gk){dGdt=(1/Cg)*(Q+In-(Gg*I*G)-Dd*G-Mu*
    (G-Gk))}
```

Note that in order to calculate the derivative $dG/dt =$ dGdt, all of the RHS variables and parameters must be defined numerically. For $t = 0$, G, I are available from the ICs set previously in the main program of Listing 2.1. For $t > 0$, G, I are available through the input argument y. All of the parameters were defined numerically in Listing 2.1.

This coding illustrates the ease of numerically including the time-dependent switch for the two forms of eqs. (2.1b) and (2.1c). Also, the nonlinear term `-(Gg*I*G)` is easily included. These features would be difficult to accommodate analytically.

- Eqs. (2.2b) and (2.2c) are programmed in a similar way, including the switch based on G0 to include the term $B_b(G - G_0)$.

```
#
# Insulin equations
  if(G< G0){dIdt=(1/Ci)*(-Aa*I)}
  if(G>=G0){dIdt=(1/Ci)*(-Aa*I+Bb*(G-G0))}
```

This is the point at which the variation in Bb (changes in the pancreas sensitivity) for the four cases ncase = 1,2,3,4 enters the numerical solution.

- The number of calls to glucose_1 is incremented

```
#
# Calls to glucose_1
  ncall <<- ncall+1
```

with the return of the value of ncall to the main program of Listing 2.1 using <<-.

- Finally, the two derivatives $dG/dt, dI/dt$ are returned as a list (as required by the ODE integrators in deSolve).

```
#
# Return derivative vector
  return(list(c(dGdt,dIdt)))
}
```

The final } concludes glucose_1.

The numerical and graphical outputs from Listings 2.1 and 2.2 follows. Abbreviated numerical output for ncase = 1,2,3,4 is in Table 2.1.

TABLE 2.1   Abbreviated output from the routines of Listings 2.1 and 2.2.

```
ncase =  1

        t      In      G       I
     0.00       0   81.14   5.671
     0.25       0   81.14   5.671
     0.50       0   81.14   5.671
     0.75       0   81.14   5.671
     1.00       0   81.14   5.671
       .                    .
       .                    .
       .                    .
  Output for t = 1.25 to 10.75 removed
       .                    .
       .                    .
       .                    .
    11.00       0   81.14   5.671
    11.25       0   81.14   5.671
    11.50       0   81.14   5.671
    11.75       0   81.14   5.671
    12.00       0   81.14   5.671

ncall =     95

ncase =  2

        t      In      G       I
     0.00   80000   81.14    5.671
     0.25   80000  201.71    7.100
     0.50   80000  286.72   10.687
     0.75       0  217.19   13.881
     1.00       0  159.88   15.265
       .                    .
       .                    .
       .                    .
```

TABLE 2.1 (*Continued*)

```
Output for t = 1.25 to 10.75 removed

       .              .
       .              .
       .              .
   11.00       0    80.90    5.681
   11.25       0    80.92    5.674
   11.50       0    80.96    5.670
   11.75       0    80.99    5.666
   12.00       0    81.03    5.664

ncall =    358

ncase =  3

       t      In       G        I
    0.00    80000    81.14    5.671
    0.25    80000   204.22    5.420
    0.50    80000   305.96    5.704
    0.75        0   265.14    6.070
    1.00        0   233.03    6.230
       .              .
       .              .
       .              .
Output for t = 1.25 to 10.75 removed

       .              .
       .              .
       .              .
   11.00       0   129.31    2.894
   11.25       0   129.31    2.900
   11.50       0   129.29    2.906
   11.75       0   129.26    2.911
   12.00       0   129.22    2.915

ncall =    297
```

(*continued*)

TABLE 2.1 *(Continued)*

```
ncase =   4

       t       In       G        I
     0.00    80000    81.14    5.671
     0.25    80000   198.66    9.167
     0.50    80000   265.50   16.454
     0.75        0   172.61   21.905
     1.00        0   108.34   23.153
      .                         .
      .                         .
      .                         .
  Output for t = 1.25 to 10.75 removed
      .                         .
      .                         .
      .                         .
    11.00        0    69.47    6.905
    11.25        0    69.49    6.911
    11.50        0    69.50    6.917
    11.75        0    69.50    6.922
    12.00        0    69.49    6.926

ncall =    422
```

We can note the following details for this output.

- For ncase = 1, the solution does not change from the ICs. This implies that the derivatives $dG/dt \approx 0, dI/dt \approx 0$ can be confirmed by numerically evaluating the RHS of eqs. (2.1c) and (2.2c) with $I_n = 0$ (no glucose infusion). First, for eq. (2.1c),

$$C_g \frac{dG}{dt} = Q + I_n - G_g IG - D_d G - M_u(G - G_k); \ G \geq G_k$$

$$\frac{dG}{dt} = \frac{1}{C_g}(Q + I_n - G_g IG - D_d G - M_u(G - G_k)); \ G \geq G_k$$

$$\frac{dG}{dt} = \frac{1}{150}(8400 + 0 - (13.9)(5.671)(81.14)$$

$$- (24.7)(81.14))$$

$$= -0.00115$$

Here, we have used the IC $G = 81.18$, $I = 5.671$, and because $G = 81.14 < G_k = 250$, the term with M_u is dropped. This small value of the derivative at $t = 0$ is actually the largest value during the solution $0 \leq t \leq 12$. So eq. (2.1c) essentially remains at the IC $G = 81.14$ as reflected in the constant (time invariant) solution for ncase = 1.

- The number of calls to ode_1, ncall = 95 is relatively small because the solution does not change.

- A similar analysis of eq. (2.2c) again indicates a small value for $\dfrac{dI}{dt}$.

$$C_i \frac{dI}{dt} = -A_a I + B_b (G - G_0), \ G \geq G_0$$

$$\frac{dI}{dt} = \frac{1}{C_i}(-A_a I + B_b (G - G_0)), \ G \geq G_0$$

$$\frac{dI}{dt} = \frac{1}{150}(-(76)(5.671) + (14.3)(81.14 - 51))$$

$$= 0.0000, \ G \geq G_0$$

so that eqs. (2.2) also remains at the IC $I = 5.671$. Note that this requires the pancreatic insulin production, $B_b(G - G_0)$, is not zero.

- The infusion of glucose will, therefore, cause the ODE system to depart from the steady state. That is, $I_n(t) \neq 0$ in eqs. (2.1b) and (2.1c) will drive the ODE system away from equilibrium. This is reflected in the solutions for ncase = 2,3,4. For ncase = 2, the abbreviated solution is

```
ncase =  2
```

t	In	G	I
0.00	80000	81.14	5.671
0.25	80000	201.71	7.100
0.50	80000	286.72	10.687
0.75	0	217.19	13.881
1.00	0	159.88	15.265

```
         .                    .
         .                    .
         .                    .
  Output for t = 1.25 to 10.75 removed
         .                    .
         .                    .
         .                    .
   11.00      0    80.90    5.681
   11.25      0    80.92    5.674
   11.50      0    80.96    5.670
   11.75      0    80.99    5.666
   12.00      0    81.03    5.664

ncall =    358
```

We can note the following details about this numerical output.

— The glucose infusion, I_n, is 80,000 for $0 \le t \le 0.5$ and zero thereafter, which follows from the programming in Listing 2.1

```
if(ncase==2){Bb=14.3; Gt=80000}
```

— The solution undergoes a transient (departure from the ICs) and then approaches the same steady state as for ncase = 1 as reflected in the output at $t = 12$: 12.0 0 81.03 5.664. In other words, the model returns to a normal condition as a response to the glucose infusion $I_n(t)$.

— The number of calls to glucose_1 is 358 which is larger than for ncase=1 because smaller steps in t are required because of the changing solution.

• For ncase = 3, the abbreviated solution is

```
ncase =   3

       t      In       G       I
    0.00   80000    81.14   5.671
    0.25   80000   204.22   5.420
    0.50   80000   305.96   5.704
    0.75       0   265.14   6.070
    1.00       0   233.03   6.230
```

.
.
.

```
Output for t = 1.25 to 10.75 removed
```

.
.
.

```
11.00        0   129.31   2.894
11.25        0   129.31   2.900
11.50        0   129.29   2.906
11.75        0   129.26   2.911
12.00        0   129.22   2.915

ncall =    297
```

We can note the following details about this numerical output.

— For ncase = 3, the insulin release rate B_b is decreased by a factor of 0.2; that is, from the main program in Listing 2.1 (Figs. 2.1 and 2.2)

```
if(ncase==3){Bb=0.2*14.3; Gt=80000}
```

— The solution undergoes a transient (departure from the ICs) and then approaches a new steady state (different than for ncase = 1,2) as reflected in the output at $t = 12$: 12.0 0 129.22 2.915. As expected (when B_b is decreased), the final glucose level $G(t)$ is higher than for ncase = 1,2 and the insulin level, $I(t)$, is lower.

— The new final equilibrium values correspond to $dG/dt \approx 0$, $dI/dt \approx 0$. This is confirmed by a numerical evaluation of the RHS of eqs. (2.1c) and (2.2c).

$$\frac{dG}{dt} = \frac{1}{150}(8400 + 0 - (13.9)(2.915)(129.22)$$
$$- (24.7)(129.22)) = -0.1836$$

This derivative at $t = 12$ is not zero but is small (and would become smaller with t beyond 12). For a comparison, the derivative $\dfrac{dG}{dt}$ at $t = 0$ is

$$\frac{dG}{dt} = \frac{1}{150}(8400 + 80000 - (13.9)(5.663)(81.027)$$
$$- (24.7)(81.027)) = 533.47$$

This large initial derivative is not unusual (frequently ODEs exhibit their largest derivatives initially), and therefore, the solution changes most rapidly at the IC.

— The insulin level $I(t)$ reaches the final value 2.915 since the derivatives is effectively zero,

$$\frac{dI}{dt} = \frac{1}{150}(-(76)(2.915) + (0.2)(14.3)(129.22 - 51))$$
$$= 0.0144, \ G \geq G_0$$

Note the reduced value of B_b used in this calculation, $(0.2)(14.3)$.

— The number of calls to glucose_1 is 297, which is different from that for ncase=2, reflecting the variable step method in lsoda of ode.

In conclusion, for ncase = 3, the reduced pancreatic sensitivity causes the glucose level $G(t)$ to reach a value higher than the normal value (because of the decreased insulin release rate B_b)—a condition of *hyperglycemia*. Similarly, the insulin level $I(t)$ reaches a value lower than the normal value.

• For ncase = 4, the abbreviated solution is

```
ncase =   4

       t       In        G       I
    0.00    80000    81.14   5.671
    0.25    80000   198.66   9.167
    0.50    80000   265.50  16.454
    0.75        0   172.61  21.905
    1.00        0   108.34  23.153
       .                       .
```

```
        .                    .
        .                    .
        .                    .
Output for t = 1.25 to 10.75 removed
        .                    .
        .                    .
        .                    .
    11.00        0    69.47   6.905
    11.25        0    69.49   6.911
    11.50        0    69.50   6.917
    11.75        0    69.50   6.922
    12.00        0    69.49   6.926

ncall =    422
```

We can note the following details about this numerical output.

— For ncase = 4, the insulin release rate B_b is increased by a factor of 2; that is, from the main program in Listing 1.1

```
if(ncase==4){Bb=2.0*14.3; Gt=80000}
```

— The solution undergoes a transient (departure from the ICs) and then then approaches a new steady state (different than for ncase = 1,2,3) as reflected in the output at $t = 12$: 12.0 0 69.49 6.926. As expected (when B_b is increased), the glucose level $G(t)$ is lower than that for ncase = 1,2,3 and the insulin level, $I(t)$, is higher.

— The new final equilibrium values correspond to $dG/dt \approx 0, dI/dt \approx 0$. This is confirmed by a numerical evaluation of the RHS of eqs. (2.1c) and (2.2c).

$$\frac{dG}{dt} = \frac{1}{150}(8400 + 0 - (13.9)(6.926)(69.49) - (24.7)(69.49))$$
$$= -0.0420$$

The derivative at $t = 0$ is the same as for ncase = 2,3 because the ICs are the same, that is,

$$\frac{dG}{dt} = \frac{1}{150}(8400 + 80000 - (13.9)(5.663)(81.027)$$
$$- (24.7)(81.027)) = 533.47$$

— The insulin level $I(t)$ reaches the final value 6.926 because the derivative is effectively zero,

$$\frac{dI}{dt} = \frac{1}{150}(-(76)(6.926) + (2)(14.3)(69.49 - 51))$$
$$= 0.0167, \ G \geq G_0$$

Note the increased value of B_b used in this calculation, (2)(14.3).

— The number of calls to glucose_1 is 422, which is different than to ncase=1,2,3 as might be expected considering the variable step algorithm in lsoda.

In conclusion, for ncase = 4, the increased pancreatic sensitivity causes the glucose level $G(t)$ to reach a value lower than the normal value (because of the increased insulin release rate B_b)—a condition of *hypoglycemia*. Similarly, the insulin level $I(t)$ reaches a value higher than the normal value.

The solutions for ncase = 1,2,3,4 can be visualized through the following composite plots produced by the main program of Listing 2.1. We observe in these plots that the solutions have the properties discussed previously: (i) for ncase = 1, $G(t), I(t)$ are unchanged with t and dG/dt, dI/dt remain at zero, and (ii) for ncase = 2,3,4, the solutions approach different final values.

These plots facilitate the overall visualization of the solutions for ncase = 1,2,3,4 and elucidate the effect of the pancreatic sensitivity, B_b. Also, all of the RHS terms in eqs. (2.1b), (2.1c), (2.2b), and (2.2c) could be computed and plotted individually to gain additional insight into the features of the solutions in Figs. 2.1 and 2.2. For example, the relative contributions of the individual RHS terms to the LHS derivatives could be investigated, and the effect of changes in the model parameters would indicate the sensitivity of the solutions to the parameter values.

We now consider an alternative numerical ODE integration using the fixed step RKF45 algorithm discussed in Chapter 1. The intent is to demonstrate that essentially the same solution is produced as the preceding solution from ode.

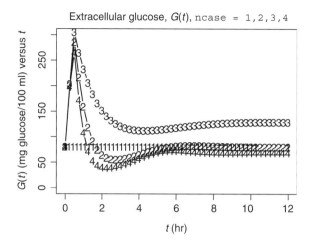

Figure 2.1 $G(t)$ for ncase = 1,2,3,4.

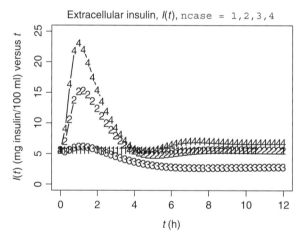

Figure 2.2 $I(t)$ for ncase = 1,2,3,4.

2.3.2   ODE Integration by RKF45

A main program with the RKF45 algorithm programmed as an in-line integrator is given in Listing 2.3.

```
#
# Glucose Tolerance Test
#
# Documentation comments removed
```

```
#
# ODE routine
  setwd("c:/R/bme_ode/chap2")
  source("glucose_2.R")
#
# Vectors, matrices for the graphical output
  nout=49
  Gplot=matrix(0,nrow=nout,ncol=4)
  Iplot=matrix(0,nrow=nout,ncol=4)
  dGplot=matrix(0,nrow=nout,ncol=4)
  dIplot=matrix(0,nrow=nout,ncol=4)
  tplot=rep(0,nout)
#
# Select rkf45 format
#
# nint = 1: No error estimation
#
# nint = 2: With error estimation
  nint=2
#
# Step through four cases
  for(ncase in 1:4){
#
# Select the case parameters
  if(ncase==1){Bb=14.3;          Gt=0}
  if(ncase==2){Bb=14.3;      Gt=80000}
  if(ncase==3){Bb=0.2*14.3; Gt=80000}
  if(ncase==4){Bb=2.0*14.3; Gt=80000}
#
# Model parameters
  Ex=15000; Cg=150; Ci=150; Q=8400; Dd=24.7;
   Gg=13.9; Gk=250;  Mu=72;  G0=51;    Aa=76;
#
# Initial condition
  t=0; ncall=0
  y=c(81.14,5.671)
  ee=c(0,0)
  cat(sprintf(
  "\n\n\n ncase = %2d \n\n            t           In          G
      I",ncase))
  if(nint==2){
```

```
  cat(sprintf("\n                                    e1
     e2" ))}
#
# Parameters for t integration
  nt=10;tout=0.25;h=tout/nt
#
# rkf45 integration
  for(i1 in 1:nout){
#
#   Glucose infusion function
    if((t>=0)&(t<=0.51)){In=Gt}
    if(t>0.51          )  {In=0}
#
#   Solution output
    cat(sprintf("\n %8.2f%10.2f%10.4f%10.4f",t,In,y[1],
       y[2]))
    if(nint==2){
    cat(sprintf("\n                         %8.4f  %8.4f",
                                           ee[1],ee[2]))}
#
#   Store solution for plotting
    Gplot[i1,ncase]=y[1]
    Iplot[i1,ncase]=y[2]
    if(ncase==1)tplot[i1]=t
#
#   nt rkf45 steps
    for(i2 in 1:nt){
    if(nint==1){
      yb=y; tb=t;
      rk1=glucose_2(tb,yb)*h
      y=yb+0.25*rk1;
      t=tb+0.25*h;
      rk2=glucose_2(t,y)*h
      y=yb+(3/32)*rk1+(9/32)*rk2;
      t=tb+(3/8)*h;
      rk3=glucose_2(t,y)*h
      y=yb+(1932/2197)*rk1-(7200/2197)*rk2+(7296/2197)
         *rk3;
      t=tb+(12/13)*h;
      rk4=glucose_2(t,y)*h
      y=yb+(439/216)*rk1-8*rk2+(3680/ 513)*rk3-(845/4104)
```

```
      *rk4;
   t=tb+h;
   rk5=glucose_2(t,y)*h
   y=yb-(8/27)*rk1+2*rk2-(3544/2565)*rk3+(1859/4104)
      *rk4-(11/40)*rk5;
   t=tb+0.5*h;
   rk6=glucose_2(t,y)*h
   y=yb+(16/135)*rk1+(6656/12825)*rk3+(28561/56430)
      *rk4-(9/50)*rk5+
         (2/55)*rk6;
   t=tb+h;
   }
   if(nint==2){
     yb=y; tb=t;
     rk1=glucose_2(tb,yb)*h
     y=yb+0.25*rk1;
     t=tb+0.25*h;
     rk2=glucose_2(t,y)*h
     y=yb+(3/32)*rk1+(9/32)*rk2;
     t=tb+(3/8)*h;
     rk3=glucose_2(t,y)*h
     y=yb+(1932/2197)*rk1-(7200/2197)*rk2+(7296/2197)
        *rk3;
     t=tb+(12/13)*h;
     rk4=glucose_2(t,y)*h
     y=yb+(439/216)*rk1-8*rk2+(3680/ 513)*rk3-( 845/4104)
        *rk4;
     t=tb+h;
     rk5=glucose_2(t,y)*h
     y=yb-(8/27)*rk1+2*rk2-(3544/2565)*rk3+(1859/4104)
        *rk4-(11/40)*rk5;
     t=tb+0.5*h;
     rk6=glucose_2(t,y)*h
#
#      Fourth order step
     y4=yb+(25/216)*rk1+( 1408/2565)*rk3+(2197/4104)
        *rk4-(1/5)*rk5;
#
#      Fifth order step
     y=yb+(16/135)*rk1+(6656/12825)*rk3+(28561/56430)
        *rk4-(9/50)*rk5+
```

```
          (2/55)*rk6;
      t=tb+h;
#
#     Truncation error estimate
      ee=y-y4
    }
    }
 }
#
# Store derivatives for plotting
  cat(sprintf("\n\n Derivatives, ncase = %2d\n",ncase))
  cat(sprintf("\n        t    dG/dt    dI/dt"))
  for(it in 1:nout){
    dgdi=glucose_2(tplot[it],c(Gplot[it,ncase],Iplot[it,
      ncase]))
    cat(sprintf("\n %8.2f%8.2f%8.2f",tplot[it],dgdi[1],
      dgdi[2]))
    dGplot[it,ncase]=dgdi[1]
    dIplot[it,ncase]=dgdi[2]
  }
#
# Next case
}
#
# Single plot for G
  par(mfrow=c(1,1))
#
# G, ncase = 1
  plot(tplot,Gplot[,1],xlab="t (hr)",
  ylab="G(t) (mg glucose/100 ml) vs t",
  xlim=c(0,12),ylim=c(0,300),type="b",lty=1,pch="1",
    lwd=2,
  main="Extracellular glucose, G(t), ncase = 1,2,3,4")
#
# G, ncase = 2
  lines(tplot,Gplot[,2],type="b",lty=1,pch="2",lwd=2)
#
# G, ncase = 3
  lines(tplot,Gplot[,3],type="b",lty=1,pch="3",lwd=2)
#
# G, ncase = 4
```

```
  lines(tplot,Gplot[,4],type="b",lty=1,pch="4",lwd=2)
#
# Single plot for I
  par(mfrow=c(1,1))
#
# I, ncase = 1
  plot(tplot,Iplot[,1],xlab="t (hr)",
  ylab="I(t) (mg insulin/100 ml) vs t",
  xlim=c(0,12),ylim=c(0,25),type="b",lty=1,pch="1",lwd=2,
  main="Extracellular insulin, I(t), ncase = 1,2,3,4")
#
# I, ncase = 2
  lines(tplot,Iplot[,2],type="b",lty=1,pch="2",lwd=2)
#
# I, ncase = 3
  lines(tplot,Iplot[,3],type="b",lty=1,pch="3",lwd=2)
#
# I, ncase = 4
  lines(tplot,Iplot[,4],type="b",lty=1,pch="4",lwd=2)
#
# Single plot for dG/dt
  par(mfrow=c(1,1))
#
# dG/dt, ncase = 1
  plot(tplot,dGplot[,1],xlab="t (hr)",
  ylab="dG(t)/dt (mg glucose/100 ml)/hr vs t",
  xlim=c(0,12),ylim=c(-400,600),type="b",lty=1,pch="1",
      lwd=2,
  main="dG(t)/dt, ncase = 1,2,3,4")
#
# dG/dt, ncase = 2
  lines(tplot,dGplot[,2],type="b",lty=1,pch="2",lwd=2)
#
# dG/dt, ncase = 3
  lines(tplot,dGplot[,3],type="b",lty=1,pch="3",lwd=2)
#
# dG/dt, ncase = 4
  lines(tplot,dGplot[,4],type="b",lty=1,pch="4",lwd=2)
#
# Single plot for dI/dt
  par(mfrow=c(1,1))
```

```
#
# dI/dt, ncase = 1
  plot(tplot,dIplot[,1],xlab="t (hr)",
  ylab="dI(t)/dt (mg Insulin/100 ml)/hr vs t",
  xlim=c(0,12),ylim=c(-10,40),type="b",lty=1,pch="1",
      lwd=2,
  main="dI(t)/dt, ncase = 1,2,3,4")
#
# dI/dt, ncase = 2
  lines(tplot,dIplot[,2],type="b",lty=1,pch="2",lwd=2)
#
# dI/dt, ncase = 3
  lines(tplot,dIplot[,3],type="b",lty=1,pch="3",lwd=2)
#
# dI/dt, ncase = 4
  lines(tplot,dIplot[,4],type="b",lty=1,pch="4",lwd=2)
```

Listing 2.3 Main program with in-line RKF45 for the numerical integration of eqs. (2.1) and (2.2).

Listing 2.3 is similar to Listing 1.11. Therefore, only the details that are different are considered next.

- The documentation at the beginning of Listing 2.1 has been removed to conserve space.
- A series of vector and matrices are declared (preallocated) for plotting the solution.

```
#
# Vectors, matrices for the graphical output
  nout=49
  Gplot=matrix(0,nrow=nout,ncol=4)
  Iplot=matrix(0,nrow=nout,ncol=4)
  dGplot=matrix(0,nrow=nout,ncol=4)
  dIplot=matrix(0,nrow=nout,ncol=4)
  tplot=rep(0,nout)
```

The use of these arrays was explained with Listings 1.11 and 2.1. Briefly, dGplot, dIplot have been added to plot the derivatives dG/dt of eqs. (2.1b) and (2.1c) and dI/dt of eqs. (2.2b) and (2.2c).

- The estimated RKF45 error ee is computed and displayed numerically with `nint=2`, as discussed in Listing 1.11. This estimated error is also initialized to zero as part of the ICs (ee=c(0,0)).
- The ODE integration using ode (and lsoda of Listing 2.1) is replaced with the RKF45 integration of Listing 1.11.

```
#
# Parameters for t integration
  nt=10;tout=0.25;h=tout/nt
#
# rkf45 integration
  for(i1 in 1:nout){
#
#   Glucose infusion function
    if((t>=0)&(t<=0.51)){In=Gt}
    if(t>0.51         )  {In=0}
#
#   Solution output
    cat(sprintf("\n %8.2f%10.2f%10.4f%10.4f",t,In,
       y[1],y[2]))
    if(nint==2){
    cat(sprintf("\n                          %8.4f  %8.4f",
                                     ee[1],ee[2]))}
#
#   Store solution for plotting
    Gplot[i1,ncase]=y[1]
    Iplot[i1,ncase]=y[2]
    if(ncase==1)tplot[i1]=t
#
#   nt rkf45 steps
    for(i2 in 1:nt){
    if(nint==1){
      yb=y; tb=t;
      rk1=glucose_2(tb,yb)*h
        .
        .
        .
    Complete RKF45 coding is in Listing 2.3
        .
        .
        .
#
#     Fifth order step
```

```
      y=yb+(16/135)*rk1+(6656/12825)*rk3+(28561/56430)
          *rk4-(9/50)*rk5+
            (2/55)*rk6;
      t=tb+h;
#
#      Truncation error estimate
      ee=y-y4
    }
    }
  }
```

Note the following in particular.

— The use of the two for loops with indices i1 and i2 (as discussed with Listing 1.11).

— The output interval in t is 0.25 and the integration step is, therefore, h = tout/nt = 0.25/10 = 0.025. This integration step was selected through nt to give good resolution in t (enough plotted points in t, e.g., 49 set previously) and a stable and accurate numerical solution (with $h = 0.025$).

— The use of glucose_2 rather than glucose_1 in RKF45 (these two routines differ in only the return statement with the inclusion of list for glucose_1). glucose_2 is in Listing 2.6.

— After nt integration steps, the derivatives $dG/dt, dI/dt$ are computed by a call to the ODE routine glucose_2 and displayed numerically (note in particular the input arguments to glucose_2 which follow from the first line of Listing 2.2). These derivatives are also stored for subsequent plotting.

```
  #
  # Store derivatives for plotting
    cat(sprintf("\n\n Derivatives, ncase = %2d\n",
        ncase))
    cat(sprintf("\n          t    dG/dt    dI/dt"))
    for(it in 1:nout){
      dgdi=glucose_2(tplot[it],c(Gplot[it,ncase],
          Iplot[it,ncase]))
      cat(sprintf("\n %8.2f%8.2f%8.2f",tplot[it],
```

```
            dgdi[1],dgdi[2]))
         dGplot[it,ncase]=dgdi[1]
         dIplot[it,ncase]=dgdi[2]
       }
   #
   # Next case
   }
```

- Plots are added for dG/dt and dI/dt.

```
  #
  # dG/dt, ncase = 1
    plot(tplot,dGplot[,1],xlab="t (hr)",
    ylab="dG(t)/dt (mg glucose/100 ml)/hr vs t",
    xlim=c(0,12),ylim=c(-400,600),type="b",lty=1,
        pch="1",lwd=2,
    main="dG(t)/dt, ncase = 1,2,3,4")
            .                    .
              .                    .
  #
  # dI/dt, ncase = 1
    plot(tplot,dIplot[,1],xlab="t (hr)",
    ylab="dI(t)/dt (mg Insulin/100 ml)/hr vs t",
    xlim=c(0,12),ylim=c(-10,40),type="b",lty=1,pch="1",
        lwd=2,
    main="dI(t)/dt, ncase = 1,2,3,4")
            .                    .
              .                    .
```

The ODE routine glucose_2 differs from glucose_1 of Listing 2.2 in one line.

```
Glucose 1
#
# Return derivative vector
  return(list(c(dGdt,dIdt)))


Glucose 2
#
# Return derivative vector
  return(c(dGdt,dIdt))
```

list is required by ode (which calls glucose_1 in Listing 2.1) and is not required by RKF45 (which calls glucose_2 in Listing 2.3).

Abbreviated numerical output from Listing 2.3 is in Table 2.2. We can note the following details of this output.

- For ncase = 1, $G(t)$ and $I(t)$ are constant and the derivatives $dG(t)/dt$ and $dI(t)/dt$ are zero as expected (see also Table 2.1).
- For all four solutions (ncase=1,2,3,4), the estimated error is zero to four figures after the decimal. This implies that the solutions are accurate to four figures after the decimal.
- All four solutions appear to have reached an equilibrium condition for $t \to 12$ (note the small derivatives).

The graphical output for $G(t)$ and $I(t)$ (Figs. 2.3 and 2.4) is the same as in Figs. 2.1 and 2.2. The graphical output for the derivatives follows in Figs. 2.3 and 2.4.

A comparison of the solutions from Listings 2.1 and 2.3 (Table 2.3) gives an indication of the accuracy of the preceding numerical solutions (in Tables 2.1 and 2.2).

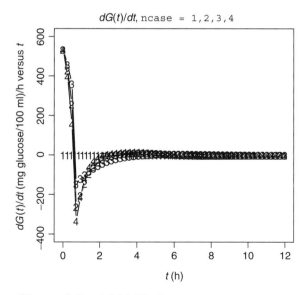

Figure 2.3 $dG(t)/dt$ for ncase = 1,2,3,4.

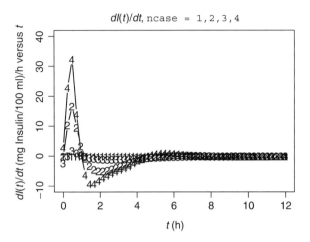

Figure 2.4 $dI(t)/dt$ for ncase = 1,2,3,4.

TABLE 2.2   Abbreviated output from of Listing 2.3.

ncase =   1

t	In	G	I
		e1	e2
0.00	0.00	81.1400	5.6710
		0.0000	0.0000
0.25	0.00	81.1397	5.6710
		-0.0000	0.0000
0.50	0.00	81.1395	5.6710
		-0.0000	0.0000
0.75	0.00	81.1393	5.6710
		-0.0000	0.0000
1.00	0.00	81.1392	5.6710
		-0.0000	0.0000
.		.	
.		.	
.		.	

Output for t = 1.25 to 10.75 removed

.		.	
.		.	
.		.	
11.00	0.00	81.1392	5.6709

TABLE 2.2 (*Continued*)

		0.0000	-0.0000
11.25	0.00	81.1392	5.6709
		0.0000	0.0000
11.50	0.00	81.1392	5.6709
		0.0000	0.0000
11.75	0.00	81.1392	5.6709
		-0.0000	0.0000
12.00	0.00	81.1392	5.6709
		0.0000	-0.0000

Derivatives, ncase = 1

t	dG/dt	dI/dt
0.00	-0.00	0.00
0.25	-0.00	0.00
0.50	-0.00	-0.00
0.75	-0.00	-0.00
1.00	-0.00	-0.00
.		.
.		.
.		.

Output for t = 1.25 to 10.75 removed

.		.
.		.
.		.
11.00	0.00	-0.00
11.25	0.00	-0.00
11.50	0.00	-0.00
11.75	0.00	0.00
12.00	0.00	0.00

ncase = 2

t	In	G	I
		e1	e2
0.00	80000.00	81.1400	5.6710
		0.0000	0.0000

(*continued*)

TABLE 2.2   (*Continued*)

0.25	80000.00	201.7138	7.0999
		0.0000	-0.0000
0.50	80000.00	286.7212	10.6868
		0.0000	-0.0000
0.75	0.00	222.5755	14.0297
		-0.0000	0.0000
1.00	0.00	162.8538	15.4879
		-0.0000	0.0000

.
.
.

Output for t = 1.25 to 10.75 removed

.
.
.

11.00	0.00	80.8916	5.6812
		-0.0000	-0.0000
11.25	0.00	80.9191	5.6748
		-0.0000	-0.0000
11.50	0.00	80.9520	5.6697
		0.0000	-0.0000
11.75	0.00	80.9871	5.6661
		0.0000	-0.0000
12.00	0.00	81.0219	5.6637
		0.0000	-0.0000

Derivatives, ncase = 2

t	dG/dt	dI/dt
0.00	533.33	0.00
0.25	423.41	10.77
0.50	240.55	17.06
0.75	-270.02	9.25
1.00	-204.55	2.82

.
.
.

Output for t = 1.25 to 10.75 removed

TABLE 2.2   (*Continued*)

	.	.
	.	.
	.	.
11.00	0.09	-0.03
11.25	0.12	-0.02
11.50	0.14	-0.02
11.75	0.14	-0.01
12.00	0.14	-0.01

ncase =   3

t	In	G	I
		e1	e2
0.00	80000.00	81.1400	5.6710
		0.0000	0.0000
0.25	80000.00	204.2189	5.4200
		0.0000	0.0000
0.50	80000.00	305.9657	5.7036
		0.0000	0.0000
0.75	0.00	271.4036	6.1015
		-0.0000	-0.0000
1.00	0.00	237.6941	6.2824
		-0.0000	0.0000
.		.	
.		.	
.		.	

Output for t = 1.25 to 10.75 removed

		.	
		.	
		.	
11.00	0.00	129.3243	2.8929
		0.0000	0.0000
11.25	0.00	129.3232	2.8994
		-0.0000	0.0000
11.50	0.00	129.3050	2.9051
		-0.0000	0.0000
11.75	0.00	129.2737	2.9100
		-0.0000	0.0000

(*continued*)

TABLE 2.2 (*Continued*)

| 12.00 | 0.00 | 129.2328 | 2.9141 |
| | | -0.0000 | 0.0000 |

Derivatives, ncase = 3

t	dG/dt	dI/dt
0.00	533.33	-2.30
0.25	453.14	0.18
0.50	350.37	1.97
0.75	-152.42	1.11
1.00	-121.52	0.38
.	.	.
.	.	.
.	.	.

Output for t = 1.25 to 10.75 removed

	.	.
	.	.
	.	.
11.00	0.04	0.03
11.25	-0.04	0.02
11.50	-0.10	0.02
11.75	-0.15	0.02
12.00	-0.18	0.02

ncase = 4

t	In	G	I
		e1	e2
0.00	80000.00	81.1400	5.6710
		0.0000	0.0000
0.25	80000.00	198.6589	9.1666
		0.0000	-0.0000
0.50	80000.00	265.5024	16.4543
		0.0000	-0.0000
0.75	0.00	177.1371	22.1836
		-0.0000	0.0000
1.00	0.00	110.0692	23.5312
		0.0000	-0.0000

TABLE 2.2   (*Continued*)

```
        .                    .
        .                    .
        .                    .
Output for t = 1.25 to 10.75 removed
        .                    .
        .                    .
        .                    .
  11.00      0.00    69.4686      6.9036
                      0.0000     -0.0000
  11.25      0.00    69.4911      6.9097
                      0.0000      0.0000
  11.50      0.00    69.5005      6.9158
                      0.0000      0.0000
  11.75      0.00    69.4998      6.9213
                      0.0000      0.0000
  12.00      0.00    69.4917      6.9259
                      0.0000      0.0000

Derivatives, ncase =  4

     t    dG/dt    dI/dt
  0.00   533.33     2.87
  0.25   387.87    23.51
  0.50   133.34    32.56
  0.75  -337.31    12.81
  1.00  -202.14    -0.66
     .        .
     .        .
     .        .
Output for t = 1.25 to 10.75 removed
     .        .
     .        .
     .        .
  11.00    0.12     0.02
  11.25    0.06     0.02
  11.50    0.02     0.02
  11.75   -0.02     0.02
  12.00   -0.04     0.02
```

TABLE 2.3   Comparison of the solutions from Listings 2.1 and 2.3.

Table 2.1, ncase=4 (Listing 2.1) $t = 0.5$ $G(t) = 265.50$
  $I(t) = 16.454$
Table 2.2, ncase=4 (Listing 2.3) $t = 0.5$ $G(t) = 265.5024$
  $I(t) = 16.4543$
Table 2.1, ncase=4 (Listing 2.1) $t = 12$ $G(t) = 69.49$
  $I(t) = 6.926$
Table 2.2, ncase=4 (Listing 2.3) $t = 12$ $G(t) = 69.4917$
  $I(t) = 6.9259$

This comparison suggests that the numerical solutions are accurate to at least four figures. In the case of the RKF45 solutions (Table 2.2), this accuracy is achieved with $h = 0.025$ and there was no indication of impending instability. To investigate this further, Listing 2.2 is modified by changing nt=10 to nt=1 so that $h = 0.025$ is changed to $h = 0.25$. The abbreviated numerical output is in Table 2.4.

The details listed in Table 2.5 are obtained by comparing the solutions in Tables 2.2 and 2.4.

The beginning results in Table 2.5 are for $t = 0.75$ rather than for $t = 0.50$ of Table 2.3 because the estimated errors ee(1),ee(2) are larger (see Table 2.4, ncase=4).

Table 2.3 suggests that the nt=10 solution from Listing 2.3 is of relatively high accuracy. If we consider it to be essentially an exact solution, then the exact error $G(t)$ for the nt=1 solution at $t = 0.75$ is $177.1371 - 170.7425 = 6.3946$. The estimated error is $ee(1) = 1.7644$ so that the error is underestimated. This is not entirely unexpected because of the large step for nt=1, $h = 0.25$, which is the output interval, that is, there is only one integration step for each output where the solution is changing most rapidly. An important point to note is that the error is only estimated by comparing the fourth-order and fifth-order solutions from RKF45, and the error estimate might be unreliable if h is large. Experience has indicated that when h is small enough to produce an accurate solution, the error estimate is also accurate and is reliable enough to adjust the integration step (in a variable step method such as RKF45 in ode of deSolve).

TABLE 2.4   Abbreviated output from Listing 2.3, nt=1.

```
ncase =  1

        t         In         G          I
                            e1         e2
     0.00       0.00    81.1400     5.6710
                         0.0000     0.0000
     0.25       0.00    81.1397     5.6710
                        -0.0000     0.0000
     0.50       0.00    81.1395     5.6710
                        -0.0000     0.0000
     0.75       0.00    81.1393     5.6710
                        -0.0000     0.0000
     1.00       0.00    81.1392     5.6710
                        -0.0000     0.0000
       .                    .
       .                    .
       .                    .
  Output for t = 1.25 to 10.75 removed
       .                    .
       .                    .
       .                    .
    11.00       0.00    81.1392     5.6709
                         0.0000    -0.0000
    11.25       0.00    81.1392     5.6709
                         0.0000    -0.0000
    11.50       0.00    81.1392     5.6709
                         0.0000    -0.0000
    11.75       0.00    81.1392     5.6709
                         0.0000    -0.0000
    12.00       0.00    81.1392     5.6709
                         0.0000    -0.0000

Derivatives, ncase =  1

        t    dG/dt    dI/dt
     0.00    -0.00     0.00
     0.25    -0.00     0.00
```

(continued)

TABLE 2.4 (*Continued*)

```
    0.50   -0.00   -0.00
    0.75   -0.00   -0.00
    1.00   -0.00   -0.00
            .       .
            .       .
            .       .
 Output for t = 1.25 to 10.75 removed
            .       .
            .       .
            .       .
   11.00    0.00   -0.00
   11.25    0.00   -0.00
   11.50    0.00   -0.00
   11.75    0.00    0.00
   12.00    0.00    0.00

ncase =   2
```

t	In	G	I
		e1	e2
0.00	80000.00	81.1400	5.6710
		0.0000	0.0000
0.25	80000.00	201.7134	7.1000
		0.0046	-0.0001
0.50	80000.00	286.7229	10.6879
		0.0307	-0.0003
0.75	0.00	222.0304	14.1499
		0.8084	0.0183
1.00	0.00	162.1029	15.5785
		-0.0014	0.0002
.	.	.	.
.	.	.	.
.	.	.	.

```
 Output for t = 1.25 to 10.75 removed
```

t	In	G	I
.	.	.	.
.	.	.	.
.	.	.	.
11.00	0.00	80.8909	5.6811
		-0.0000	-0.0000

TABLE 2.4   (*Continued*)

11.25	0.00	80.9186	5.6747
		-0.0000	-0.0000
11.50	0.00	80.9518	5.6696
		-0.0000	-0.0000
11.75	0.00	80.9871	5.6660
		0.0000	-0.0000
12.00	0.00	81.0220	5.6636
		0.0000	-0.0000

Derivatives, ncase = 2

t	dG/dt	dI/dt
0.00	533.33	0.00
0.25	423.40	10.77
0.50	240.52	17.06
0.75	-271.69	9.14
1.00	-204.71	2.70
.	.
.	.
.	.

Output for t = 1.25 to 10.75 removed

.	.
.	.
.	.
11.00	0.09	-0.03
11.25	0.12	-0.02
11.50	0.14	-0.02
11.75	0.14	-0.01
12.00	0.14	-0.01

ncase = 3

t	In	G	I
		e1	e2
0.00	80000.00	81.1400	5.6710
		0.0000	0.0000
0.25	80000.00	204.2186	5.4200
		0.0010	0.0000

(continued)

TABLE 2.4   (*Continued*)

```
 0.50  80000.00  306.1217     5.7042
                   0.0033    -0.0000
 0.75      0.00  275.8744     6.1299
                   0.3163     0.0039
 1.00      0.00  240.8850     6.3242
                   0.0011     0.0000
    .                    .
    .                    .
    .                    .
Output for t = 1.25 to 10.75 removed
    .                    .
    .                    .
    .                    .
11.00      0.00  129.3329     2.8922
                   0.0000     0.0000
11.25      0.00  129.3327     2.8988
                   0.0000     0.0000
11.50      0.00  129.3150     2.9046
                   0.0000     0.0000
11.75      0.00  129.2838     2.9096
                  -0.0000     0.0000
12.00      0.00  129.2428     2.9138
                  -0.0000     0.0000


Derivatives, ncase =  3

       t    dG/dt    dI/dt
    0.00   533.33    -2.30
    0.25   453.14     0.18
    0.50   350.17     1.97
    0.75  -158.55     1.18
      .              .
      .              .
      .              .
Output for t = 1.25 to 10.75 removed
      .              .
      .              .
      .              .
   11.00    0.04     0.03
```

TABLE 2.4   (*Continued*)

11.25	-0.04	0.02
11.50	-0.10	0.02
11.75	-0.15	0.02
12.00	-0.18	0.02

ncase =   4

t	In	G	I
		e1	e2
0.00	80000.00	81.1400	5.6710
		0.0000	0.0000
0.25	80000.00	198.6600	9.1672
		0.0084	-0.0007
0.50	80000.00	265.4178	16.4550
		0.0276	-0.0017
0.75	0.00	170.7245	22.3869
		1.7644	0.0303
1.00	0.00	106.3199	23.4860
		-0.0014	0.0003
.		.	
.		.	
.		.	

Output for t = 1.25 to 10.75 removed

.		.	
.		.	
.		.	
11.00	0.00	69.4710	6.9041
		0.0000	-0.0000
11.25	0.00	69.4923	6.9102
		0.0000	-0.0000
11.50	0.00	69.5008	6.9163
		0.0000	-0.0000
11.75	0.00	69.4993	6.9217
		0.0000	0.0000
12.00	0.00	69.4908	6.9263
		0.0000	0.0000

(*continued*)

TABLE 2.4   (*Continued*)

```
Derivatives, ncase =  4

         t    dG/dt    dI/dt
      0.00   533.33     2.87
      0.25   387.86    23.51
      0.50   133.51    32.55
      0.75  -326.28    11.48
      1.00  -192.90    -1.35
         .             .
         .             .
         .             .
    Output for t = 1.25 to 10.75 removed
         .             .
         .             .
         .             .
     11.00    0.11     0.02
     11.25    0.06     0.02
     11.50    0.01     0.02
     11.75   -0.02     0.02
     12.00   -0.04     0.02
```

2.3.3   ODE Integration with RKF45 in a Separate Routine

We now consider a variation of Listing 2.3 in which RKF45 is placed in a separate routine. This is a worthwhile approach as it makes the programming easier to follow (more modular). First, the main program that parallels Listing 2.3 is in Listing 2.4.

```
#
# Glucose Tolerance Test
#
# Documentation comments removed
#
# ODE routine
  setwd("c:/R/bme_ode/chap2")
  source("glucose_2.R")
  source("rkf45.R")
#
```

TABLE 2.5   Comparison of the solutions from Listing 2.3, nt=1,10.

Table 2.2, ncase=4, nt=10	$t = 0.75$	$G(t) = 177.1371$	$I(t) = 22.1836$
		$ee(1) = -0.0000$	$ee(2) = 0.0000$
Table 2.4, ncase=4, nt=1	$t = 0.75$	$G(t) = 170.7245$	$I(t) = 22.3869$
		$ee(1) = 1.7644$	$ee(2) = 0.0303$
Table 2.2, ncase=4, nt=10	$t = 12$	$G(t) = 69.4917$	$I(t) = 6.9259$
		$ee(1) = 0.0000$	$ee(2) = 0.0000$
Table 2.4, ncase=4, nt=1	$t = 12$	$G(t) = 69.4908$	$I(t) = 6.9263$
		$ee(1) = 0.0000$	$ee(2) = 0.0000$

```
# Select RKF45 method
#
# nint = 1: No error estimation
#
# nint = 2: With error estimation
  nint=2
#
# Vectors, matrices for the graphical output
  nout=49
  Gplot=matrix(0,nrow=nout,ncol=4)
  Iplot=matrix(0,nrow=nout,ncol=4)
  tplot=rep(0,nout)
#
# Step through four cases
  for(ncase in 1:4){
#
# Select the case parameters
  if(ncase==1){Bb=14.3;          Gt=0}
  if(ncase==2){Bb=14.3;      Gt=80000}
  if(ncase==3){Bb=0.2*14.3; Gt=80000}
  if(ncase==4){Bb=2.0*14.3; Gt=80000}
#
# Model parameters
  Ex=15000; Cg=150; Ci=150; Q=8400; Dd=24.7;
   Gg=13.9; Gk=250;  Mu=72;  G0=51;    Aa=76;
#
# Initial condition
  t=0; ncall=0
```

```
  y=c(81.14,5.671)
  ee=c(0,0)
  cat(sprintf(
  "\n ncase = %2d \n\n            t         In         G
    I",ncase))
  if(nint==2){
  cat(sprintf("\n                                         e1
    e2" ))}
#
# Parameters, functions for t integration
  nt=1;tout=0.25;h=tout/nt
#
# rkf45 integration
  for(i1 in 1:nout){
#
#   Glucose infusion function
    if((t>=0)&(t<=0.5)){In=Gt}
    if(t>0.5           )   {In=0}
#
#   Solution output
    cat(sprintf("\n %8.2f%10.2f%10.4f%10.4f",t,In,y[1],
      y[2]))
    if(nint==2){
    cat(sprintf("\n                              %8.4f  %8.4f",
                                       ee[1],ee[2]))}
#
#
#   Store solution for plotting
    Gplot[i1,ncase]=y[1]
    Iplot[i1,ncase]=y[2]
    if(ncase==1)tplot[i1]=t
#
#   rkf45 integration over nt points
    yout=rkf45(nt,h,t,y)
    y=yout; t=t+tout
  }
#
# Calls to glucose_2
  cat(sprintf("\n\n ncall = %5d\n\n",ncall))
#
# Next case
```

```
}
#
# Single plot for G
  par(mfrow=c(1,1))
#
# G, ncase = 1
  plot(tplot,Gplot[,1],xlab="t (hr)",
  ylab="G(t) (mg glucose/100 ml) vs t",
  xlim=c(0,12),ylim=c(0,300),type="b",lty=1,pch="1",lwd=2,
  main="Extracellular glucose, G(t), ncase = 1,2,3,4")
#
# G, ncase = 2
  lines(tplot,Gplot[,2],type="b",lty=1,pch="2",lwd=2)
#
# G, ncase = 3
  lines(tplot,Gplot[,3],type="b",lty=1,pch="3",lwd=2)
#
# G, ncase = 4
  lines(tplot,Gplot[,4],type="b",lty=1,pch="4",lwd=2)
#
# Single plot for I
  par(mfrow=c(1,1))
#
# I, ncase = 1
  plot(tplot,Iplot[,1],xlab="t (hr)",
  ylab="I(t) (mg insulin/100 ml) vs t",
  xlim=c(0,12),ylim=c(0,25),type="b",lty=1,pch="1",lwd=2,
  main="Extracellular insulin, I(t), ncase = 1,2,3,4")
#
# I, ncase = 2
  lines(tplot,Iplot[,2],type="b",lty=1,pch="2",lwd=2)
#
# I, ncase = 3
  lines(tplot,Iplot[,3],type="b",lty=1,pch="3",lwd=2)
#
# I, ncase = 4
  lines(tplot,Iplot[,4],type="b",lty=1,pch="4",lwd=2)
```

Listing 2.4 Main program with call to a separate ODE integration routine for RKF45.

Listing 2.4 is the same as Listing 2.3 except for the call to the separate ODE integration routine, rkf45, and the display of the number of calls to the ODE routine glucose_2.

```
#
#    rkf45 integration over nt points
     yout=rkf45(nt,h,t,y)
     y=yout; t=t+tout
 }
#
# Calls to glucose_2
   cat(sprintf("\n\n ncall = %5d\n\n",ncall))
```

$G(t)$ and $I(t)$ are again programmed as y[1] and y[2], which are computed as the vector yout returned by rkf45 (these are equated as y=yout right after the call to rkf45).

rkf45 is listed in Listing 2.5.

```
     rkf45=function(nt,h,t,y) {
#
#    Function rkf45 implements a fourth order Runge Kutta
#    method embedded in a fifth order Runge Kutta method.
#    The ODE routine has to be renamed for a new
#    application.
#
#    The arguments are
#
#      Input
#
#        nt - number of rkf45 steps between the starting
#             and final points along the solution
#
#        h  - integration step (constant)
#
#        t  - initial value of the independent variable
#
#        y  - initial dependent variable vector
#
#      Output
#
#        y  - solution vector after nt integration steps
```

```
#
#    nt rkf45 steps
     for(i2 in 1:nt){
     if(nint==1){
       yb=y; tb=t;
       rk1=glucose_2(tb,yb)*h
       y=yb+0.25*rk1;
       t=tb+0.25*h;
       rk2=glucose_2(t,y)*h
       y=yb+(3/32)*rk1+(9/32)*rk2;
       t=tb+(3/8)*h;
       rk3=glucose_2(t,y)*h
       y=yb+(1932/2197)*rk1-(7200/2197)*rk2+(7296/2197)
          *rk3;
       t=tb+(12/13)*h;
       rk4=glucose_2(t,y)*h
       y=yb+(439/216)*rk1-8*rk2+(3680/ 513)*rk3-( 845/4104)
          *rk4;
       t=tb+h;
       rk5=glucose_2(t,y)*h
       y=yb-(8/27)*rk1+2*rk2-(3544/2565)*rk3+(1859/4104)
          *rk4-(11/40)*rk5;
       t=tb+0.5*h;
       rk6=glucose_2(t,y)*h
       y=yb+(16/135)*rk1+(6656/12825)*rk3+(28561/56430)
          *rk4-(9/50)*rk5+
            (2/55)*rk6;
       t=tb+h;
     }
     if(nint==2){
       yb=y; tb=t;
       rk1=glucose_2(tb,yb)*h
       y=yb+0.25*rk1;
       t=tb+0.25*h;
       rk2=glucose_2(t,y)*h
       y=yb+(3/32)*rk1+(9/32)*rk2;
       t=tb+(3/8)*h;
       rk3=glucose_2(t,y)*h
       y=yb+(1932/2197)*rk1-(7200/2197)*rk2+(7296/2197)
          *rk3;
       t=tb+(12/13)*h;
```

```
        rk4=glucose_2(t,y)*h
        y=yb+(439/216)*rk1-8*rk2+(3680/ 513)*rk3-( 845/4104)
           *rk4;
        t=tb+h;
        rk5=glucose_2(t,y)*h
        y=yb-(8/27)*rk1+2*rk2-(3544/2565)*rk3+(1859/4104)
           *rk4-(11/40)*rk5;
        t=tb+0.5*h;
        rk6=glucose_2(t,y)*h
#
#       Fourth order step
        y4=yb+(25/216)*rk1+( 1408/2565)*rk3+(   2197/4104)
           *rk4-( 1/5)*rk5;
#
#       Fifth order step
        y=yb+(16/135)*rk1+(6656/12825)*rk3+(28561/56430)
           *rk4-(9/50)*rk5+
              (2/55)*rk6;
        t=tb+h;
#
#       Truncation error estimate
        ee=y-y4
        ee <<- ee
      }
   }
      return(c(y))
}
```

Listing 2.5 Routine `rkf45`.

We can note the following details about `rkf45`.

- The input (RHS) arguments follow directly from Listing 2.4.

  ```
  rkf45=function(nt,h,t,y)
  ```

- nt integration steps are taken within each call to `rkf45`. Two options are programmed: `nint=1` without error estimation and `nint=2` with error estimation.

  ```
  for(i2 in 1:nt){
    if(nint==1){
  ```

- The programming of the RKF45 algorithm is the same as in Listing 2.3.
- The estimated error `ee` is returned to the main program of Listing 2.4 (note the use of `<<-` to provide the return to the higher level main program).

```
ee <<- ee
```

- The solution vector is returned after `nt` steps along the solution.

```
      }
    }
        return(c(y))
  }
```

The first brace `}` completes the `nint=2` option. The second brace completes the `for` in `i2`. The third brace completes `rkf45`.

- `rkf45` of Listing 2.5 can be considered to be a library routine that can be applied to other ODE systems. However, it does require the specification of an ODE routine, in this case `glucose_2`. Changing this name is easily accomplished with an editor. An alternative would be to pass the ODE routine to `rkf45` as an argument, as was done with `ode` (`func=glucose_1` in Listing 2.1).

The ODE routine `glucose_2` is in Listing 2.6.

```
glucose_2=function(t,y) {
#
# Assign state variables:
  G=y[1];
  I=y[2];
#
# Glucose infusion function
  if((t>=0)&(t<=0.51)){In=Gt}
  if(t>0.51           ){In=0}
#
# ODEs
#
# Glucose equations
```

```
  if(G< Gk){dGdt=(1/Cg)*(Q+In-(Gg*I*G)-Dd*G)}
  if(G>=Gk){dGdt=(1/Cg)*(Q+In-(Gg*I*G)-Dd*G-Mu*(G-Gk))}
#
# Insulin equations
  if(G< G0){dIdt=(1/Ci)*(-Aa*I)}
  if(G>=G0){dIdt=(1/Ci)*(-Aa*I+Bb*(G-G0))}
#
# Calls to glucose_2
  ncall <<- ncall+1
#
# Return derivative vector
  return(c(dGdt,dIdt))
}
```

Listing 2.6 ODE routine glucose_2.

The essential detail is the return, that is, return(list(c(dGdt, dIdt))) in glucose_1 of Listing 2.2 and return(c(dGdt,dIdt)) in glucose_2 of Listing 2.6. The output from Listings 2.4–2.6 is the same as in Table 2.2, with the addition of the number of calls to glucose_2.

```
ncall =  2940
```

This number (which is the same for ncase=1,2,3,4) comes from the six derivative evaluations in rkf45 of Listing 2.5, that is, 6*nout*nt = (6)(49)(10) = 2940. This modest number of calls indicates that eqs. (2.1) and (2.2) are nonstiff (in contrast with 240000 for eqs. (1.1)).

If the main program in Listing 2.4 is executed with nt=1, the solution of Table 2.4 is produced, with the number of calls to glucose_2

```
ncall =   294
```

as expected (2940/10). In the case of eqs. (2.1) and (2.2), h was determined by accuracy rather than stability; even with the large value $h = 0.25$ for nt=1, the solution was stable but inaccurate (consider again Table 2.5). In order words, eqs. (2.1) and (2.2) are not stiff.

In the case of eqs. (1.1), h was constrained by stability to a small value because eqs. (1.1) are stiff. The small value of h then produced excessive accuracy (very small errors) and clearly the use of a stiff (implicit) integrator (such as `lsoda`) was very efficient in the sense that the stiff integrator required far fewer calls to the ODE routine than the nonstiff integrators such as the explicit Euler method through the RKF45 integrator.

In conclusion, the stiffness of an ODE system generally is not apparent and some experimentation with the choice of an integrator and the integration step is usually required. Physical considerations may immediately indicate that an ODE system is stiff, for example, some chemical kinetic models (with fast and slow reactions) have stiffness ratios of $10^9 - 10^{12}$ so that the required use of a stiff integrator is immediately apparent.

2.3.4 *h* Refinement

The preceding error analysis in which the investigation of h was carried out through the variation in `nt` is termed as *h refinement*. Generally, h is varied and the observed effect on the solution is used to infer the accuracy of the solution. This can be done without using an analytical solution (only the ODE is required, and it does not have to be differentiated to include additional terms in the Taylor series that represents the solution). However, the accuracy can only be inferred even with explicit error estimates such as from an embedded method. Also, as h is varied, instability may occur indicating that the stability limit of the method has been exceeded. In this case, h is determined by stability and not by accuracy, and the use of a stiff integrator may be required.

2.3.5 *p* Refinement

The preceding error analysis also indicates that varying the order of the integration method can provide an estimate of the integration error. As the order of a method is typically designated as $O(h^p)$, comparing solutions from algorithms of different orders is usually termed as *p refinement*. In the case of RKF45, the solutions for a fourth-order method and a fifth-order method were compared through the estimated error (`ee` in Listing 2.4).

Library integrators such as `lsoda` perform h and p refinement simultaneously and are, therefore, generally more complicated than the preceding explicit methods. Also, the source code is not readily available to study the details. Therefore, the basic explicit integrators considered previously (explicit Euler method through RKF45) can be useful as an introduction and can also be used to calculate solutions to nonstiff ODEs with good accuracy.

2.4 Conclusions

This concludes the discussion of the numerical integration of eqs. (2.1) and (2.2) by a variety of algorithms, both nonstiff (explicit) and stiff (implicit). An error analysis was performed in several ways without the use of an exact solution. Some experimentation, for example, with the step h (h refinement), was suggested by the results.

This need for numerical experimentation is generally true for a new ODE application. For example, additional tests could include changes in the method (p refinement) and variation of the error tolerances for a variable step method such as the BDF (backward differentiation formula methods) in `lsoda`. The solutions for a new ODE application should be viewed critically and tested thoroughly with some form of error analysis.

Once a solution of acceptable accuracy is computed, experimentation with the model can proceed, which is the ultimate objective of computer-based mathematical modeling. We, therefore, should keep in mind the famous statement by Richard Hamming [1]: *The purpose of computing is insight, not numbers.*

Eqs. 2.1 and 2.2 are an early model of the dynamics of the glucose tolerance test [3]. This test has been the subject of a series of papers and remains an active area of research. An example is given in [5].

References

[1] Hamming, R. W. (1962), *Numerical Methods for Scientists and Engineers*, McGraw-Hill Book Co., New York.

[2] Lee, H.J., and W.E. Schiesser (2004), *Ordinary and Partial Differential Equation Routines, in C, C++, Fortran, Java, Maple and Matlab*, CRC Press, Boca Raton, FL.

[3] Randall, J.E. (1980), *Microcomputers and Physiological Simulation*, Addison-Wesley Publishing Company, Inc., Reading, MA.

[4] Shampine, L.F., and S. Thompson (2007), Stiff systems, Scholarpedia, vol. 2, no. 3, p 2855; available at: `http://www.scholarpedia.org/article/Stiff_systems`.

[5] Vahidi, O., K.E. Kwok, R.B. Gopaluni, and L. Sum (2011), Developing a physiological model for type II diabetes mellitus, *Biochem. Eng. J.*, **55** (1), pp 7–16.

CHAPTER 3

Apoptosis

3.1 Introduction

This case study has a four-fold purpose:

1. An introduction to the analysis of apoptosis, that is, naturally occurring cell death that is also linked to cancer.
2. Application of an ODE model to apoptosis.
3. Integration (solution) of the model equations by a library ODE integrator `lsoda` of `ode` in `deSolve` and an explicit Runge Kutta integrator, RKF45.
4. Consideration of features of the model and its numerical solutions that illustrate some basic properties of ODE models.

Thus, the intent is to illustrate the use of computer-based ODE analysis of apoptosis through an example application. The source code for the R routines that implement the model is discussed in detail and is available as a download.

3.2 Mathematical Model

This application is based on the paper by Laise et al. [1]. To start, the excellent summary statement explaining apoptosis in [1] is repeated here:

Differential Equation Analysis in Biomedical Science and Engineering: Ordinary Differential Equation Applications with R, First Edition. William E. Schiesser.
© 2014 John Wiley & Sons, Inc. Published 2014 by John Wiley & Sons, Inc.

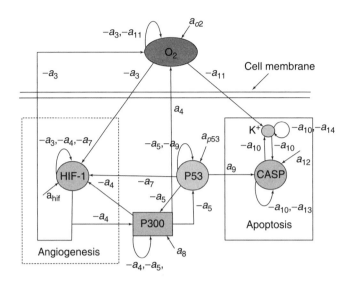

Figure 3.1 Diagram for the apoptosis model of eqs. (3.1)–(3.6).

Apoptosis can be envisaged as a complex machinery of reactions aimed to eliminate damaged (unwanted) single cells inside a whole organism. The entire process is mediated by the activation of specific gene products and occurs in different situations. Indeed apoptosis occurs during development, as well as when the homeostatic maintenance of a cell population within a tissue is needed, or as a defense strategy in the reactions of the immune system to external pathogens and during aging. Moreover, apoptosis is responsible for many pathological conditions; in fact, it may be caused by a different damaging stimulus such as heat, radiation, cytotoxic antineoplastic drugs and hypoxia.

The structure of the ODE model is summarized in Fig. 3.1 [1], with particular emphasis on apoptosis, hypoxia, and angiogenesis.

The six ODEs for the model follow.

$$\frac{dy_{hif}}{dt} = a_{hif} - a_3 y_{o2} y_{hif} - a_4 y_{hif} y_{p300} - a_7 y_{p53} y_{hif} \qquad (3.1)$$

$$\frac{dy_{o2}}{dt} = a_{o2} - a_3 y_{o2} y_{hif} + a_4 y_{hif} y_{p300} - a_{11} y_{o2} \qquad (3.2)$$

$$\frac{dy_{p300}}{dt} = -a_4 y_{hif} y_{p300} - a_5 y_{p300} y_{p53} + a_8 \tag{3.3}$$

$$\frac{dy_{p53}}{dt} = a_{p53} - a_5 y_{p300} y_{p53} - a_9 y_{p53} \tag{3.4}$$

$$\frac{dy_{casp}}{dt} = a_9 y_{p53} + a_{12} - a_{13} y_{casp} \tag{3.5}$$

$$\frac{dy_{kp}}{dt} = -a_{10} y_{casp} y_{kp} + a_{11} y_{o2} - a_{14} y_{kp} \tag{3.6}$$

The six concentrations (dependent variables) of eqs. (3.1)–(3.6) are summarized in Table 3.1.

TABLE 3.1   Variables of eqs. (3.1)–(3.6).

Variable	Interpretation
y_{hif}	hypoxia inducible factor concentration
y_{o2}	oxygen concentration
y_{p300}	hypoxia coactivator concentration
y_{p53}	tumor suppressor gene concentration
y_{casp}	caspase concentration
y_{kp}	potassium ion concentration
t	time

To complete the definition of the mathematical model, we require (i) an initial (IC) vector for eqs. (3.1)–(3.6) and (ii) a parameter set basically for the constants in eqs. (3.1)–(3.6). These requirements are stated in Tables 3.2 and 3.3.

TABLE 3.2   IC vector for eqs. (3.1)–(3.6).

$y_{hif}(t=0) = 1$	$y_{o2}(t=0) = 0$	$y_{p300}(t=0) = 0$
$y_{p53}(t=0) = 0$	$y_{casp}(t=0) = 0$	$y_{kp}(t=0) = 0$

Note that five of the six dependent variables have a homogeneous (zero) IC, while the sixth dependent variable, y_{hif}, has a unit IC. These ICs are rather artificial (would not correspond directly to a realistic physical condition). This IC vector is used because, in the study by Laise et al. [1], the final steady-state or equilibrium condition was of primary interest and therefore the IC could be selected arbitrarily. This presupposes that the final condition is not determined by the IC, which might not be necessarily true, particularly because eqs. (3.1)–(3.6) are nonlinear as discussed subsequently; that is, for a nonlinear ODE system, the final condition is not necessarily unique so that multiple final conditions are possible depending on the particular initial condition that is specified. These important details will be considered when the numerical solution of eqs. (3.1)–(3.6) is discussed subsequently.

The parameter set for eqs. (3.1)–(3.6) is given in Table 3.3.

TABLE 3.3   Parameter set for eqs. (3.1)–(3.6).[a]

$a_{hif} = 1.52$	$a_{o2} = 1.8$	$a_{p53} = 0.05$	$a_3 = 0.9$
$a_4 = 0.2$	$a_5 = 0.001$	$a_7 = 0.7$	$a_8 = 0.06$
$a_9 = 0.1$	$a_{10} = 0.7$	$a_{11} = 0.2$	$a_{12} = 0.1$
$a_{13} = 0.1$	$a_{14} = 0.05$		

[a] Taken from [1].

The role of these parameters is illustrated in Fig. 3.1, and their precise use in the model is given by the RHS of eqs. (3.1)–(3.6). For the given numerical values of Tables 3.2 and 3.3, the numerical solution to eqs. (3.1)–(3.6) is programmed in the R routines that follow.

Before proceeding to the R programming, we consider briefly the terms in the RHS of eqs. (3.1)–(3.6). When considering these terms, keep in mind that all of the parameters in Table 3.3 are nonnegative (zero or positive).

- **Eq. (3.1)**

    1. a_{hif} is a constant value (see Table 3.3) that serves to move the solution of eqs. (3.1) to (3.6) away from the ICs of Table 3.2. As $a_{hif} \geq 0$, y_{hif} will tend to increase with t (dy_{hif}/dt will be more positive according to eq. (3.1)).

    2. $-a_3 y_{o2} y_{hif}$ is the rate of depletion of y_{hif} (as eq. (3.1) is the ODE for y_{hif}) because of the combination of y_{o2} and

y_{hif} (note the product $y_{o2}y_{hif} \geq 0$ with $y_{o2} \geq 0$ and $y_{hif} \geq 0$ because concentrations must be nonnegative). Thus, if either y_{o2} or y_{hif} increases, the rate of depletion of y_{hif} will increase (dy_{hif}/dt will be more negative according to eq. (3.1), recalling that $a_3 > 0$).

3. $-a_4 y_{hif} y_{p300}$ is the rate of depletion of y_{hif} (as eq. (3.1) is the ODE for y_{hif}) because of the combination of y_{hif} and y_{p300} (note the product $y_{hif} y_{p300} \geq 0$ with $y_{hif} \geq 0$ and $y_{p300} \geq 0$ because concentrations must be nonnegative). Thus, if either y_{hif} or y_{p300} increases, the rate of depletion of y_{hif} will increase (dy_{hif}/dt will be more negative according to eq. (3.1), recalling that $a_4 > 0$).

4. $-a_7 y_{p53} y_{hif}$ is the rate of depletion of y_{hif} (as eq. (3.1) is the ODE for y_{hif}) because of the combination of y_{p53} and y_{hif} (note the product $y_{p53}y_{hif} \geq 0$ with $y_{p53} \geq 0$ and $y_{hif} \geq 0$ because concentrations must be nonnegative). Thus, if either y_{p53} or y_{hif} increases, the rate of depletion of y_{hif} will increase (dy_{hif}/dt will be more negative according to eq. (3.1), recalling that $a_7 > 0$).

In summary, the RHS of eq. (3.1) determines how y_{hif} changes with t according to the current values of the four variables y_{hif}, y_{o2}, y_{p300}, and y_{p53}. These variables appear in RHS terms that can be interpreted, analyzed, evaluated, and possibly revised using basic physical, chemical, and biological principles and criteria; ideally, these terms can also be evaluated through comparisons with experimental observations. In other words, the RHS terms are the essence of the mathematical model, and in particular, they determine how the model responds in t because they define the ODE derivatives in t through eqs. (3.1)–(3.6). The contributions of the RHS terms of eq. (3.1) can be visualized by referring to Fig. 3.1 (note in particular the circle labeled hif).

As a specific example of how this formulation and analysis of ODE RHS terms might proceed, consider the second term of eq. (3.1), $-a_7 y_{p53} y_{hif}$. We can note the following points about this term:

- The multiplication function, $y_{p53}y_{hif}$, will have a significant (substantially greater than zero) value only if the two concentrations, y_{p53} **and** y_{hif}, have significant values. The key word here, in bold face, is **and**. In other words, this function acts similarly to an and gate requiring both conditions to be true in order for the function to be true. This seems logical if, for example, the term represents the rate of a biochemical reaction and both reactants must be present in significant concentrations for the reaction to proceed. Generally, this multiplication function implies a (physical or chemical) interaction between $p53$ and hif, and the precise nature of this interaction comes from an understanding of the phenomena occurring in the modeled system.
- Multiplication functions of this type are commonplace in the mathematical modeling of biochemical systems. They have the important property that they are nonlinear. That is, although the individual concentrations are to the first power, their product makes the function nonlinear. This has important implications because nonlinear equations
  — have properties not shared by linear equations, for example, multiple or nonunique solutions;
  — are relatively difficult to solve mathematically; the usual recourse then is to use numerical methods as we will do in the subsequent analysis.
- An alternative to the multiplication function is to use a linear function of the form $c_1 y_{p53} + c_2 y_{hif}$. This function will have a significant value if either $c_1 y_{p53}$ **or** $c_2 y_{hif}$ has a significant value (this will depend to some extend on the values of the constants c_1 and c_2). The key word here, in bold face, is **or**, so this linear function acts as an or gate. That is, it will have a significant value if either concentration is significant.
- The choice between multiplication and linear functions will depend on the circumstances of the application, that is, the particular phenomenon that a function is intended to represent. Thus, some judgment, perhaps based on experience and

experimental evidence, is required in selecting which of the two forms is used in the RHS of the ODE.

- In addition, other functions can be considered, for example, $y_{p53}^a y_{hif}^b$ where constants a and b are selected for a particular application. Typically, in chemical kinetics, these constants are integers or even fractions with specific values determined possibly by some theory about the reaction and perhaps confirmed experimentally. Still other functions could be considered, for example, division, exponential, and logarithmic. The point is that the form of the RHS functions is usually defined by a combination of available theory and experimental data. This selection is as much an art as a science and is directed by the background, experience, and insight of the analyst. Ideally, the choice of a RHS function will produce model solutions that confirm observations. If this can be achieved, then the model can be used to study the modeled system with some assurance that the computed solutions are realistic.

  Also, a trial-and-error investigation of RHS functions can be performed because high speed computers will quickly produce numerical solutions to the proposed equations (as demonstrated subsequently for eqs. (3.1)–(3.6)).

  Ideally, this process will converge to a useful model that provides insight into the phenomena and features of the problem system, and can then be used to modify the problem system to achieve a desired outcome, for example, a therapy that effectively treats a disease. Virtually, any form of the RHS functions can be investigated because the available computer-based numerical methods of solution are quite general and robust.

We now continue the discussion of the RHS functions for eqs. (3.2)–(3.6).

- **Eq. (3.2)**

  1. a_{o2} is a constant value (see Table 3.3) that serves to move the solution of eqs. (3.1)–(3.6) away from the ICs of Table 3.2.

As $a_{o2} \geq 0$, y_{o2} will tend to increase with t (dy_{o2}/dt will be more positive according to eq. (3.2)).

2. $-a_3 y_{o2} y_{hif}$ is the rate of depletion of y_{o2} (because eq. (3.2) is the ODE for y_{o2}) because of the combination of y_{o2} and y_{hif}; again, note the product $y_{o2} y_{hif} \geq 0$ with $y_{o2} \geq 0$ and $y_{hif} \geq 0$ (because concentrations must be nonnegative); also this term is the same as in eq. (3.1) so that it produces the same change in y_{hif} and y_{o2} (from eqs. (3.1) and (3.2)); this might be interpreted as an interaction between y_{o2} and y_{hif} that consumes y_{o2} and y_{hif} at the same rate (consumes because $a_3 > 0$ and therefore the term is negative).

3. $+a_4 y_{hif} y_{p300}$ is the term of the same magnitude as in eq. (3.1) but of opposite sign. This can be interpreted as consumption of *hif* from the negative sign in eq. (3.1) and production of O_2 from the positive sign in eq. (3.2). Rates of equal magnitude but opposite in sign is a common situation when modeling physical and chemical phenomena.

4. $-a_{11} y_{o2}$ is the linear rate of depletion of y_{o2} (because eq. (3.2) is the ODE for y_{o2}). Note that $a_{11} > 0$. The source of this consumption would be determined by the phenomena occurring within a cell, for example, metabolism.

In summary, the RHS of eq. (3.2) determines how y_{o2} changes with t according to the current values of the three variables y_{hif}, y_{o2}, and y_{p300} (the reader might also refer to the additional comments at the analogous point for eq. (3.1)). The contributions of the RHS terms of eq. (3.2) can be visualized by referring to Fig. 3.1 (note in particular the circle labeled O_2).

- **Eq. (3.3)**

  1. $-a_4 y_{hif} y_{p300}$ is the same *hif*-$p300$ interaction term as in eq. (3.2) of equal magnitude but opposite sign. This term corresponds to a depletion of $p300$ (because eq. (3.3) is the ODE for y_{p300}). Note that $a_4 > 0$ (from Table 3.3).

  2. $-a_5 y_{p300} y_{p53}$ is a $p300$-$p53$ interaction term as in eq. (3.2) of equal magnitude but opposite sign. This term corresponds to

a depletion of $p300$ (because eq. (3.3) is the ODE for y_{p300}). Note that $a_5 > 0$ (from Table 3.3).

3. $+a_8$ is a constant value (see Table 3.3) that serves to move the solution of eqs. (3.1)–(3.6) away from the ICs of Table 3.2. As $+a_8 \geq 0$, y_{p300} will tend to increase with t (dy_{p300}/dt will be more positive according to eq. (3.3)).

In summary, the RHS of eq. (3.3) determines how y_{p300} changes with t according to the current values of the three variables y_{hif}, y_{p300}, and y_{p53}. The contributions of the RHS terms of eq. (3.3) can be visualized by referring to Fig. 3.1 (note in particular the circle labeled $p300$). The reader can also refer to the comments in the analogous position for eq. (3.1).

- **Eq. (3.4)**

  1. a_{p53} is a constant value (see Table 3.3) that serves to move the solution of eqs. (3.1)–(3.6) away from the ICs of Table 3.2. As $a_{p53} \geq 0$, y_{p53} will tend to increase with t (dy_{p53}/dt will be more positive according to eq. (3.4)).

  2. $-a_5 y_{p300} y_{p53}$ is the same $p300$–$p53$ interaction term as in eq. (3.3). This term corresponds to a depletion of $p53$ (because eq. (3.4) is the ODE for y_{p53}). Note that $a_5 > 0$ (from Table 3.3).

  3. $-a_9 y_{p53}$ is a linear term in $p53$. This term corresponds to a depletion of $p53$ (because eq. (3.4) is the ODE for y_{p53}). Note that $a_9 > 0$ (from Table 3.3).

  In summary, the RHS of eq. (3.4) determines how y_{p53} changes with t according to the current values of the two variables y_{53} and y_{p300}. The contributions of the RHS terms of eq. (3.4) can be visualized by referring to Fig. 3.1 (note in particular the circle labeled $p53$). The reader can also refer to the comments in the analogous position for eq. (3.1).

- **Eq. (3.5)**

  1. $a_9 y_{p53}$ is the linear term in $p53$ of eq. (3.4), equal in magnitude but opposite in sign so that it is a production term for casp (because eq. (3.5) is the ODE for y_{casp}). Note that $a_9 > 0$ (from Table 3.3).

2. a_{12} is a constant value (see Table 3.3) that serves to move the solution of eqs. (3.1)–(3.6) away from the ICs of Table 3.2. As $a_{12} \geq 0$, y_{casp} will tend to increase with t (because eq. (3.5) is the ODE for y_{casp}).

3. $-a_{13}y_{casp}$ is a linear term in *casp*. This term corresponds to the depletion of *casp* (because eq. (3.5) is the ODE for y_{casp}). Note that $a_{13} > 0$ (from Table 3.3).

In summary, the RHS of eq. (3.5) determines how y_{casp} changes with t according to the current values of the two variables y_{53} and y_{casp}. The contributions of the RHS terms of eq. (3.5) can be visualized by referring to Fig. 3.1 (note in particular the circle labeled *casp*). The reader can also refer to the comments in the analogous position for eq. (3.1).

- **Eq. (3.6)**

  1. $-a_{10}y_{casp}y_{kp}$ is a *casp-kp* interaction term. This term corresponds to a depletion of *kp* (because eq. (3.6) is the ODE for y_{kp}). Note that $a_{11} > 0$ (from Table 3.3).

  2. $+a_{11}y_{O2}$ is a linear term in $O2$. This term corresponds to a production of *kp* (because eq. (3.6) is the ODE for y_{kp}). Note that $a_{11} > 0$ (from Table 3.3).

  3. $-a_{13}y_{casp}$ is a linear term in *casp* that corresponds to a depletion of *kp* (because eq. (3.6) is the ODE for y_{kp}). Note that $a_{13} > 0$ (from Table 3.3).

  4. $-a_{14}y_{kp}$ is a linear term in *kp* that corresponds to a depletion of *kp* (because eq. (3.6) is the ODE for y_{kp}). Note that $a_{14} > 0$ (from Table 3.3).

  In summary, the RHS of eq. (3.6) determines how y_{kp} changes with t according to the current values of the three variables y_{casp}, y_{kp}, and y_{o2}. The contributions of the RHS terms of eq. (3.6) can be visualized by referring to Fig. 3.1 (note in particular the circle labeled *kp*). The reader can also refer to the comments in the analogous position for eq. (3.1).

We can also observe that the various RHS terms of eqs. (3.1)–(3.6) represent a rather complicated combination of constant terms (sources), linear terms, and nonlinear terms. An analytical solution to eqs. (3.1)–(3.6) is therefore essentially impossible and a numerical approach is necessary. Also, Laise et al. [1] developed an approximate analytical analysis by first linearizing eqs. (3.1)–(3.6), but this approach probably circumvented some important nonlinear effects.

3.3 Main Program

We now consider the programming of eqs. (3.1)–(3.6) with the ICs of Table 3.2 and the parameters of Table 3.3. We start with a main program listed next.

```
#
# Apoptosis model
#
# Library of R ODE solvers
  library("deSolve")
#
# ODE routine
  setwd("c:/R/bme_ode/chap3")
  source("apoptosis_1.R")
#
# Multiple cases
  for(ncase in 1:1){
#
# Model parameters
  if(ncase==1){
  a_hif=1.52;   a_o2=1.8; a_p53=0.05; a_3=0.9 ; a_4=0.2 ;
    a_5=0.001;
  a_7  =0.7 ;   a_8=0.06; a_9  =0.1 ; a_10=0.7; a_11=0.2;
    a_12=0.1 ;
  a_13=0.1   ; a_14=0.05;}
#
# Initial condition
  nout=101; ncall=0
  yini=c(1,0,0,0,0,0)
#
# t interval
  times=seq(from=0,to=100,by=100/(nout-1))
#
```

```
# ODE integration
  out=ode(y=yini,times=times,func=apoptosis_1,parms=NULL)
#
# ODE numerical solution
  cat(sprintf("\n\n ncase = %2d",ncase))
  for(it in 1:nout){
  if((it==1)|(it==26)|(it==51)|(it==101)){
  cat(sprintf("\n\n t = %4.1f",out[it,1]))
  cat(sprintf("\n   y_hif  = %8.4f   y_o2  = %8.4f",
    out[it,2],out[it,3]))
  cat(sprintf("\n   y_p300 = %8.4f   y_p53 = %8.4f",
    out[it,4],out[it,5]))
  cat(sprintf("\n   y_casp = %8.4f   y_kp  = %8.4f",
    out[it,6],out[it,7]))
  }
  }
#
# Calls to apoptosis_1
  cat(sprintf("\n\n ncall = %5d\n\n",ncall))
#
# Six plots for y_hif,y_o2,y_p300,y_p53,y_casp,y_kp vs t
  par(mfrow=c(3,2))
#
# y_hif
  plot(out[,1],out[,2],xlab="t",ylab="y_hif(t)",
    xlim=c(0,100),
  type="l",lwd=2,main="Hypoxia inducible factor")
#
# y_o2
  plot(out[,1],out[,3],xlab="t",ylab="y_o2(t)",
    xlim=c(0,100),
  type="l",lwd=2,main="Oxygen level")
#
# y_p300
  plot(out[,1],out[,4],xlab="t",ylab="y_p300(t)",
    xlim=c(0,100),
  type="l",lwd=2,main="Co-activator")
#
# y_p53
  plot(out[,1],out[,5],xlab="t",ylab="y_p53(t)",
    xlim=c(0,100),
```

```
    type="l",lwd=2,main="Tumor suppressor gene")
#
# y_casp
  plot(out[,1],out[,6],xlab="t",ylab="y_casp(t)",
    xlim=c(0,100),
  type="l",lwd=2,main="Caspases")
#
# y_k
  plot(out[,1],out[,7],xlab="t",ylab="y_kp(t)",
    xlim=c(0,100),
  type="l",lwd=2,main="Potassium ions")
#
# Next case
}
```

Listing 3.1 Main program for the numerical integration of eqs. (3.1)–(3.6).

We can note the following points about Listing 3.1.

- The R library of integrators, deSolve, and the ODE routine apoptosis_1 are accessed.

```
#
# Apoptosis model
#
# Library of R ODE solvers
  library("deSolve")
#
# ODE routine
  setwd("c:/R/bme_ode/chap3")
  source("apoptosis_1.R")
```

- A for is used for multiple runs of the main program (e.g., to change parameters) using the index ncase. Here, only one value of ncase is used but this could be increased by setting a larger value for the upper limit of the for loop. An example of the use of the for loop for more than one case is discussed subsequently.

```
#
# Multiple cases
  for(ncase in 1:1){
```

- The parameters in Table 3.3 are defined numerically.

```
#
# Model parameters
  if(ncase==1){
  a_hif=1.52;  a_o2=1.8; a_p53=0.05; a_3=0.9 ;
     a_4=0.2 ; a_5=0.001;
  a_7  =0.7 ;   a_8=0.06; a_9  =0.1 ; a_10=0.7;
     a_11=0.2; a_12=0.1 ;
  a_13=0.1   ; a_14=0.05;}
```

Note that this set of parameters is defined for ncase=1 (the only values programmed, but other sets of parameter values could be added here).

- The IC vector of Table 3.2 is defined.

```
#
# Initial condition
  nout=101; ncall=0
  yini=c(1,0,0,0,0,0)
```

Also, the number of output points for the numerical solution and the counter for the calls to the ODE routine apoptosis_1 are initialized.

- The time scale, $0 \leq t \leq 100$ is selected to display a full solution, that is, one for which the solution eventually reaches an equilibrium (this will be demonstrated when the numerical and graphical output is considered). The units of time have not been specified and can be considered as arbitrary (dimensionless) because none of the parameters in Table 3.3 have been assigned units of time. This is in accordance with the original statement of the model equations [1].

```
#
# t interval
  times=seq(from=0,to=100,by=100/(nout-1))
```

- The numerical solution of eqs. (3.1)–(3.6) is by ode (accessed through deSolve).

```
#
# ODE integration
  out=ode(y=yini,times=times,func=apoptosis_1,
      parms=NULL)
```

Note the inputs to ode, the IC vector, yini, the vector of output values of t, times, and the specification of the ODE routine, apoptosis_1. parms, an argument for passing parameters to apoptosis_1, is unused. The integration is by lsoda, the default for ode.

- The numerical solution is displayed through the use of the ode output array out, including the value of t, out[it,1]. The formatting of out is discussed in some detail in Chapter 1.

```
#
# ODE numerical solution
  cat(sprintf("\n\n ncase = %2d",ncase))
  for(it in 1:nout){
  if((it==1)|(it==26)|(it==51)|(it==101)){
  cat(sprintf("\n\n t = %4.1f",out[it,1]))
  cat(sprintf("\n   y_hif  = %8.4f   y_o2  = %8.4f",
      out[it,2],out[it,3]))
  cat(sprintf("\n   y_p300 = %8.4f   y_p53 = %8.4f",
      out[it,4],out[it,5]))
  cat(sprintf("\n   y_casp = %8.4f   y_kp  = %8.4f",
      out[it,6],out[it,7]))
  }
  }
```

In order to keep the output at a manageable volume, the solution only at $t = 0, 25, 50, 100$ is displayed (corresponding to it=1,26,51,101). In the if, | is the or operator.

- At the end of the solution, the number of calls to apoptosis_1 is displayed.

```
#
# Calls to apoptosis_1
  cat(sprintf("\n\n ncall = %5d\n\n",ncall))
```

- The solutions to eqs. (3.1)–(3.6) are displayed as a 3 × 2 array (3 rows, 2 columns) of separate plots.

```
#
# Six plots for y_hif,y_o2,y_p300,y_p53,y_casp,y_kp
#    vs t
  par(mfrow=c(3,2))
#
# y_hif
  plot(out[,1],out[,2],xlab="t",ylab="y_hif(t)",
     xlim=c(0,100),
  type="l",lwd=2,main="Hypoxia inducible factor")
#
# y_o2
  plot(out[,1],out[,3],xlab="t",ylab="y_o2(t)",
     xlim=c(0,100),
  type="l",lwd=2,main="Oxygen level")
#
# y_p300
  plot(out[,1],out[,4],xlab="t",ylab="y_p300(t)",
     xlim=c(0,100),
  type="l",lwd=2,main="Co-activator")
#
# y_p53
  plot(out[,1],out[,5],xlab="t",ylab="y_p53(t)",
     xlim=c(0,100),
  type="l",lwd=2,main="Tumor suppressor gene")
#
# y_casp
  plot(out[,1],out[,6],xlab="t",ylab="y_casp(t)",
     xlim=c(0,100),
  type="l",lwd=2,main="Caspases")
#
# y_k
  plot(out[,1],out[,7],xlab="t",ylab="y_kp(t)",
     xlim=c(0,100),
  type="l",lwd=2,main="Potassium ions")
#
# Next case
}
```

The parameters of the plot utility are described in some detail in Chapter 1. Note in particular the use of the solution array out for the independent variable t (out[,1]) and the six dependent variables of eqs. (3.1)–(3.6) (out[,2],...,out[,7]). Also, automatic scaling of the ordinate (vertical) scale is used so that ylim is not used. The use of the other parameters will be clear when the graphical output is discussed subsequently. The final } concludes the for in ncase.

3.4   ODE Routine

The ODE routine, apoptosis_1, called by ode is in Listing 3.2.

```
  apoptosis_1=function(t,y,parms) {
#
# Transfer dependent variable vector to problem variables
  y_hif =y[1];
  y_o2  =y[2];
  y_p300=y[3];
  y_p53 =y[4];
  y_casp=y[5];
  y_kp  =y[6];
#
# Apoptosis model ODEs
  yt_hif =a_hif-a_3*y_o2*y_hif-a_4*y_hif*y_p300-a_7*y_p53*
    y_hif;
  yt_o2  =a_o2 -a_3*y_o2*y_hif+a_4*y_hif*y_p300-a_11*y_o2;
  yt_p300=a_8                 -a_4*y_hif*y_p300-a_5*
    y_p300*y_p53;
  yt_p53 =a_p53-a_9*y_p53                      -a_5*
    y_p300*y_p53;
  yt_casp=a_12 +a_9*y_p53-a_13*y_casp;
  yt_kp  =-a_10*y_casp*y_kp-a_14*y_kp          +a_11*y_o2;
#
# Increment calls to apoptosis_1
  ncall <<- ncall+1
#
# Return derivative vector
```

```
    return(list(c(yt_hif,yt_o2,yt_p300,yt_p53,yt_casp,
      yt_kp)))
}
```

Listing 3.2 ODE routine `apoptosis_1` for the numerical integration of eqs. (3.1)–(3.6).

We can note the following points about `apoptosis_1`.

- The function is defined.

  ```
  apoptosis_1=function(t,y,parms) {
  ```

- The second input argument of `apoptosis_1`, `y`, a vector of six values, is placed in six scalar variables that reflect the dependent variables of eqs. (3.1)–(3.6). This renaming facilitates the programming of eqs. (3.1)–(3.6) in terms of the six dependent variables.

  ```
  %
  % Transfer dependent variable vector to problem
        variables
    y_hif =y(1);
    y_o2  =y(2);
    y_p300=y(3);
    y_p53 =y(4);
    y_casp=y(5);
    y_kp  =y(6);
  ```

- Eqs. (3.1)–(3.6) are programmed.

  ```
  #
  # Apoptosis model ODEs
    yt_hif =a_hif-a_3*y_o2*y_hif-a_4*y_hif*y_p300-a_7*
      y_p53*y_hif;
    yt_o2  =a_o2 -a_3*y_o2*y_hif+a_4*y_hif*y_p300-a_11*
      y_o2;
    yt_p300=a_8                    -a_4*y_hif*y_p300-a_5*
      y_p300*y_p53;
    yt_p53 =a_p53-a_9*y_p53                        -a_5*
      y_p300*y_p53;
  ```

```
yt_casp=a_12 +a_9*y_p53-a_13*y_casp;
yt_kp  =-a_10*y_casp*y_kp-a_14*y_kp                  +a_11*
   y_o2;
```

For example, eq. (3.1) is programmed as

```
yt_hif =a_hif-a_3*y_o2*y_hif-a_4*y_hif*y_p300-a_7*
   y_p53*y_hif;
```

The close correspondence between the mathematical statement of eq. (3.1) and the programming is clear. Note in particular that the derivative of eq. (3.1), dy_{hif}/dt, is named yt_hif in order to provide a valid programming variable name.

The spacing in the RHS programming was selected to emphasize the common terms of the ODEs as suggested by Fig. 3.1. For example, eqs. (3.1) and (3.2) have the common function $a_3 y_{o2} y_{hif}$ and eqs. (3.1)–(3.3) have the common function $a_4 y_{hif} y_{p300}$, which is emphasized by aligning these functions vertically in the programming (note that the signs of these terms can be + for an increase with t and - for a decrease with t because all of the concentrations are positive). Similarly, -a_11*y_02 appears in eq. (3.2) and +a_11*y_o2 appears in the eq. (3.6), reflecting a decrease of O_2 and an increase of kp, respectively.

- The counter for the number of calls to apoptosis is incremented.

```
#
# Increment calls to apoptosis_1
  ncall <<- ncall+1
```

Note the use of <<- to pass the new value of ncall back to the main program of Listing 3.1.

- Finally, the six derivatives in t are returned to the ODE integrator lsoda as a list (as required by the ODE integrators in deSolve).

```
#
# Return derivative vector
  return(list(c(yt_hif,yt_o2,yt_p300,yt_p53,yt_casp,
    yt_kp)))
}
```

This completes the discussion of the programming of eqs. (3.1)–(3.6). The numerical and graphical output produced by the main program and the ODE routine of Listings 3.1 and 3.2 is now considered.

3.5 Base Case Output

The numerical output is in Table 3.4.

We can note the following points about this output.

- The solution starts at the ICs of Table 3.2, t=0.0. This is an important check because if the IC vector is not correct, the subsequent solution (t > 0) will not be correct.

TABLE 3.4   Numerical output from Listings 3.1 and 3.2.

```
ncase =  1

t =  0.0
   y_hif  =    1.0000    y_o2  =    0.0000
   y_p300 =    0.0000    y_p53 =    0.0000
   y_casp =    0.0000    y_kp  =    0.0000

t = 25.0
   y_hif  =    0.5420    y_o2  =    2.6645
   y_p300 =    0.4706    y_p53 =    0.4576
   y_casp =    1.2735    y_kp  =    0.5706

t = 50.0
   y_hif  =    0.5038    y_o2  =    2.8407
   y_p300 =    0.5771    y_p53 =    0.4940
   y_casp =    1.4708    y_kp  =    0.5267

t = 100.0
   y_hif  =    0.4991    y_o2  =    2.8646
   y_p300 =    0.5978    y_p53 =    0.4970
   y_casp =    1.4968    y_kp  =    0.5219

ncall =    506
```

- The solution approaches an equilibrium (constant or time-invariant) condition for which the six dependent variables do not change with t (that is more obvious in the graphical output). This is an important property as reflected in the following details.

  — The system modeled by eqs. (3.1)–(3.6) is inherently stable. In other words, it does not continue to change, perhaps ultimately becoming unbounded, as t increases. This stability results from the complex interplay of the various RHS terms of eqs. (3.1) and (3.6) (to lead to a stable equilibrium or stable point). These terms are constant, linear, and nonlinear, and each may depend on one or two of the dependent variables as discussed previously.

  — If the solution turned out to be unstable (which it is not), this would suggest a fundamental deficiency of the mathematical model because the physical system is not expected to be unstable, for example, one or more concentrations increasing without bound.

  — As a related point, all six dependent variables are nonnegative, which is an important check, because they represent concentrations (and therefore physically cannot be negative).

  — The equilibrium solution results from the six LHS derivatives of eqs. (3.1)–(3.6) approaching zero. This property will be examined in some detail later.

  — As a related point, when the LHS derivatives of eqs. (3.1)–(3.6) are zero (at equilibrium), the solution is for a set of nonlinear algebraic equations that are the RHS functions of eqs. (3.1)–(3.6) set to zero. In fact, this suggests a method for solving a nonlinear algebraic system, that is, add a derivative to each equation, then integrate the resulting system of ODEs to an equilibrium condition. This can be considered to be a form of continuation in which the IC vector (arbitrarily selected) is continued to an equilibrium solution. t in this case is a continuation parameter (and may not be part of the original problem of interest, such as in a nonlinear algebraic system).

— The equilibrium solution may depend on the choice of ICs, particularly because eqs. (3.1)–(3.6) are nonlinear. This point will be examined in some detail later.

— The equilibrium solution is dependent on the choice of a particular parameter set. In other words, the solution of Table 3.4 corresponds to the parameter set of Table 3.3. For another parameter set, the equilibrium solution will in general be different. In fact, how sensitive the solution is to changes in particular parameters is often an important consideration (or result) when formulating and using a mathematical model.

• The six dependent variables all remain within a rather narrow band or interval, typically $0 \leq y \leq 5$. This results from the form of the ODEs and the choice of ICs in Table 3.2 and parameters in Table 3.3. An alternative would be to use physical variables that might have a much broader range of variation (orders of magnitude are not unusual). The present formulation can be considered informative in the sense that it indicates how the six dependent variables vary relative to each other (even though their absolute values may result from a normalization process such as the ICs of Table 3.2 normalized with respect to unity).

• Thus, the choice of variable types is an important consideration in the formulation of a mathematical model, that is, whether to use absolute variables (possibly with units that reflect the physical, chemical, and biological basis of the model such as, for example, the model in Chapters 1 and 2) or relative (possibly normalized) variables as in the present case.

• The computational effort to produce the solution of Table 3.4 is quite modest (with `ncall = 506`).

The six plots produced by Listings 3.1 and 3.2 appear next as shown in Fig. 3.2.

We can note the following details of Fig. 3.2.

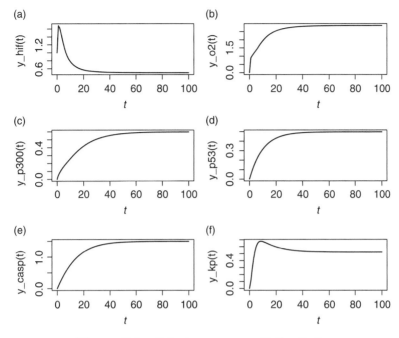

Figure 3.2   Solutions to eqs. (3.1)–(3.6).

- $y_{hif}(t)$ undergoes a relatively sharp transient at $t = 0$ as it moves away from the IC $y_{hif}(t = 0) = 1$ (from Table 3.2). This is rather typical of solutions of ODEs, that is, the greatest variation is usually at the beginning of the solution. Also, the transient at the beginning remains nonnegative; if an excursion to negative values occurred, even for a brief interval in t, the model would be considered invalid (because negative concentrations are not possible).
- These same conclusions apply to the solutions for eqs. (3.2)–(3.6).
- All six solutions approach constant (equilibrium) values, as reflected in the numerical solution of Table 3.4.

3.6   Base Case with Variation in ICs

The ICs of Table 3.2 produce a stable, equilibrium solution as demonstrated in Fig. 3.2. However, the equilibrium solution might change with the ICs and may even become unstable (primarily because eqs. (3.1)–(3.6) are nonlinear). We now investigate through one example how the ICs affect the equilibrium solution. This is done using the for loop in ncase of Listing 3.1 which is now executed for two cases.

.
.
.

```
#
# Multiple cases
  for(ncase in 1:2){
#
# Model parameters
  a_hif=1.52;  a_o2=1.8; a_p53=0.05; a_3=0.9 ; a_4=0.2 ;
    a_5=0.001;
  a_7  =0.7 ;  a_8=0.06; a_9  =0.1 ; a_10=0.7; a_11=0.2;
    a_12=0.1 ;
  a_13=0.1  ; a_14=0.05;
#
# Initial condition
  nout=101; ncall=0
  if(ncase==1){yini=c(1,0,0,0,0,0)}
  if(ncase==2){yini=c(0,0,0,0,0,0)}
```

.
.
.

Listing 3.3 Changes in the code for a new IC vector.

We can note the following points.

- ncase=1 is the base case of Table 3.2.
- For ncase=2, a homogeneous (zero) IC is used for y_{hif} (everything else remains unchanged).

The numerical output for ncase=2 is listed in Table 3.5. We can note the following points about this output.

- The IC (t = 0.0) for ncase=2 is correct (always a good check).

TABLE 3.5   Numerical output from Listing 3.3, ncase=2.

```
ncase =  2

t =  0.0
  y_hif  =   0.0000    y_o2  =   0.0000
  y_p300 =   0.0000    y_p53 =   0.0000
  y_casp =   0.0000    y_kp  =   0.0000

t = 25.0
  y_hif  =   0.5392    y_o2  =   2.6779
  y_p300 =   0.4800    y_p53 =   0.4575
  y_casp =   1.2735    y_kp  =   0.5740

t = 50.0
  y_hif  =   0.5036    y_o2  =   2.8419
  y_p300 =   0.5783    y_p53 =   0.4940
  y_casp =   1.4708    y_kp  =   0.5269

t = 100.0
  y_hif  =   0.4991    y_o2  =   2.8646
  y_p300 =   0.5978    y_p53 =   0.4970
  y_casp =   1.4968    y_kp  =   0.5219

ncall =    463
```

- Even though the transient solutions are different (consider y_hif that starts at 1 for ncase=1 and at 0 for ncase=2), the equilibrium solutions are the same, for example, at $t = 100$,

```
ncase =  1 (Table 3.4)

t = 100.0
  y_hif  =   0.4991    y_o2  =   2.8646
  y_p300 =   0.5978    y_p53 =   0.4970
  y_casp =   1.4968    y_kp  =   0.5219

ncase =  2 (Table 3.5)

t = 100.0
```

```
y_hif   =    0.4991    y_o2  =    2.8646
y_p300 =    0.5978    y_p53 =    0.4970
y_casp =    1.4968    y_kp  =    0.5219
```

Thus, the change in the IC for h_{hif} is inconsequential for large t.
- The computational effort for the two cases is approximately the same.

```
ncase = 1, ncall =    506

ncase = 2, ncall =    463
```

Thus, the performance of lsoda was unaffected by the change in the IC.

In summary, the change in the h_{hif} IC affected only the transient part of the solution of eqs. (3.1)–(3.6).

The graphical output for ncase=2 is in Fig. 3.3.

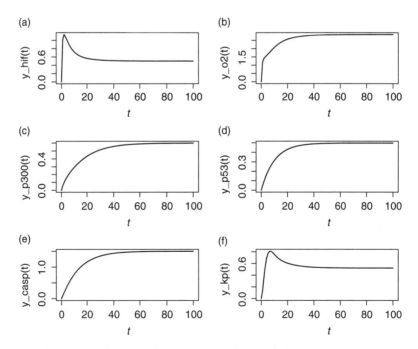

Figure 3.3   Solutions to eqs. (3.1)–(3.6) for ncase=2.

3.7 Variation in ODEs

We now consider another variation of the basic model (in addition to the variation of the IC in Section 3.6). Specifically, the ODEs can be changed, in this case as a function of t. As the concentration of the caspaces is a fundamental factor in regulating apoptosis, we consider a variation in eq. (3.5), namely, the effect of a reduction in the production rate constant a_{12}. To this end, we use a modified version of Listing 3.2 (Listing 3.4).

```
  apoptosis_1=function(t,y,parms) {
#
# Transfer dependent variable vector to problem variables
  y_hif =y[1];
  y_o2  =y[2];
  y_p300=y[3];
  y_p53 =y[4];
  y_casp=y[5];
  y_kp  =y[6];
#
# Apoptosis model ODEs
  yt_hif =a_hif-a_3*y_o2*y_hif-a_4*y_hif*y_p300-a_7*y_p53*
    y_hif;
  yt_o2  =a_o2 -a_3*y_o2*y_hif+a_4*y_hif*y_p300-a_11*
    y_o2;
  yt_p300=a_8                 -a_4*y_hif*y_p300-a_5*
    y_p300*y_p53;
  yt_p53 =a_p53-a_9*y_p53                      -a_5*
    y_p300*y_p53;
  if(ncase==1){
    yt_casp=+a_9*y_p53+a_12-a_13*y_casp;}
  if(ncase==2){
    yt_casp=+a_9*y_p53+a_12*exp(-0.1*t)-a_13*y_casp;}
  yt_kp  =-a_10*y_casp*y_kp-a_14*y_kp           +a_11*
    y_o2;
#
# Increment calls to apoptosis_1
  ncall <<- ncall+1
#
# Return derivative vector
```

```
return(list(c(yt_hif,yt_o2,yt_p300,yt_p53,yt_casp,
    yt_kp))))
}
```

Listing 3.4 ODE routine for eqs. (3.1) to (3.6) with variation in a_12.

We can note the following points about Listing 3.4.

- The programming up to eq. (3.5) is the same as in Listing 3.2 and therefore is not repeated here (up to and including eq. (3.4) with the derivative yt_p53).
- Two forms of eq. (3.5) are programmed, as selected by ncase (set in the main program of Listing 3.1 with the ICs of Table 3.2).

```
if(ncase==1){
  yt_casp=+a_9*y_p53+a_12-a_13*y_casp;}
if(ncase==2){
  yt_casp=+a_9*y_p53+a_12*exp(-0.1*t)-a_13*y_casp;}
```

For ncase=1, eq. (3.5) is programmed as in Listing 3.2, that is, for the base case of the model.

For ncase==2, a_12 is programmed as an exponential function of t, a_12*exp(-0.1*t). The exponential function, exp(-0.1*t), starts at an initial value of 1 (for $t = 0$, exp(0)=1); note that the value of t is available as the first RHS input argument of apoptosis_1. As t increases, the exponential function decreases. When $t = 100$ at the end of the solution, the exponential function has decreased to $e^{-0.1(100)} = 4.45 \times 10^{-5}$ so that the constant caspase source term in the RHS of eq. (3.5) is (with $a_{12} = 0.1$) $a_{12}e^{0.1(100)} = (0.1)(4.45 \times 10^{-5})$, a small value as we shall see in the subsequent analysis. In other words, the factor 0.1 in $e^{0.1t}$ was selected so that $e^{0.1(100)}$ is small.

- The remainder of the programming, starting with eq. (3.6), is the same as in apoptosis_1 of Listing 3.2 and is not repeated here.

The programming of the a_{12} term in eq. (3.5) demonstrates the ease of programming the RHS functions of the ODEs as a function of the independent variable t. This approach can be applied to any function such as the constant term a_12, a linear term, a nonlinear term, or any combination of these. Further, any RHS term can be programmed as a function (condition) of any of the ODE-dependent variables as well as the independent variable t (because all of the dependent variables are available through the second RHS (input) argument of apoptosis_1). In other words, complete flexibility is available in programming the ODE RHS functions which is one of the principal features of the numerical approach to the ODE integration (an example of the programming of the ODE RHS functions as a function of the dependent variables is given in glucose_1 of Chapter 2).

Execution of the main program of Listing 3.1 (with for(ncase in 1:2)) gives the following numerical output.

We can note the following details of this output.

- The output for ncase=1 is the same as the base output in Table 3.4 as expected.
- The output for ncase=2 is substantially changed for y_casp,y_kp because the exponentially varying a_12 in Listing 3.4 appears in the ODEs for these two variables, that is, in the RHS of eqs. (3.5) and (3.6). In particular, y_casp decreased relative to the base case of ncase=1, while y_kp increased. These changes have important implications for apoptosis.

The graphical output is in Fig. 3.4.

A comparison of Fig. 3.2 and Fig. 3.4 clearly indicates the differences in y_casp as discussed for Table 3.6. The effect of the variation of a_12 could be further analyzed by computing and plotting the individual RHS terms of eqs. (3.5) and (3.6). This could be done easily by a call to apoptosis_1 of Listing 3.4. The use of the ODE derivative routine in this way to further explain the contributions of the individual ODE RHS terms is illustrated in Chapter 2. This is a very effective way to understand the observed characteristics of a computed ODE solution.

TABLE 3.6   Numerical output with exponential variation of a_12 in Listing 3.4.

```
ncase =   1

t =   0.0
   y_hif  =   1.0000    y_o2  =   0.0000
   y_p300 =   0.0000    y_p53 =   0.0000
   y_casp =   0.0000    y_kp  =   0.0000

t =  25.0
   y_hif  =   0.5420    y_o2  =   2.6645
   y_p300 =   0.4706    y_p53 =   0.4576
   y_casp =   1.2735    y_kp  =   0.5706

t =  50.0
   y_hif  =   0.5038    y_o2  =   2.8407
   y_p300 =   0.5771    y_p53 =   0.4940
   y_casp =   1.4708    y_kp  =   0.5267

t = 100.0
   y_hif  =   0.4991    y_o2  =   2.8646
   y_p300 =   0.5978    y_p53 =   0.4970
   y_casp =   1.4968    y_kp  =   0.5219

ncall =    506


ncase =   2

t =   0.0
   y_hif  =   0.0000    y_o2  =   0.0000
   y_p300 =   0.0000    y_p53 =   0.0000
   y_casp =   0.0000    y_kp  =   0.0000

t =  25.0
   y_hif  =   0.5392    y_o2  =   2.6779
   y_p300 =   0.4800    y_p53 =   0.4575
   y_casp =   0.5608    y_kp  =   1.1832
```

TABLE 3.6   (*Continued*)

```
t = 50.0
   y_hif  =   0.5036    y_o2  =   2.8419
   y_p300 =   0.5783    y_p53 =   0.4940
   y_casp =   0.5112    y_kp  =   1.3837

t = 100.0
   y_hif  =   0.4991    y_o2  =   2.8646
   y_p300 =   0.5978    y_p53 =   0.4970
   y_casp =   0.4973    y_kp  =   1.4390

ncall =    477
```

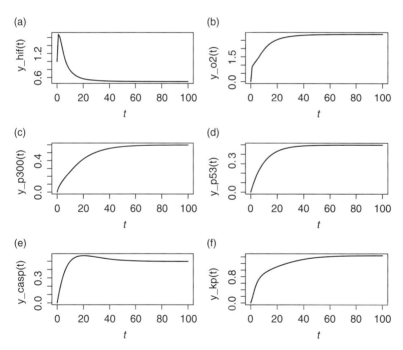

Figure 3.4   Solution with exponential variation of a_12.

3.8 Selection of Units

The discussion so far has been in terms of eqs. (3.1)–(3.6) without a consideration of units. We now consider briefly how units (physical, chemical, biological) can be included in the analysis. Also, Chapters 1 and 2 have a discussion of a model with units.

The ICs of Table 3.2 are based on the unit concentration for y_{hif}, that is, $y_{hif}(t = 0) = 1$. The unit value can be considered as dimensionless (based on the approach in the previous discussion), so that, for example, if $y_{hif} = 1.2$ at some point along the solution (specific value of t), we can conclude that y_{hif} increased by 20% from its initial value in Table 3.2.

However, the unit value in the IC can also be considered a physical concentration, with typical values of 1 g mol/l, $0.001 = 10^{-3}$ g mol/l = 1 mg mol/l, $0.000001 = 10^{-6}$ g mol/l = 1 μg mol/l, $0.000000001 = 10^{-9}$ g mol/l = 1 ng mol/l, and $0.000000000001 = 10^{-12}$ g mol/l = 1 pg mol/l. This wide range of values (12 orders of magnitude) is not unusual for concentrations in biochemical engineering applications. Other possibilities are (with 1 l = 1000 cubic centimeters (cc) = 1000 ml) 1 mg mol/l = 0.001 mg mol/cc = 0.001 mg mol/ml.

The choice of a particular set of units will be determined by the application and circumstances, with a choice frequently based on the unit value (e.g., 1 ng mol/ml is somewhat more convenient to use than 10^{-9} g mol/ml). Also, g (grams) might be used in place of g mol through a conversion based on the molecular weight, for example, 1 g mol of H_2O = 18 g of H_2O (assuming gram molars, g mols).

Also, there is the matter of a timescale with units. Previously, we used $0 \leq t \leq 100$ without a consideration of time units. But we could consider $0 \leq t \leq 100$ seconds (s), minutes (min), hours (hr), days, or months, for example. Again, wide variations in the units of time are typical in BMSE applications.

Whatever units we choose, they must then be reflected consistently in the model parameters, such as in Table 3.4. For example, if we choose concentration units of μg mols/ml (typically abbreviated as μmols/ml or μmols/cc, assuming gram molars or g mol rather than, for example, kilogram molars, kg mols), and time units of days, then the terms in eq. (3.1) will have the following units:

$$\frac{dy_{hif}}{dt}: (\mu mol/ml)(1/days)$$

a_{hif}: $\mu mol/(ml\ days)$

$-a_3 y_{o2} y_{hif}$: $(1/\mu mol/ml)(1/days)(\mu mol/ml)(\mu mol/ml)$

$-a_4 y_{hif} y_{p300}$: $(1/\mu mol/ml)(1/days)(\mu mol/ml)(\mu mol/ml)$

$-a_7 y_{p53} y_{hif}$: $(1/\mu mols/ml)(1/days)(\mu mols/ml)(\mu mols/ml)$

Thus, a_{hif} has the units $\mu mol/(ml\ days)$ and a_3, a_4, and a_7 (in Table 3.3) have the units of $(1/\mu mol/ml)(1/days)$. Similar reasoning applies to all of the other parameters in Table 3.3.

In summary, any consistent set of units can be selected, but it must be consistent throughout the ODE and between all of the ODEs. This may seem like an obvious point, but units can easily be mixed incorrectly when using parameters taken from the literature. Also, the parameters with time define the timescale of the solution. Thus, the solutions of eqs. (3.1)–(3.6) will have t in days because, for example, the numerical integration of dy_{hif}/dt with the units $(\mu mol/ml)(1/days)$ will produce $y_{hif}(t)$ with t in days.

3.9   Model Solution with RKF45

We conclude this discussion of the apoptosis model of eqs. (3.1)–(3.6) with a numerical solution computed with the RKF45 algorithm (detailed in Chapters 1 and 2). A main program that includes this algorithm is in Listing 3.5.

```
#
# Apoptosis model
#
# ODE routine
  setwd("c:/R/bme_ode/chap3")
  source("rkf45.R")
  source("apoptosis_2.R")
#
# Vectors, matrices for the graphical output
```

```
  nout=101
  plot_hif =matrix(0,nrow=nout,ncol=1)
  plot_o2  =matrix(0,nrow=nout,ncol=1)
  plot_p300=matrix(0,nrow=nout,ncol=1)
  plot_p53 =matrix(0,nrow=nout,ncol=1)
  plot_casp=matrix(0,nrow=nout,ncol=1)
  plot_kp  =matrix(0,nrow=nout,ncol=1)
  tplot=rep(0,nout)
#
# Select rkf45 format
#
# nint = 1: No error estimation
#
# nint = 2: With error estimation
  nint=2
#
# Multiple cases
  for(ncase in 1:1){
#
# Model parameters
  if(ncase==1){
  a_hif=1.52;  a_o2=1.8; a_p53=0.05; a_3=0.9 ; a_4=0.2 ;
    a_5=0.001;
  a_7  =0.7 ;  a_8=0.06; a_9  =0.1 ; a_10=0.7; a_11=0.2;
    a_12=0.1 ;
  a_13=0.1  ; a_14=0.05;}
#
# Initial condition
  t=0;ncall=0;
  y=c(1,0,0,0,0,0)
  cat(sprintf("\n\n t = %4.1f",t))
  cat(sprintf("\n   y_hif  = %8.4f   y_o2  = %8.4f",y[1],
    y[2]))
  cat(sprintf("\n   y_p300 = %8.4f   y_p53 = %8.4f",y[3],
    y[4]))
  cat(sprintf("\n   y_casp = %8.4f   y_kp  = %8.4f",y[5],
    y[6]))
  if(nint==2){
  ee=c(0,0,0,0,0,0)
  cat(sprintf("\n   e_hif  = %8.4f   e_o2  = %8.4f",ee[1],
    ee[2]))
```

```
    cat(sprintf("\n    e_p300 = %8.4f    e_p53 = %8.4f",ee[3],
      ee[4]))
    cat(sprintf("\n    e_casp = %8.4f    e_kp   = %8.4f",ee[5],
      ee[6]))}
#
# Store solution for plotting
  plot_hif[1,ncase] =y[1]
  plot_o2[1,ncase]  =y[2]
  plot_p300[1,ncase]=y[3]
  plot_p53[1,ncase] =y[4]
  plot_casp[1,ncase]=y[5]
  plot_kp[1,ncase]  =y[6]
  if(ncase==1)tplot[1]=t
#
# Parameters for t integration
  tout=1;nt=10;h=tout/nt
#
# rkf45 integration
  for(i1 in 2:nout){
#
#    rkf45 integration over nt points
    yout=rkf45(nt,h,t,y)
    y=yout; t=t+tout
#
#    Solution after nt rkf45 steps
    if((i1==1)|(i1==26)|(i1==51)|(i1==101)){
    cat(sprintf("\n\n t = %4.1f",t))
    cat(sprintf("\n    y_hif  = %8.4f    y_o2  = %8.4f",
      y[1],y[2]))
    cat(sprintf("\n    y_p300 = %8.4f    y_p53 = %8.4f",
      y[3],y[4]))
    cat(sprintf("\n    y_casp = %8.4f    y_kp  = %8.4f",
      y[5],y[6]))
    if(nint==2){
    cat(sprintf("\n    e_hif  = %8.4f    e_o2  = %8.4f",
      ee[1],ee[2]))
    cat(sprintf("\n    e_p300 = %8.4f    e_p53 = %8.4f",
      ee[3],ee[4]))
    cat(sprintf("\n    e_casp = %8.4f    e_kp  = %8.4f",
      ee[5],ee[6]))}
    }
```

```
#
#   Store solution for plotting
    plot_hif[i1,ncase] =y[1]
    plot_o2[i1,ncase]  =y[2]
    plot_p300[i1,ncase]=y[3]
    plot_p53[i1,ncase] =y[4]
    plot_casp[i1,ncase]=y[5]
    plot_kp[i1,ncase]  =y[6]
    if(ncase==1)tplot[i1]=t
 }
#
# Calls to apoptosis_1
  cat(sprintf("\n\n ncall = %5d\n\n",ncall))
#
# Six plots for y_hif,y_o2,y_p300,y_p53,y_casp,y_kp vs t
  par(mfrow=c(3,2))
#
# y_hif
  plot(tplot,plot_hif[,ncase],xlab="t",ylab="y_hif(t)",
     xlim=c(0,100),
  type="l",lwd=2,main="Hypoxia inducible factor")
#
# y_o2
  plot(tplot,plot_o2[,ncase],xlab="t",ylab="y_o2(t)",
     xlim=c(0,100),
  type="l",lwd=2,main="Oxygen level")
#
# y_p300
  plot(tplot,plot_p300[,ncase],xlab="t",ylab="y_p300(t)",
     xlim=c(0,100),
  type="l",lwd=2,main="Co-activator")
#
# y_p53
  plot(tplot,plot_p53[,ncase],xlab="t",ylab="y_p53(t)",
     xlim=c(0,100),
  type="l",lwd=2,main="Tumor suppressor gene")
#
# y_casp
  plot(tplot,plot_casp[,ncase],xlab="t",ylab="y_casp(t)",
     xlim=c(0,100),
  type="l",lwd=2,main="Caspases")
```

```
#
# y_k
  plot(tplot,plot_kp[,ncase],xlab="t",ylab="y_kp(t)",
     xlim=c(0,100),
  type="l",lwd=2,main="Potassium ions")
#
# Next case
}
```

Listing 3.5 Main program for eqs. (3.1)–(3.6) based on RKF45 integration.

Listing 3.5 is similar to Listing 3.1, with the important difference of a call to rkf45 rather than ode. The differences are listed next.

- rkf45 of Listing 2.5 and apoptosis_2 of Listing 3.5 are accessed. (glucose_2 of Listing 2.5 was changed to apoptosis_2 in rkf45).

  ```
  #
  # Apoptosis model
  #
  # ODE routine
    setwd("c:/R/bme_ode/chap3")
    source("rkf45.R")
    source("apoptosis_2.R")
  ```

- A set of vectors and matrices is declared (preallocated) for plotting the numerical solution.

  ```
  #
  # Vectors, matrices for the graphical output
    nout=101
    plot_hif =matrix(0,nrow=nout,ncol=1)
    plot_o2  =matrix(0,nrow=nout,ncol=1)
    plot_p300=matrix(0,nrow=nout,ncol=1)
    plot_p53 =matrix(0,nrow=nout,ncol=1)
    plot_casp=matrix(0,nrow=nout,ncol=1)
    plot_kp  =matrix(0,nrow=nout,ncol=1)
    tplot=rep(0,nout)
  ```

Note that `nout=101` specifies the number of output values in the plotted solution.

- The explicit error estimate of `rkf45` can be used with `nint=2`.

```
#
# Select rkf45 format
#
# nint = 1: No error estimation
#
# nint = 2: With error estimation
  nint=2
```

- The base case parameters of Listing 3.1 are used.

```
#
# Multiple cases
  for(ncase in 1:1){
#
# Model parameters
  if(ncase==1){
  a_hif=1.52;  a_o2=1.8; a_p53=0.05; a_3=0.9 ;
    a_4=0.2 ; a_5=0.001;
  a_7  =0.7 ;  a_8=0.06; a_9  =0.1 ; a_10=0.7;
    a_11=0.2; a_12=0.1 ;
  a_13=0.1  ; a_14=0.05;}
```

- The base case IC of Table 3.2 is used ($y=c(1,0,0,0,0,0)$). Also, the estimated error vector, ee, is initialized, $ee=c(0,0,0,0,0,0)$. These six errors are zero because the IC is prescribed as the ODE solution at $t = 0$ (the numerical solution has no error at $t = 0$).

```
#
# Initial condition
  t=0;ncall=0;
  y=c(1,0,0,0,0,0)
  cat(sprintf("\n\n t = %4.1f",t))
  cat(sprintf("\n   y_hif   = %8.4f y_o2   = %8.4f",
    y[1],y[2]))
  cat(sprintf("\n   y_p300 = %8.4f y_p53 = %8.4f",
    y[3],y[4]))
```

```
cat(sprintf("\n    y_casp = %8.4f  y_kp   = %8.4f",
    y[5],y[6]))
if(nint==2){
ee=c(0,0,0,0,0,0)
cat(sprintf("\n    e_hif  = %8.4f  e_o2   = %8.4f",
    ee[1],ee[2]))
cat(sprintf("\n    e_p300 = %8.4f  e_p53  = %8.4f",
    ee[3],ee[4]))
cat(sprintf("\n    e_casp = %8.4f  e_kp   = %8.4f",
    ee[5],ee[6]))}
```

Also, the counter for the calls to the ODE routine, apoptosis_2, is initialized (ncall=0).

- The IC is placed in the arrays for plotting.

```
#
# Store solution for plotting
  plot_hif[1,ncase] =y[1]
  plot_o2[1,ncase]  =y[2]
  plot_p300[1,ncase]=y[3]
  plot_p53[1,ncase] =y[4]
  plot_casp[1,ncase]=y[5]
  plot_kp[1,ncase]  =y[6]
  if(ncase==1)tplot[1]=t
```

Note that the first subscript for the arrays is 1 corresponding to $t = 0$, for example, plot_hif[1,ncase]. The second subscript has only the value ncase=1 because of the preceding for(ncase in 1:1). This arrangement facilitates multiple case solutions of eqs. (3.1)–(3.6).

- The parameters for the RKF45 integration are specified.

```
#
# Parameters for t integration
  tout=1;nt=10;h=tout/nt
```

$h = 1/10 = 0.1$ was selected to give a stable, accurate solution (as confirmed by the subsequent output).

- The solution is computed over nt steps by a call to rkf45.

```
#
# rkf45 integration
  for(i1 in 2:nout){
#
#    rkf45 integration over nt points
     yout=rkf45(nt,h,t,y)
     y=yout; t=t+tout
```

The arguments and use of rkf45 are discussed in some detail in Chapter 2.

- The solution and integration error after nt steps are displayed.

```
#
#    Solution after nt rkf45 steps
     if((i1==1)|(i1==26)|(i1==51)|(i1==101)){
     cat(sprintf("\n\n t = %4.1f",t))
     cat(sprintf("\n   y_hif  = %8.4f    y_o2   = %8.4f",
       y[1],y[2]))
     cat(sprintf("\n   y_p300 = %8.4f    y_p53  = %8.4f",
       y[3],y[4]))
     cat(sprintf("\n   y_casp = %8.4f    y_kp   = %8.4f",
       y[5],y[6]))
     if(nint==2){
     cat(sprintf("\n   e_hif  = %8.4f    e_o2   = %8.4f",
       ee[1],ee[2]))
     cat(sprintf("\n   e_p300 = %8.4f    e_p53  = %8.4f",
       ee[3],ee[4]))
     cat(sprintf("\n   e_casp = %8.4f    e_kp   = %8.4f",
       ee[5],ee[6]))}
     }
```

The error vector ee is available from rkf45. Again, the output is for only $t = 0, 25, 50, 100$.

- The ODE solution from rkf45 (y,t) is placed in arrays for subsequent plotting.

```
#
#    Store solution for plotting
```

```
    plot_hif[i1,ncase] =y[1]
    plot_o2[i1,ncase]  =y[2]
    plot_p300[i1,ncase]=y[3]
    plot_p53[i1,ncase] =y[4]
    plot_casp[i1,ncase]=y[5]
    plot_kp[i1,ncase]  =y[6]
    if(ncase==1)tplot[i1]=t
  }
```

Note the use of the first subscript i1 corresponding to a particular point along the solution (particular value of t).

- The 3×2 array of plots is produced as before (see Listing 3.1))

```
#
# Calls to apoptosis_1
  cat(sprintf("\n\n ncall = %5d\n\n",ncall))
#
# Six plots for y_hif,y_o2,y_p300,y_p53,y_casp,y_kp
#    vs t
  par(mfrow=c(3,2))
#
# y_hif
  plot(tplot,plot_hif[,ncase],xlab="t",
      ylab="y_hif(t)",xlim=c(0,100),
    type="l",lwd=2,main="Hypoxia inducible factor")
#
# y_o2
  plot(tplot,plot_o2[,ncase],xlab="t",
      ylab="y_o2(t)",xlim=c(0,100),
    type="l",lwd=2,main="Oxygen level")
#
# y_p300
  plot(tplot,plot_p300[,ncase],xlab="t",
      ylab="y_p300(t)",xlim=c(0,100),
    type="l",lwd=2,main="Co-activator")
#
# y_p53
  plot(tplot,plot_p53[,ncase],xlab="t",
      ylab="y_p53(t)",xlim=c(0,100),
    type="l",lwd=2,main="Tumor suppressor gene")
```

```
  #
  # y_casp
    plot(tplot,plot_casp[,ncase],xlab="t",
        ylab="y_casp(t)",xlim=c(0,100),
    type="l",lwd=2,main="Caspases")
  #
  # y_k
    plot(tplot,plot_kp[,ncase],xlab="t",ylab="y_kp(t)",
        xlim=c(0,100),
    type="l",lwd=2,main="Potassium ions")
  #
  # Next case
  }
```

The concluding } terminates the for in ncase.

ODE routine apoptosis_2 is in Listing 3.6.

```
apoptosis_2=function(t,y,parms) {
#
# Transfer dependent variable vector to problem variables
  y_hif =y[1];
  y_o2  =y[2];
  y_p300=y[3];
  y_p53 =y[4];
  y_casp=y[5];
  y_kp  =y[6];
#
# Apoptosis model ODEs
  yt_hif =a_hif-a_3*y_o2*y_hif-a_4*y_hif*y_p300-a_7*y_p53*
    y_hif;
  yt_o2  =a_o2 -a_3*y_o2*y_hif+a_4*y_hif*y_p300-a_11*y_o2;
  yt_p300=a_8                    -a_4*y_hif*y_p300-a_5*
    y_p300*y_p53;
  yt_p53 =a_p53-a_9*y_p53                         -a_5*
    y_p300*y_p53;
  yt_casp=a_12 +a_9*y_p53-a_13*y_casp;
  yt_kp  =-a_10*y_casp*y_kp-a_14*y_kp            +a_11*y_o2;
#
# Increment calls to apoptosis_1
  ncall <<- ncall+1
```

```
#
# Return derivative vector
  return(c(yt_hif,yt_o2,yt_p300,yt_p53,yt_casp,yt_kp))
}
```

Listing 3.6 ODE routine `apoptosis_2` for the numerical integration of eqs. (3.1)–(3.6).

`apoptosis_2` has the final return

```
return(c(yt_hif,yt_o2,yt_p300,yt_p53,yt_casp,yt_kp))
```

whereas `apoptosis_1` (Listing 3.2) has the return

```
return(list(c(yt_hif,yt_o2,yt_p300,yt_p53,yt_casp,
  yt_kp)))
```

The only difference between the two routines is the use of `list` in `apoptosis_1`.

The numerical output from Listings (3.5) and (3.6) (and `rkf45` of Listing 2.5) is in Table 3.7.

We can note the following details of this output.

- The IC of Table 3.2 (`t = 0.0`) is correct.
- The estimated error vector `ee` is zero throughout the solution to four figures after the decimal. This suggests the solution is correct to four figures after the decimal, which is inferred by the agreement with the `ode` solution of Tables 3.4 and 3.7. This agreement is illustrated subsequently in Table 3.8.
- `ncall = 6000` results from the six-derivative evaluations of `rkf45`. Thus,

  ```
  (6)(nout-1)(nt) = (6)(100)(10) = 6000
  ```

- `ncall = 6000` compares with the lower value of `ncall = 504` for `ode` in Table 3.4. This suggests that `ode` is computationally more efficient than `rkf45`. However, two points can be kept in mind: (i) `lsoda` of `ode` may require more calculations at each

TABLE 3.7 Numerical solution from Listings 3.6 and 3.7.

```
t =   0.0
   y_hif  =   1.0000    y_o2  =   0.0000
   y_p300 =   0.0000    y_p53 =   0.0000
   y_casp =   0.0000    y_kp  =   0.0000
   e_hif  =   0.0000    e_o2  =   0.0000
   e_p300 =   0.0000    e_p53 =   0.0000
   e_casp =   0.0000    e_kp  =   0.0000

t =  25.0
   y_hif  =   0.5420    y_o2  =   2.6645
   y_p300 =   0.4706    y_p53 =   0.4576
   y_casp =   1.2735    y_kp  =   0.5706
   e_hif  =   0.0000    e_o2  =   0.0000
   e_p300 =   0.0000    e_p53 =  -0.0000
   e_casp =  -0.0000    e_kp  =  -0.0000

t =  50.0
   y_hif  =   0.5038    y_o2  =   2.8407
   y_p300 =   0.5771    y_p53 =   0.4940
   y_casp =   1.4708    y_kp  =   0.5267
   e_hif  =   0.0000    e_o2  =   0.0000
   e_p300 =   0.0000    e_p53 =  -0.0000
   e_casp =  -0.0000    e_kp  =   0.0000

t = 100.0
   y_hif  =   0.4991    y_o2  =   2.8646
   y_p300 =   0.5978    y_p53 =   0.4970
   y_casp =   1.4968    y_kp  =   0.5219
   e_hif  =   0.0000    e_o2  =   0.0000
   e_p300 =  -0.0000    e_p53 =   0.0000
   e_casp =   0.0000    e_kp  =   0.0000

ncall =   6000
```

step than rkf45 and (ii) h for rkf45 could possibly be increased, which would reduce the value of ncall.

A comparison of the numerical solutions in Table 3.4 or 3.6 (ode) and Table 3.7 (rkf45) is given in Table 3.8

**TABLE 3.8   Comparison of numerical solutions from
ode (Table 3.4 or 3.6) and rkf45 (Table 3.7).**

```
ode solution (Table 3.6)

t = 100.0
    y_hif  =    0.4991    y_o2  =    2.8646
    y_p300 =    0.5978    y_p53 =    0.4970
    y_casp =    1.4968    y_kp  =    0.5219

ncall =    506

rkf45 solution (Table 3.7)

t = 100.0
    y_hif  =    0.4991    y_o2  =    2.8646
    y_p300 =    0.5978    y_p53 =    0.4970
    y_casp =    1.4968    y_kp  =    0.5219
    e_hif  =    0.0000    e_o2  =    0.0000
    e_p300 =   -0.0000    e_p53 =    0.0000
    e_casp =    0.0000    e_kp  =    0.0000

ncall =   6000
```

The two solutions agree to four figures after the decimal. This is a
form of p refinement in which the solutions from the variable order
lsoda and the 4–5 order RKF45 are compared.

In summary, eqs. (3.1)–(3.6) are nonstiff as reflected in ncall =
6000 for RKF45 compared with 240000 for RKF45 in Chapter 1.

3.10   Conclusion

In the preceding discussion of the apoptosis model of eqs. (3.1)–(3.6),
we have considered some of the basic properties of ODEs models,
for example, the effect of the ICs and the approach to an equilibrium
solution. Implicit in this model is the assumption that variations in
the concentrations of the six dependent variables with spatial position

are not considered. This leads to the consideration of only one independent variable, time, and thus, to ODEs. If spatial variations in the dependent variables are an essential requirement in the development of the model, then PDEs would be used with time and one or more spatial coordinates as independent variables. For example, the rate of diffusion of one or more of the dependent variable concentrations might be important in determining the characteristics of the apoptosis system. Then, a diffusion equation, generally Fick's second law, plus reaction, and possibly other terms, would be the starting point for the analysis. ODE models are generally very useful, but this restriction to only temporal variations should be recognized and considered.

Reference

[1] Laise, P., D. Fanelli, and A. Arcangeli (2012), A dynamical model of apoptosis and its role in tumor progression, *Commun. Nonlinear Sci. Numer. Simulat.*, **17**, pp 1795–1804.

## CHAPTER 4

Dynamic Neuron Model

4.1 Introduction

The dynamic electrical properties of neurons have been studied extensively with a series of ODE models proposed such as the Hodgkin–Huxley and Fitzhugh–Nagumo models [1]. In this chapter, we consider a 2×2 (two ODEs in two unknowns) dynamic neuron model (DNM) that has been described in detail by Izhikevich [3]. This model reproduces a spectrum of dynamic neuron effects that have been observed experimentally and discussed extensively in the literature ([2], pp 279–280).

This case study has a four-fold purpose:

1. An introduction to a 2×2 ODE DNM.
2. Consideration of some of the solution properties of the DNM equations for selected special cases.
3. Review of a series of well-established algorithms for the numerical integration (solution) of ODEs with particular application to the DNM equations.
4. Discussion of the computer implementation of the integration algorithms in R [7]. The source code for the R routines is discussed in detail and is available as a download.

Differential Equation Analysis in Biomedical Science and Engineering: Ordinary Differential Equation Applications with R, First Edition. William E. Schiesser.
© 2014 John Wiley & Sons, Inc. Published 2014 by John Wiley & Sons, Inc.

4.2 The Dynamic Neuron Model

The DNM ODEs to be considered are [2, pp 272–277]

$$C\frac{dv}{dt} = k(v - v_r)(v - v_t) - w + In \tag{4.1}$$

$$\frac{dw}{dt} = a[b(v - v_r) - w] \tag{4.2}$$

Eqs. (4.1) and (4.2) are first order ODEs and therefore, each requires an IC that will be stated in general form here and made specific later on.

$$v(t = 0) = v_0 \tag{4.3}$$

$$w(t = 0) = w_0 \tag{4.4}$$

v_0, w_0 are constants to be specified.

The variables of eqs. (4.1) and (4.2) are [3]

$\quad\quad v\quad\quad$ neuron membrane potential
$\quad\quad w\quad\quad$ recovery current
$\quad\quad t\quad\quad$ time

The role of the parameters $C, v_r, v_t, k, a, b, c,$ and d is explained subsequently. *In* in eq. (4.1) is a specified function of time, t; the details of this function are explained when the programming of eqs. (4.1) and (4.2) is discussed.

The individual RHS terms of eqs. (4.1) and (4.2) are discussed next to give some insight into the observed features of the equation solutions.

- v is a voltage-like variable that allows regenerative self-excitation via a positive feedback. The RHS terms of eq. (4.1) have the following general characteristics.
  - The first RHS nonlinear term $k(v - v_r)(v - v_t)$ is positive if $k > 0, v - v_r > 0, v - v_t > 0$ (which are the conditions during execution of the model). Thus, this term will tend to cause the derivative dv/dt to be positive and therefore v will increase with t (the source of the positive feedback effect).

— The second RHS term $-kw$ contributes to a decrease $(w > 0)$ or an increase $(w < 0)$ in v (again, with $k > 0$).
— The third RHS term I is a prescribed function of t. In the specific case to be discussed next, I switches from a zero initial value to a constant positive value at a particular point along the solution (particular value of t).

The response of $v(t)$ from the integration of eq. (4.1) will be due to a balancing of these three RHS terms.

- w is a recovery variable having linear dynamics that provides a slower negative feedback. The RHS terms of eq. (4.2) have the following general characteristics.
  — The first RHS term $(a)(b)(v - v_r)$ is negative if $a > 0$, $b < 0$, $(v - v_r) > 0$ and therefore provides negative feedback.
  — The second RHS term $-aw$ (with $a > 0$) has a similar effect on w as in eq. (4.1) (negative or positive feedback depending on the sign of w).

The response of $w(t)$ from the integration of eq. (4.2) will be due to a balancing of these two RHS terms. The overall model response $(v(t)$ and $w(t))$ is therefore rather complicated but can be investigated and explained through computed special case solutions of eqs. (4.1) and (4.2).

4.3   ODE Numerical Integration

We now consider a numerical solution to eqs. (4.1) and (4.2) (to give $v(t)$ and $w(t)$ in numerical form). To start, we consider the following translation of code taken from [3] for a regular spiking (RS) DNM (the RS will be evident when the numerical solution of eqs. (4.1) and (4.2) is observed graphically).

4.3.1   Explicit Euler Integration

The code in Listing 4.1 implements the explicit Euler integration of eqs. (4.1) and (4.2).

```
#
# ODE routine
  setwd("c:/R/bme_ode/chap4")
  source("euler.R")
  source("neuron_1.R")
#
# Model parameters
  C=100;   vr=-60; vt=-40;   k=0.7;    # parameters used
     for RS
  an=0.03; bn=-2; cn=-50; dn=100;    # neocortical
     pyramidal neurons
  vpeak=35                           # spike cutoff
#
# Pulse of input DC current
  nout=1000;
  In=rep(0,nout+1);
  for(i in 1:nout+1){
  if(i< 101)In[i]=0;
  if(i>=101)In[i]=70;}
#
# Initial condition
  v=rep(0,nout+1);
  w=rep(0,nout+1);
  v[1]=vr;w[1]=0;
  t0=seq(from=0,to=nout,by=1);
  ncall=0;
#
# Parameters for t integration
  nt=1;h=1;
#
# Euler integration
  for(i in 1:nout){
  yout=euler(nt,h,t0[i],c(v[i],w[i]))
  v[i+1]=yout[1];
  w[i+1]=yout[2];
  if(v[i+1]>=vpeak){                 # a spike is fired
    v[i]=vpeak;                      # padding the spike
                                          amplitude

    v[i+1]=cn;                       # membrane voltage
                                          reset
```

```
    w[i+1]=w[i+1]+dn;}                    # recovery variable
                                                reset
}
#
# Selected output to evaluate solution
  cat(sprintf("\n\n     t           v          w"
    ));
  cat(sprintf("\n %5.1f%10.4f%10.4f",t0[1]    ,v[1]
    ,w[1]   ));
  cat(sprintf("\n %5.1f%10.4f%10.4f",t0[251] ,v[251]
    ,w[251] ));
  cat(sprintf("\n %5.1f%10.4f%10.4f",t0[501] ,v[501]
    ,w[501] ));
  cat(sprintf("\n %5.1f%10.4f%10.4f",t0[751] ,v[751]
    ,w[751] ));
  cat(sprintf("\n %5.1f%10.4f%10.4f",t0[1001],v[1001]
    ,w[1001]));
  cat(sprintf("\n\n"));
#
# Calls to neuron_1
  cat(sprintf("\n\n ncall = %5d\n\n",ncall))
#
# Three plots for v(t),w(t) vs t, w(t) vs v(t)
#
# v(t)
  par(mfrow=c(1,1))
  plot(t0,v,xlab="t",ylab="v(t)",xlim=c(0,1000),
  type="l",lwd=2,main="v(t), Euler integration")
#
# w(t)
  par(mfrow=c(1,1))
  plot(t0,w,xlab="t",ylab="w(t)",xlim=c(0,1000),
  type="l",lwd=2,main="w(t), Euler integration")
#
# w(t) vs v(t) (phase plane plot)
  par(mfrow=c(1,1))
  plot(v,w,xlab="v(t)",ylab="w(t)",
  type="l",lwd=2,main="w(t) vs v(t), Euler integration")
```

Listing 4.1: Main program for a regular spiking (RS) DNM.

We can note the following details about this code.

- The Euler routine (discussed in Chapter 2), euler.R, and the ODE routine called by euler.R, neuron_1.R, are accessed by setwd and source statements.

```
#
# ODE routine
  setwd("c:/R/bme_ode/chap4")
  source("euler.R")
  source("neuron_1.R")
```

Note in setwd the use of / rather than \. neuron_1.R and euler.R are subsequently discussed through Listings 4.2 and 4.3, respectively.

- The model parameters are defined numerically. The names of the parameters follow directly from eqs. (4.1) and (4.2).

```
#
# Model parameters
  C=100;   vr=-60; vt=-40;   k=0.7;   # parameters used
      for RS
  an=0.03; bn=-2; cn=-50; dn=100;   # neocortical
      pyramidal neurons
  vpeak=35                             # spike cutoff
```

Also, explanatory comments set off by # are included. Note that in R names are case sensitive, so that, for example, C and c represent different entities (C is a variable name and c is the R vector utility).

- The input current In in eq. (4.1) is defined as a function of t.

```
#
# Pulse of input DC current
  nout=1000;
  In=rep(0,nout+1);
  for(i in 1:nout+1){
  if(i< 101)In[i]=0;
  if(i>=101)In[i]=70;}
```

In switches from 0 to 70 after 101 points in t (counting $t = 0$).

- ICs (4.3) and (4.4) are defined after v and w of eqs. (4.1) and (4.2) are declared (preallocated) as (nout+1)-vectors with rep statements.

```
#
# Initial condition
  v=rep(0,nout+1);
  w=rep(0,nout+1);
  v[1]=vr;w[1]=0;
  t0=seq(from=0,to=nout,by=1);
  ncall=0;
```

t is also declared as a vector for the interval $0 \le t \le 1000$ with $t = 0, 1, 2, \ldots, 1000$ ms. Finally, the number of calls to neuron_1 is initialized.

- The parameters of the Euler integration are set, that is, nt=1 Euler steps of length h=1 in each call to euler.

```
#
# Parameters for t integration
  nt=1;h=1;
```

- The solution is computed by repeated calls to euler in a for.

```
#
# Euler integration
  for(i in 1:nout){
  yout=euler(nt,h,t0[i],c(v[i],w[i]))
  v[i+1]=yout[1];
  w[i+1]=yout[2];
  if(v[i+1]>=vpeak){          # a spike is fired
    v[i]=vpeak;               # padding the spike
                                  amplitude
    v[i+1]=cn;               # membrane voltage
                                  reset
    w[i+1]=w[i+1]+dn;}       # recovery variable
                                  reset
}
```

The four arguments of `euler` are discussed in detail in Chapter 2 and in Listing 4.3 that follows. Note in particular the fourth argument is a 2-vector of the dependent variables $v(t)$, $w(t)$ at the base (starting) point of the Euler step with index i. The numerical solution at the next point in t with index i+1 is returned in yout, and this solution is placed in v[i+1] and w[i+1]. Also, the ODE routine must be explicitly named neuron_1 in `euler` (see Listing 4.3). After each Euler step, a test is made to determine if a spike has fired (using vpeak). If so, v and w are reset according to the code from [3]. The final } concludes the `for`.

- After completion of the Euler integration, the solution, $v(t)$ and $w(t)$ from eqs. (4.1) and (4.2), is displayed for $t = 0$, $250, 500, 750, 1000$.

```
#
# Selected output to evaluate solution
  cat(sprintf("\n\n    t           v          w"
    ));
  cat(sprintf("\n %5.1f%10.4f%10.4f",t0[1]    ,v[1]
    ,w[1]   ));
  cat(sprintf("\n %5.1f%10.4f%10.4f",t0[251] ,v[251]
    ,w[251] ));
  cat(sprintf("\n %5.1f%10.4f%10.4f",t0[501] ,v[501]
    ,w[501] ));
  cat(sprintf("\n %5.1f%10.4f%10.4f",t0[751] ,v[751]
    ,w[751] ));
  cat(sprintf("\n %5.1f%10.4f%10.4f",t0[1001],v[1001]
    ,w[1001]));
  cat(sprintf("\n\n"));
```

These five values of t were selected merely to limit the output to a reasonable size.

- At the completion of the solution, the number of calls to neuron_1 is displayed (as an indication of the total computational effort to generate the numerical solution).

```
#
# Calls to neuron_1
  cat(sprintf("\n\n ncall = %5d\n\n",ncall))
```

- Three individual plots of the solution, (i) $v(t)$ versus t, (ii) $w(t)$ versus t, and (iii) $v(t)$ versus $w(t)$ (a phase plane plot) are produced by plot.

```
#
# Three plots for v(t),w(t) vs t, w(t) vs v(t)
#
# v(t)
  par(mfrow=c(1,1))
  plot(t0,v,xlab="t",ylab="v(t)",xlim=c(0,1000),
  type="l",lwd=2,main="v(t), Euler integration")
#
# w(t)
  par(mfrow=c(1,1))
  plot(t0,w,xlab="t",ylab="w(t)",xlim=c(0,1000),
  type="l",lwd=2,main="w(t), Euler integration")
#
# w(t) vs v(t) (phase plane plot)
  par(mfrow=c(1,1))
  plot(v,w,xlab="v(t)",ylab="w(t)",
  type="l",lwd=2,main="w(t) vs v(t), Euler
      integration")
```

The ODE routine neuron_1 called by euler is listed as follows.

```
neuron_1=function(t,y) {
#
# Transfer dependent variable vector to problem variables
  vn=y[1];
  wn=y[2];
#
# Neuron model ODEs
  dvndt=(k*(vn-vr)*(vn-vt)-wn+In[i])/C;
  dwndt=an*(bn*(vn-vr)-wn);
#
# Increment calls to neuron_1
  ncall <<- ncall+1
#
# Return derivative vector
  return(c(dvndt,dwndt))
}
```

Listing 4.2. ODE routine neuron_1.

We can note the following details in `neuron_1`.

- The function is defined.

```
neuron_1=function(t,y) {
```

- The input dependent variable vector y is placed in two scalars, vn,wn, to facilitate the programming of eqs. (4.1) and (4.2).

```
#
# Transfer dependent variable vector to problem
#    variables
  vn=y[1];
  wn=y[2];
```

The variable names vn,wn are used to avoid a conflict with v,w used in the main program of Listing 4.1 (a characteristic of R is the global nature of variables that are shared by name with subordinate routines so that care is required to avoid unintended conflicts).

- Eqs. (4.1) and (4.2) are programmed.

```
#
# Neuron model ODEs
  dvndt=(k*(vn-vr)*(vn-vt)-wn+In[i])/C;
  dwndt=an*(bn*(vn-vr)-wn);
```

All of the parameters defined in Listing 4.1 are available numerically for use in neuron_1, that is, k,vr,vt,C,an,bn. Also, note the use of i in In[i]; the particular value of i is set by the for in the main program of Listing 4.1.

- The number of calls to neuron_1 is incremented and returned to the main program of Listing 4.1 by the <<-.

```
#
# Increment calls to neuron_1
  ncall <<- ncall+1
```

- The RHS vectors of eqs. (4.1) and (4.2), $dv/dt, dw/dt$, are returned as a vector (to euler) for the next Euler step along the solution.

```
#
# Return derivative vector
  return(c(dvndt,dwndt))
}
```

The final } completes function neuron_1.

To complete the discussion of the coding, euler is in Listing 4.3.

```
euler=function(nt,h,t,y) {
#
#   Function euler implements the first order Euler
#      method.
#   The ODE routine has to be renamed for a new
#      application.
#
#   The arguments are
#
#     Input
#
#       nt - number of Euler steps between the starting
#             and final points along the solution
#
#       h  - integration step (constant)
#
#       t  - initial value of the independent variable
#
#       y  - initial dependent variable vector
#
#     Output
#
#       y  - solution vector after nt integration steps
#
#
#   nt Euler steps
    for(i2 in 1:nt){
      yt=neuron_1(t,y)
```

```
        y=y+yt*h;  t=t+h}
#
#    Return Euler solution
     return(c(y))
}
```

Listing 4.3 `euler` for the numerical integration of eqs. (4.1) and (4.2).

We can note the following details of `euler`.

- The function is defined.

  ```
  euler=function(nt,h,t,y) {
  ```

  The input arguments of `euler` are discussed in detail in Chapter 2.

- `neuron_1` is called for the Euler integration over `nt` steps of length `h`.

  ```
  #
  #    nt Euler steps
       for(i2 in 1:nt){
          yt=neuron_1(t,y)
          y=y+yt*h;  t=t+h}
  ```

- The dependent variable (solution) vector `y` is returned to the calling program of Listing 4.1.

  ```
  #
  #    Return Euler solution
       return(c(y))
  }
  ```

  The final } concludes `euler`.

The output from Listings 4.1 to 4.3 is considered next.

4.3.2   Numerical and Graphical Solutions

The numerical output from Listing 4.1 is in Table 4.1.

TABLE 4.1   Numerical solution from listing 4.1.

t	v	w
0.0	-60.0000	0.0000
250.0	-54.4819	6.2834
500.0	-50.6154	59.0910
750.0	-49.5530	-12.4763
1000.0	-53.6973	1.5649
ncall =	1000	

This abbreviated output reflects only approximately the limits of the $v(t), w(t)$ variation. Also, the number of calls to neuron_1 has the expected value (nt)(nout)=(1)(1000), from the Euler algorithm in euler of Listing 4.3. The graphical output in Figs. 4.1–4.3 reflects the characteristics of the solutions to eqs. (4.1) and (4.2).

We can note the following details from Figs. 4.1–4.3.

- The oscillatory characteristic of $v(t)$ and $w(t)$ of Figs. 4.1 and 4.2 is clear. This is due to the use of vpeak in Listing 4.1 immediately after the call to euler.

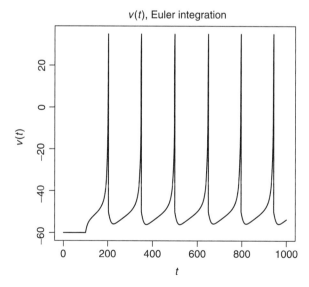

Figure 4.1 $v(t)$ from eq. (4.1).

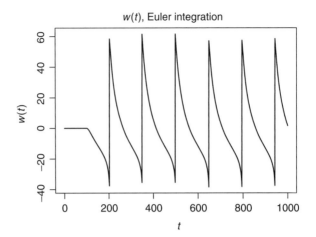

Figure 4.2 $w(t)$ from eq. (4.2).

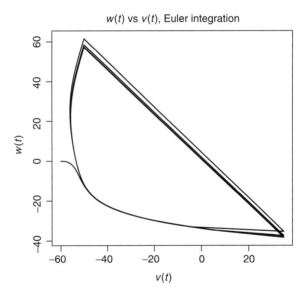

Figure 4.3 $v(t)$ vs $w(t)$.

- The sharp peaks ("spikes" is perhaps a better description) indicate why a large number of integration steps (nout=1000) is required to resolve the solution in t. Also, the sharp variation in the solutions precluded the use of h refinement to investigate the convergence of the solution. For example, the four cases (i) nt=1,h=1 (in Table 4.1); (ii) nt=2,h=0.5; (iii) nt=4,h=0.25; and

(4) `nt=10,h=0.1` did not indicate convergence of the numerical solution to well-defined values.

As an explanation of this apparent lack of convergence, the solutions in Figs. 4.1 and 4.2 do not have a smoothness in the derivatives required by the Taylor series that is the basis for the ODE integration algorithms. For example, the Euler method is based on the first-order polynomial, the Taylor series truncated after the linear term in h, and this linear function will give different results as h is varied where the solution is changing so rapidly, that is, within the spikes of Figs. 4.1 and 4.2 where the derivatives are essentially discontinuous.

- The limit cycle in Fig. 4.3 is evident ($v(t)$ and $w(t)$ eventually follow the same path, starting from the ICs of eqs. (4.3) and (4.4), $v(t = 0) = v_r = -60$, $w(t = 0) = 0$).

4.3.3   Evaluation and Plotting of the ODE Derivative Vector

The solutions in Figs. 4.1 and 4.2 were computed by the numerical integration of eqs. (4.1) and (4.2). The sharp, periodic variation of these solutions raises the question of the form of the derivatives that were integrated numerically. To address this question, we can compute and plot the derivatives (LHS of eqs. (4.1) and (4.2)) by using a direct call to the ODE routine, `neuron_1`. This procedure is implemented in the main program of Listing 4.1 (just before the plotting of the solutions).

```
#
# Analysis of derivatives
  dvdt=rep(0,nout+1);
  dwdt=rep(0,nout+1);
  out=rep(0,2);
  for(i in 1:nout+1){
    out=neuron_1(t0[i],c(v[i],w[i]));
    dvdt[i]=out[1];
    dwdt[i]=out[2];
  }
```

Listing 4.4a Calculation of the derivative vector.

We can note the following details about Listing 4.4a.

- Two vectors, dvdt,dwdt, are defined for the derivatives $dv/dt, dw/dt$ of eqs. (4.1) and (4.2).

```
dvdt=rep(0,nout+1);
dwdt=rep(0,nout+1);
out=rep(0,2);
```

A 2-vector, out, is also defined for temporary storage of the derivative vector returned by neuron_1.

- The derivatives $dv/dt, dw/dt$ are computed through $0 \le t \le 1000$ with a for. At each value of t $(t = 0, 1, 2, \ldots, 1000)$, neuron_1 is called to compute $dv/dt, dw/dt$ (returned in out). Note in particular the input arguments to neuron_1, that is, the independent variable t and the corresponding solution, $v(t), w(t)$ (formed as a vector with c).

```
for(i in 1:nout+1){
  out=neuron_1(t0[i],c(v[i],w[i]));
  dvdt[i]=out[1];
  dwdt[i]=out[2];
}
```

The derivatives are placed in two vectors dvdt,dwdt for subsequent plotting. The final } concludes the for in t.

The derivative vectors dvdt,dwdt can now be plotted. This is done with the following statements added to the plotting of Listing 4.1.

```
#
# Two plots for dv(t)/dt, dw(t)/dt vs t
#
# dv/dt(t) vs v(t)
  par(mfrow=c(1,1))
  plot(t0,dvdt,xlab="t",ylab="dv(t)/dt",
  type="l",lwd=2,main="dv(t)/dt, Euler integration")
#
# dw/dt(t) vs v(t)
```

```
par(mfrow=c(1,1))
plot(t0,dwdt,xlab="t",ylab="dw(t)/dt",
type="l",lwd=2,main="dw(t)/dt, Euler integration")
```

Listing 4.4b Plotting of the derivative vector.

The plots from Listing 4.4b are in Figs. 4.4 and 4.5.

We can note in Figs. 4.4 and 4.5 the sharp variations in the derivatives $dv/dt, dw/dt$ as expected from the solutions in Figs. 4.1 and 4.2. In fact, the successful numerical integration of these derivatives to produce the solutions of Figs. 4.1 and 4.2 is perhaps better than can be expected. The sharp variations in the derivatives explain why the h refinement mentioned previously ($h = 1, 0.5, 0.25, 0.1$ for the Euler method) did not lead to a well-defined convergence of numerical solution values. To investigate this latter point a bit further, we next consider p refinement by using $O(h^2), O(h^4), O(h^5)$ (so that $p = 2, 4, 5$) integration algorithms.

4.3.4 *p* Refinement

The constant step, classical fourth-order integration algorithm in Chapter 1, can be applied to eqs. (4.1) and (4.2) by calling neuron_1

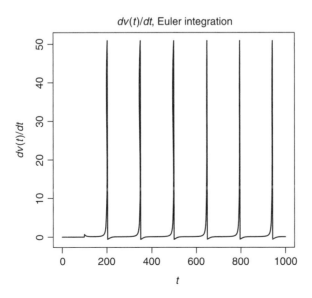

Figure 4.4 $dv(t)/dt$ from eq. (4.1).

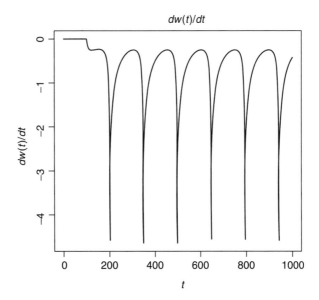

Figure 4.5 *dw*(*t*)/*dt* from eq. (4.2).

from rkc4 (in Listing 4.8). The programming is the same as in Listing 4.1 except that the call to euler is replaced with a call to rkc4, that is,

```
yout=rkc4(nt,h,t0[i],c(v[i],w[i]))
```

in place of

```
yout=euler(nt,h,t0[i],c(v[i],w[i]))
```

The numerical output that results for nt=1,h=1 is given in Table 4.2.

TABLE 4.2   Numerical solution from Listing 4.1 with rkc4 in place of euler.

t	v	w
0.0	-60.0000	0.0000
250.0	-54.2040	4.8130
500.0	-54.4605	41.1540
750.0	-48.0395	-15.0560
1000.0	-52.5168	-3.8444

ncall =   4000

A comparison of Tables 4.1 and 4.2 indicates that the solutions from euler and rkc4 are substantially different. Thus, this attempt at p refinement (by changing p from $p = 1$ in euler to $p = 4$ in rkc4) did not produce a well-defined convergence of the numerical solution. This is probably to be expected considering the sharp variation of the derivatives in Figs. 4.4 and 4.5 and the substantial change in the order of the algorithms ($p = 1$ to $p = 4$).

We can investigate this attempt at p refinement further by using other integration algorithms. For example, if the modified Euler method discussed in Chapter 1 is placed in a routine meuler, Listing 4.1 can be modified as given in Listing 4.5.

```
#
# modified Euler integration
  nint=1;
  for(i in 1:nout){
  yout=meuler(nt,h,t0[i],c(v[i],w[i]))
  v[i+1]=yout[1];
  w[i+1]=yout[2];
  if(v[i+1]>=vpeak){                    # a spike is fired
    v[i]=vpeak;                         # padding the spike
                                          amplitude
    v[i+1]=cn;                          # membrane voltage
                                          reset
    w[i+1]=w[i+1]+dn;}                  # recovery variable
                                          reset
}
```

Listing 4.5 Modification of Listing 4.1 for meuler in place of euler.

nint=1 is used so that the modified Euler method without error estimation is used (see meuler in Listing 4.7). The output from meuler is given in Table 4.3a.

The solution in Table 4.3a indicates an approach to convergence as the $O(h^2)$ of the modified Euler method in meuler (in Listing 4.7) is replaced with the $O(h^4)$ of the classical Runge Kutta method in rkc4 (in Listing 4.8). To investigate this further, rkf45 for RKF45 (from Chapter 2) can be used in Listing 4.1 as

```
#
# rkf45 integration
  nint=1;
  for(i in 1:nout){
  yout=rkf45(nt,h,t0[i],c(v[i],w[i]))
  v[i+1]=yout[1];
  w[i+1]=yout[2];
  if(v[i+1]>=vpeak){          # a spike is fired
    v[i]=vpeak;               # padding the spike
                                  amplitude
    v[i+1]=cn;                # membrane voltage
                                  reset
    w[i+1]=w[i+1]+dn;}        # recovery variable
                                  reset
}
```

Listing 4.6 Modification of Listing 4.1 for rkf45 in place of euler.

**TABLE 4.3a   Numerical solution from
Listing 4.1 with meuler in place of euler.**

t	v	w
0.0	-60.0000	0.0000
250.0	-54.3451	5.5790
500.0	-54.2916	44.2500
750.0	-48.6740	-14.0479
1000.0	-52.8457	-2.4395
ncall =	2000	

The output from rkf45 is given in Table 4.3b.

A comparison of Tables 4.2, 4.3a, and 4.3b suggests an apparent approach to convergence as the order of the algorithms increases as $O(h^2), O(h^4), O(h^5)$ (meuler, rkc4, rkf45, respectively). This convergence could then be investigated further with h refinement (for $p = 2, 4, 5$) by decreasing the integration step below $h = 1$, but in any case, the numerical solutions of Tables 4.1–4.3 suggest an approximately 2–3 figure convergence; the corresponding plots are (visually) identical.

**TABLE 4.3b   Numerical solution from
Listing 4.1 with `rkf45` in place of `euler`.**

t	v	w
0.0	-60.0000	0.0000
250.0	-54.1941	4.7611
500.0	-54.7910	40.3858
750.0	-48.3264	-14.6183
1000.0	-52.8739	-2.3479

ncall = 6000

Finally, to complete this discussion, meuler and rkc4 are listed next (rkf45 is listed in Chapter 2).

```
    meuler=function(nt,h,t,y) {
#
#   Function meuler implements the second order modified
#   Euler method.  The ODE routine has to be renamed for
#   a new application.
#
#   The arguments are
#
#     Input
#
#       nt - number of modified Euler steps between the
#            starting and final points along the solution
#
#       h  - integration step (constant)
#
#       t  - initial value of the independent variable
#
#       y  - initial dependent variable vector
#
#     Output
#
#       y  - solution vector after nt integration steps
#
#   nt modified Euler steps
    for(i2 in 1:nt){
```

```
if(nint==1){
  yb=y
  rk1=neuron_1(t,y)*h
  y1=yb+rk1; t=t+h
  rk2=neuron_1(t,y1)*h
  y=yb+(rk1+rk2)/2
  ee=y-y1
}
if(nint==2){
  yb=y
  rk1=neuron_1(t,y)*h
  y1=yb+rk1; t=t+h
  rk2=neuron_1(t,y1)*h
  ee=(rk2-rk1)/2
  y=y1+ee
}
}
#
#   Return modified Euler solution
    return(c(y))
}
```

Listing 4.7 Integration routine meuler.

```
rkc4=function(nt,h,t,y) {
#
#   Function rkc4 implements a second order Runge Kutta
#   method embedded in a fourth order Runge Kutta method.
#   The ODE routine has to be renamed for a new
#   application.
#
#   The arguments are
#
#     Input
#
#       nt - number of rkc4 steps between the starting
#            and final points along the solution
#
#       h  - integration step (constant)
#
#       t  - initial value of the independent variable
#
```

```
#       y  - initial dependent variable vector
#
#    Output
#
#       y  - solution vector after nt integration steps
#
#    nt rkc4 steps
     for(i2 in 1:nt){
     if(nint==1){
       yb=y; tb=t
       rk1=neuron_1(tb,yb)*h
       y=yb+0.5*rk1; t=tb+0.5*h
       rk2=neuron_1(t,y)*h
       y=yb+0.5*rk2; t=tb+0.5*h
       rk3=neuron_1(t,y)*h
       y=yb+rk3; t=tb+h
       rk4=neuron_1(t,y)*h
       y=yb+(1/6)*(rk1+2*rk2+2*rk3+rk4)
     }
     if(nint==2){
       yb=y; tb=t
       rk1=neuron_1(tb,yb)*h
       y=yb+0.5*rk1; t=tb+0.5*h
       rk2=neuron_1(t,y)*h
       y2=yb+rk2
       y=yb+0.5*rk2; t=tb+0.5*h
       rk3=neuron_1(t,y)*h
       y=yb+rk3; t=tb+h
       rk4=neuron_1(t,y)*h
       y=yb+(1/6)*(rk1+2*rk2+2*rk3+rk4)
       ee=y-y2
       ee <<- ee
     }
   }
     return(c(y))
}
```

Listing 4.8 Integration routine rkc4.

The mathematical details of the numerical integration algorithms programmed in Listings 4.7 and 4.8 are discussed in Chapter 1.

In conclusion, eqs. (4.1) and (4.2) are a stringent test of ODE numerical integration as reflected in the derivatives of Figs. 4.4 and 4.5, but the classical, constant step, explicit algorithms that were considered appear to give a solution of acceptable (approximately 2–3 figure) accuracy. Also, the use of a variable step ODE integrator might not produce a clear convergence to a numerical solution. This point is discussed in [3], pp 60–64, in terms of an ODE application with sharp, periodic solutions similar to the solutions of eqs. (4.1) and (4.2). We will not consider here the possibility of using a variable step ODE integrator, but this could be done by replacing the use of euler, meuler, rkc4 and rkf45 with one of the integrators in deSolve, e.g., rkf45, lsode.

4.4 Conclusions

From the preceding discussion, we can state the following conclusions.

- The periodic solution to eqs. (4.1) and (4.2) based on the threshold value of $v(t)$ for switching (vpeak in Listing 4.1) could be easily implemented numerically. This is an illustration of the generality of the numerical approach applied to an ODE system that would be difficult to study analytically.
- The sharp variation in the derivative vector and the corresponding solution could be handled numerically and p refinement provided an acceptable degree of convergence. The graphical agreement of the solutions from the various explicit, constant step algorithms also suggests that the solutions have acceptable accuracy.
- The preceding routines (in Listings 4.1–4.4) can now be used for the investigation of the parameters of the DNM. This should provide some insight into the features and characteristics of the model.
- Numerous detailed discussions of neuron dynamics appear in the literature. The books by Keener and Sneyd [4], Izhikevich [3],

and Murray [5] and the online articles by FitzHugh [1] and Okun [6] are a good starting point. The neuron model of eqs. (4.1) and (4.2) does not include spatial variations of the dependent variables $v(t)$ and $w(t)$. If spatial variations are important, for example, due to diffusion, then PDEs with space and time as independent variables are required rather than ODEs with just time as an independent variable. For example, the Hodgkin–Huxley and Fitzhugh–Nagumo PDE models are considered in [2], Chapter 9.

References

[1] Available at: http://www.scholarpedia.org/article/FitzHugh-Nagumo_model.

[2] Griffiths, G.W., and W.E. Schiesser (2012), *Traveling Wave Analysis of Partial Differential Equations*, Cambridge University Press, Cambridge, UK.

[3] Izhikevich, E.M. (2007), *Dynamical Systems in Neuroscience: The Geometry of Excitability and Bursting*, The MIT Press, Cambridge, MA.

[4] Keener, J., and J. Sneyd (1998), *Mathematical Physiology*, Springer, NY.

[5] Murray, J.D. (2002), *Mathematical Biology, I. An Introduction*, 3rd edition, Springer, NY, Section 7.5.

[6] Available at: http://www.scholarpedia.org/article/Balance_of_excitation_and_inhibition.

[7] Soetaert, K., J. Cash, and F. Mazzia (2012), *Solving Differential Equations in R*, Springer-Verlag, Berlin.

## CHAPTER 5

Stem Cell Differentiation

5.1 Introduction

Stem cells have the distinctive characteristic of differentiation, that is, they can evolve into a specific type of cell starting from an initial or a base form. Which direction they will take, and therefore what type of cells they will eventually become, is a paramount problem in cell biology. In this chapter, we study this process at an introductory basic level using a 2×2 (two equations in two unknowns) ODE model reported in [1].

The following quotes provide an additional introduction ([1], p 450):

A stem cell is a cell that has the ability to continuously divide and differentiate (develop) into various other kinds of cells/tissues. A related concept is that of a progenitor cell that can differentiate into any of several different types. During development, the decision to leave the progenitor state, and the selection of a differentiation pathway, is regulated by transcription factors. The two transcription factors PU.1 and GATA-1 regulate the differentiation of a particular branch of blood cells.

The initial progenitor state has low level activation of both PU.1 and GATA-1 genes. This initial state is referred to as an indeterminate state in this study. Thus, the understanding of how PU.1 and GATA-1 interact is important in the study of this differentiation process, and accurate modelling of the process promises opportunities to control stem cell development for significant therapeutic benefits.

Differential Equation Analysis in Biomedical Science and Engineering: Ordinary Differential Equation Applications with R, First Edition. William E. Schiesser.
© 2014 John Wiley & Sons, Inc. Published 2014 by John Wiley & Sons, Inc.

The concentrations of the expression level of the two genes PU.1 and GATA-1 are the two dependent variables of the ODE system; time is the independent variable. Thus, we will determine how the expression-level concentrations vary with time through numerical integration (solution) of the 2×2 ODE system.

This study has three basic sections:

1. A brief description of the ODE model for the expression-level concentrations of the two genes.
2. The numerical solution of the ODE model.
3. A review of the numerical solutions produced by the routines, including the contributions of the individual RHS terms of the model ODEs.

5.2 Model Equations

Four models for stem cell differentiation reported in the literature are first reviewed in [1]. Then the authors present a fifth model that reflects recent experimental observations. The ODEs are ([1], eqs. (5))

$$\frac{d[G]}{dt} = a_1 \frac{[G]^n}{\theta_{a1}^n + [G]^n} + b_1 \frac{\theta_{b1}^m}{\theta_{b1}^m + [G]^m [P]^m} - k_1[G] \qquad (5.1a)$$

$$\frac{d[P]}{dt} = a_2 \frac{[P]^n}{\theta_{a2}^n + [P]^n} + b_2 \frac{\theta_{b2}^m}{\theta_{b2}^m + [G]^m [P]^m} - k_2[P] \qquad (5.1b)$$

where

Variable Parameter	Interpretation
G	normalized concentration of the expression level of gene GATA-1
P	normalized concentration of the expression level of gene PU.1
t	time
$a_1, b_1, \theta_{a1}, \theta_{b1}, k_1, n, m$	parameters (constants) in eq. (5.1a)
$a_2, b_2, \theta_{a2}, \theta_{b2}, k_2, n, m$	parameters (constants) in eq. (5.1b)

Eqs. (5.1) are integrated numerically for prescribed ICs taken from [1] as explained subsequently. Also, the parameter sets $a_1, b_1, \theta_{a1}, \theta_{b1}, k_1, n, m$ for eq. (5.1a) and $a_2, b_2, \theta_{a2}, \theta_{b2}, k_2, n, m$ for eq. (5.1b) are defined numerically in the routines to follow.

The following symmetry conditions $a_1 = a_2, b_1 = b_2, \theta_{a1} = \theta_{a2}, \theta_{b1} = \theta_{b2}$, and $k = k_1 = k_2$ and the definition of dependent variables and alternate parameters $x = k[G], y = k[P], a = ka_1, b = kb_1, \theta_1 = k\theta_{a1}$, and $\theta_2 = k^2\theta_{b1}$ lead to the ODE system ([1], eqs. (6)),

$$\frac{dx}{dt} = a\frac{x^n}{\theta_1^n + x^n} + b\frac{\theta_2^m}{\theta_2^m + x^m y^m} - x \qquad (5.2a)$$

$$\frac{dy}{dt} = a\frac{y^n}{\theta_1^n + y^n} + b\frac{\theta_2^m}{\theta_2^m + x^m y^m} - y \qquad (5.2b)$$

These symmetry conditions facilitate an analytical phase-plane, bifurcation analysis [1]. However, with the numerical approach to be discussed, specialization of the parameter set is not required and we therefore use eqs. (5.1) as the starting point for the following computational analysis.

5.3   R Routines

The R routines for the numerical integration of eqs. (5.1) are discussed next, starting with a main program.

5.3.1   Main Program

```
#
# Stem cell differentiation model
#
# Two cases are programmed for a variation in ODE
#    parameters.
#
# Access deSolve library (with lsodes)
  library("deSolve")
```

```
#
# ODE routine
  setwd("c:/R/bme_ode/chap5")
  source("stem_1.R")
#
# Step through cases
  for(ncase in 1:2){
#
# Model parameters
       b1=1;        b2=1;
    tha1=0.5;    tha2=0.5;
    thb1=0.07; thb2=0.07;
       k1=1;        k2=1;
        n=4;         m=1;
#
# ncase = 1
  if(ncase==1){G0=1; P0=1; a1=1; a2=1;};
#
# ncase = 2
  if(ncase==2){G0=1; P0=1; a1=5; a2=10;};
#
# Write selected parameters and heading
  cat(sprintf("\n ncase = %2d    n = %5.2f
     m = %5.2f\n\n",
                  ncase,n,m));
  cat(sprintf("    t          G          P      dG/dt
     dP/dt\n"));
#
# Initial condition
  tf=5;nout=26; ncall=0;
  G=rep(0,nout);P=rep(0,nout);
  G[1]=G0;P[1]=P0;
  tm=seq(from=0,to=tf,by=tf/(nout-1));
#
# Initial derivatives
  dG=rep(0,nout);dP=rep(0,nout);
  dydt=stem_1(tm[1],c(G[1],P[1]));
  dG[1]=dGPdt[1];dP[1]=dGPdt[2];
#
# Display initial variables
  cat(sprintf("%5.2f%10.3f%10.3f%10.3f%10.3f\n",
```

```
              tm[1],G[1],P[1],dG[1],dP[1]));
#
# lsodes ODE integration
  parms=c(rtol=1e-8,atol=1e-8)
  out=lsodes(times=tm,y=c(G[1],P[1]),func=stem_1,
     parms=parms)
  for(i in 2:nout){
  G[i]=out[i,2];
  P[i]=out[i,3];
  dydt=stem_1(tm[i],c(G[i],P[i]));
  dG[i]=dGPdt[1];dP[i]=dGPdt[2];
  cat(sprintf("%5.2f%10.3f%10.3f%10.3f%10.3f\n",
                tm[i],G[i],P[i],dG[i],dP[i]));
  }
#
# Calls to stem_1
  cat(sprintf("\n ncall = %5d\n\n",ncall))
#
# Four plots for G(t), P(t), dG(t)/dt, dP(t)/dt vs t
#
# G(t)
  par(mfrow=c(2,2))
  plot(tm,G,xlab="t",ylab="G(t)",xlim=c(0,5),
  type="l",lwd=2,main="G(t), LSODES")
#
# P(t)
  plot(tm,P,xlab="t",ylab="P(t)",xlim=c(0,5),
  type="l",lwd=2,main="P(t), LSODES")
#
# dG(t)/dt
  plot(tm,dG,xlab="t",ylab="dG(t)/dt",xlim=c(0,5),
  type="l",lwd=2,main="dG(t)/dt")
#
# dP(t)/dt
  plot(tm,dP,xlab="t",ylab="dP(t)/dt",xlim=c(0,5),
  type="l",lwd=2,main="dP(t)/dt")
#
# Next case
  }
```

Listing 5.1 Main program for eqs. (5.1).

We can note the following details about Listing 5.1.

- The library of ODE integrators (including `lsodes`), deSolve, is accessed.

```
#
# Access deSolve library (with lsodes)
  library("deSolve")
#
# ODE routine
  setwd("c:/R/bme_ode/chap5")
  source("stem_1.R")
```

Also, the ODE routine `stem_1.R` that has for the programming for eqs. (5.1) (discussed subsequently) is accessed.

- A `for` loop steps through multiple cases.

```
#
# Step through cases
  for(ncase in 1:2){
```

Two cases are programmed, `ncase=1,2`, so that a base case and a variant of it can be studied. A single case can be programmed as `ncase=1:1` or `ncase=2:2`, which might be useful to limit the output while some experimentation with the model is underway. Of course, more than two cases can also be programmed.

- A subset of the parameters of eqs. (5.1) is specified. These are taken from [1], Fig. 7a (stable progenitor).

```
#
# Model parameters
      b1=1;          b2=1;
   tha1=0.5;    tha2=0.5;
   thb1=0.07; thb2=0.07;
      k1=1;          k2=1;
       n=4;           m=1;
```

with $\theta_{a1} = $ tha1, $\theta_{a2} = $ tha2, $\theta_{b1} = $ thb1, and $\theta_{b2} = $ thb2. Note the symmetry of the parameters (they are the same for eqs. (5.1a) and (5.1b)), but with the numerical approach, they can, in principle, be set to any values.

- The parameters a1,a2 and the ICs for eqs. (5.1) are specified for each of the two cases.

```
#
# ncase = 1
  if(ncase==1){G0=1; P0=1; a1=1; a2=1;};
#
# ncase = 2
  if(ncase==2){G0=1; P0=1; a1=5; a2=10;};
```

ncase=1 corresponds to a steady-state solution for which the LHS derivatives of eqs. (5.1), $dG/dt, dP/dt$ remain at zero (this will be clear when the output is subsequently discussed). ncase=2 has different values for a1,a2 so that eqs. (5.1) moves through a transient and then approaches a steady-state solution. In this way, a second set of parameters for the unstable progenitor case of [1], Fig. 7b, can be selected.

- Selected parameters and a heading for the numerical solution are displayed.

```
#
# Write selected parameters and heading
  cat(sprintf("\n ncase = %2d    n = %5.2f
    m = %5.2f\n\n",
                 ncase,n,m));
  cat(sprintf("    t            G          P        dG/dt
    dP/dt\n"));
```

- The IC for eqs. (5.1) is specified.

```
#
# Initial condition
  tf=5;nout=26; ncall=0;
  G=rep(0,nout);P=rep(0,nout);
  G[1]=G0;P[1]=P0;
  tm=seq(from=0,to=tf,by=tf/(nout-1));
```

In particular, the interval in t is $0 \le t \le 5$ with 26 output points $t = 0, 0.2, 0.4, \ldots, 5$ (these values are placed in tm). The initial

values $G(t = 0), P(t = 0)$ are placed in the arrays G,P and the
counter for the calls to the ODE routine stem_1 is initialized.
For ncase=1, the ICs for eqs. (5.1) are defined as $G(t = 0) = 1$
(G0=1), $P(t = 0) = 1$ (P0=1), and the parameters a1=a2=1, so
that eqs. (5.1) are the same and their solutions should be identical
(this is an obvious case, but useful to check the programming in
the sense that if the two solutions are not the same, an error in
the programming requires correction).

- The initial derivatives $dG(t = 0)/dt, dP(t = 0)/dt$ are also computed by a call to the ODE routine stem_1. The 2-vector of
derivatives is returned as dGPdt and placed in the 1D arrays
dG,dP for subsequent numerical and graphical output.

```
#
# Initial derivatives
  dG=rep(0,nout);dP=rep(0,nout);
  dydt=stem_1(tm[1],c(G[1],P[1]));
  dG[1]=dGPdt[1];dP[1]=dGPdt[2];
```

The return of dGPdt from stem_1 will be clear when this routine
is discussed subsequently.

- The ICs and the initial derivatives are displayed.

```
#
# Display initial variables
  cat(sprintf("%5.2f%10.3f%10.3f%10.3f%10.3f\n",
              tm[1],G[1],P[1],dG[1],dP[1]));
```

- Eqs. (5.1) are integrated by lsodes, which is available in
deSolve.

```
#
# lsodes ODE integration
  parms=c(rtol=1e-8,atol=1e-8)
  out=lsodes(times=tm,y=c(G[1],P[1]),func=stem_1,
    parms=parms)
```

Note the inputs to lsodes, (i) the vector of t values, tm; (ii) the
ICs in y; (iii) the ODE routine stem_1; and (iv) the vector of

parameters for `lsodes`, in this case the error tolerances for the numerical integration. In other words, `times,y,func,parms` are reserved names in the call to `lsodes`.

- A `for` is used to place the numerical solution from `lsodes` in 1D arrays for subsequent numerical and graphical output (note that the index `i` of the `for` steps through the 25 values $t = 0.2, 0.4, \ldots, 5$ corresponding to `i=2,3,...,26`).

```
for(i in 2:nout){
G[i]=out[i,2];
P[i]=out[i,3];
dydt=stem_1(tm[i],c(G[i],P[i]));
dG[i]=dGPdt[1];dP[i]=dGPdt[2];
cat(sprintf("%5.2f%10.3f%10.3f%10.3f%10.3f\n",
            tm[i],G[i],P[i],dG[i],dP[i]));
}
```

The ODE integrators in `deSolve` return the solution in a 2D array, for example, `out`. The independent variable t is in `out[i,1]` (which is not used here because these values of t are also in `tm`). The first dependent variable, $G(t)$, is in `out[i,2]` (from the integration of eq. (5.1a)), and the second dependent variable, $P(t)$, is in `out[i,3]` (from the integration of eq. (5.1b)). The two dependent variables are placed in vectors `G` and `P` for subsequent numerical and graphical output. Also note the use of `stem_1` to place the derivatives $dG/dt, dP/dt$ in vectors `dG,dP` for subsequent numerical and graphical output. Again, the 2-vector of derivatives `dGPdt` is returned from `stem_1`.

The final { concludes the `for` loop in `i`.

- The number of calls to `stem_1` is displayed as a measure of the computational effort by `lsodes` to produce the numerical solution.

```
#
# Calls to stem_1
  cat(sprintf("\n ncall = %5d\n\n",ncall))
```

- The numerical solution is displayed graphically.

```
#
# Four plots for G(t), P(t), dG(t)/dt, dP(t)/dt vs t
#
# G(t)
  par(mfrow=c(2,2))
  plot(tm,G,xlab="t",ylab="G(t)",xlim=c(0,5),
  type="l",lwd=2,main="G(t), LSODES")
#
# P(t)
  plot(tm,P,xlab="t",ylab="P(t)",xlim=c(0,5),
  type="l",lwd=2,main="P(t), LSODES")
#
# dG(t)/dt
  plot(tm,dG,xlab="t",ylab="dG(t)/dt",xlim=c(0,5),
  type="l",lwd=2,main="dG(t)/dt")
#
# dP(t)/dt
  plot(tm,dP,xlab="t",ylab="dP(t)/dt",xlim=c(0,5),
  type="l",lwd=2,main="dP(t)/dt")
#
# Next case
  }
```

This programming produces a composite (one page) of four plots (as a 2×2 array from par(mfrow=c(2,2))). Note the use of tm for t and G,H,dG,dP for $G(t),P(t),dG(t)/dt,dP(t)/dt$, respectively. The final } concludes the for in ncase.

The ODE routine stem_1 is considered next.

5.3.2 ODE Routine

ODE routine stem_1 is in Listing 5.2.

```
  stem_1=function(t,y,parms) {
#
# Transfer dependent variable vector to problem variables
  G=y[1];
  P=y[2];
#
# Stem cell model ODEs
```

```
  dGdt=a1*G^n/(tha1^n+G^n)+b1*thb1^m/(thb1^m+G^m*P^m)
    -k1*G;
  dPdt=a2*P^n/(tha2^n+P^n)+b2*thb2^m/(thb2^m+G^m*P^m)
    -k2*P;
#
# Increment calls to neuron_1
  ncall <<- ncall+1;
#
# Return numerical derivative vector
  dGPdt <<- c(dGdt,dPdt);
#
# Return derivative vector as list
  return(list(c(dGdt,dPdt)))
}
```

Listing 5.2 ODE routine `stem_1` for eqs. (5.1).

We can note the following details from Listing 5.2.

- The function is defined.

  ```
  stem_1=function(t,y,parms) {
  ```

  The RHS input arguments are (i) the current value of the independent variable, t; (ii) the current vector of dependent variables $(G(t), P(t))$; and (iii) any parameters that are passed to `stem_1`. These three arguments are required, even if they are not used, for example, `parms`. The initial $(t = 0)$ values of t and y come from the ICs set in Listing 5.1. Subsequent values $(t > 0)$ come from `lsodes`.

- The RHS (input) vector, y, is placed in two scalar variables, G, P, to facilitate the programming of eqs. (5.1).

  ```
  #
  # Transfer dependent variable vector to problem
  #    variables
    G=y[1];
    P=y[2];
  ```

- Equations (5.1) are programmed.

  ```
  #
  # Stem cell model ODEs
  ```

```
dGdt=a1*G^n/(tha1^n+G^n)+b1*thb1^m/(thb1^m+G^m*P^m)
  -k1*G;
dPdt=a2*P^n/(tha2^n+P^n)+b2*thb2^m/(thb2^m+G^m*P^m)
  -k2*P;
```

The correspondence of this programming with eqs. (5.1) is clear. Also, this programming was used to calculate the LHS derivatives of eqs. (5.1) $(dG/dt, dP/dt)$ in Listing 5.1 (by a call to stem_1 in the main program as discussed previously).

- The number of calls to stem_1 is incremented and the value is returned to the main program of Listing 5.1 (note the use of <<- to effect this return to the main program).

```
#
# Increment calls to neuron_1
  ncall <<- ncall+1;
```

- The derivative vector is returned to the main program of Listing 5.1 as dGPdt.

```
#
# Return numerical derivative vector
  dGPdt <<- c(dGdt,dPdt);
```

- The derivative vector is also returned to lsodes as a list.

```
#
# Return derivative vector as list
  return(list(c(dGdt,dPdt)))
}
```

This completes the programming of eqs. (5.1). The output from Listings 5.1 and 5.2 is discussed next.

5.3.3 Numerical and Graphical Output

Abbreviated output from Listing 5.1 is given in Table 5.1.

TABLE 5.1 Abbreviated numerical output from Listing 5.1.

ncase = 1   n = 4.00   m = 1.00

t	G	P	dG/dt	dP/dt
0.00	1.000	1.000	0.007	0.007
0.20	1.001	1.001	0.006	0.006
0.40	1.002	1.002	0.005	0.005
0.60	1.003	1.003	0.004	0.004
0.80	1.004	1.004	0.003	0.003
1.00	1.004	1.004	0.003	0.003
.				.
.				.
.				.

Output for t = 1.2 to 3.8 removed

.				.
.				.
.				.
4.00	1.007	1.007	0.000	0.000
4.20	1.007	1.007	0.000	0.000
4.40	1.007	1.007	0.000	0.000
4.60	1.007	1.007	0.000	0.000
4.80	1.007	1.007	0.000	0.000
5.00	1.007	1.007	0.000	0.000

ncall =   67

ncase = 2   n = 4.00   m = 1.00

t	G	P	dG/dt	dP/dt
0.00	1.000	1.000	3.771	8.477
0.20	1.711	2.617	3.268	7.385
0.40	2.306	3.957	2.691	6.049
0.60	2.794	5.053	2.206	4.951
0.80	3.194	5.950	1.807	4.053
1.00	3.521	6.685	1.480	3.318
.				.
.				.

(continued)

TABLE 5.1   (*Continued*)

.			.	
Output for t = 1.2 to 3.8 removed				
.			.	
.			.	
.			.	
4.00	4.927	9.836	0.074	0.165
4.20	4.941	9.866	0.060	0.135
4.40	4.952	9.891	0.049	0.111
4.60	4.960	9.911	0.040	0.091
4.80	4.968	9.927	0.033	0.074
5.00	4.974	9.941	0.027	0.061
ncall = 124				

We can note the following about this output.

- The solution starts at the ICs set in the main program of Listing 5.1., that is, $G(t = 0) = P(t = 0) = 1$ (checking the ICs is a good idea; if they are not correct, the solution will not be correct).

- For ncase=1, the solution essentially remains at the IC ($t = 0$). This is evident from the nearly zero values of the derivatives $dG(t)/dt, dP(t)/dt$. This is in accordance with [1], Fig. 7a (i.e., the solutions remain at the center stable point in the figure). Also, the number of calls to stem_1 is small, ncall = 67, because the numerical integration is relatively easy for this invariant solution.

- For ncase=2, the solution moves through a transient and reaches a steady-state or equilibrium solution. Also, from eqs. (5.1), because a2 > a1 (from Listing 5.1), the derivative dP/dt is greater than dG/dt and therefore $P(t)$ undergoes a larger change than $G(t)$. The calls to stem_1 remain quite modest (ncall = 124) indicating the efficiency of lsodes, a stiff integrator (an attempted solution with one of the explicit integrators, e.g., euler, did not move past the IC). Clearly, for this application of eqs. (5.1), a stiff integrator is essential.

The graphical output from Listing 5.1 is in Figs. 5.1 and 5.2.

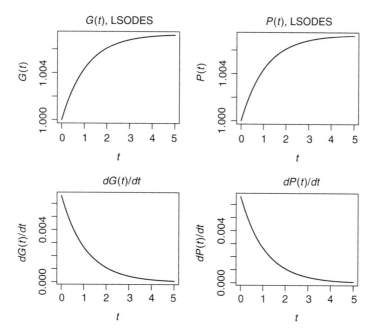

Figure 5.1 $G(t), P(t), dG/dt, dP/dt$ from eqs. (5.1) for ncase=1.

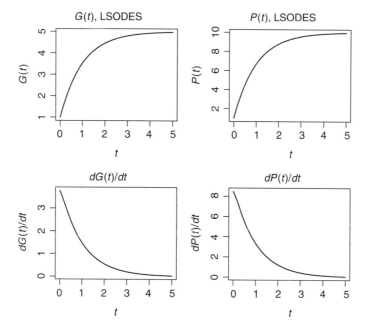

Figure 5.2 $G(t), P(t), dG/dt, dP/dt$ from eqs. (5.1) for ncase=2.

Figure 5.1 appears to indicate a variation of the solution with t. Note, however, that the ordinate (vertical) scale has little variation. Figure 5.2 clearly indicates the approach to the steady state for ncase=2 apparent in Table 5.1.

5.3.4 Analysis of the Terms in the ODEs

An important aspect of the numerical analysis of an ODE system is the investigation of the individual terms in the ODEs to gain a better understanding of the origin of the solution characteristics. We illustrate this procedure by investigating the RHS terms of eqs. (5.1).

As the solution for $G(t), P(t)$ is already available in Listing 5.1, calculating the RHS terms in eqs. (5.1) that are a function of the solution is straightforward. To do this, we add some programming at the end of Listing 5.1 (after the plotting) (Listing 5.3).

```
#
# Declare (preallocate) additional arrays for ODE
#    analysis
  Gterm1=rep(0,nout);Gterm2=rep(0,nout);Gterm3=rep(0,
    nout);
  Pterm1=rep(0,nout);Pterm2=rep(0,nout);Pterm3=rep(0,
    nout);
#
# Compute and save the RHS terms of the ODEs
  for(i in 1:nout){
  Gterm1[i]=a1*G[i]^n/(tha1^n+G[i]^n);
  Gterm2[i]=b1*thb1^m/(thb1^m+G[i]^m*P[i]^m);
  Gterm3[i]=-k1*G[i];
  Pterm1[i]=a2*P[i]^n/(tha2^n+P[i]^n);
  Pterm2[i]=b2*thb2^m/(thb2^m+G[i]^m*P[i]^m);
  Pterm3[i]=-k2*P[i];
  }
#
# Plot the terms of the G(t) ODE
#
# Single graph
  par(mfrow=c(1,1))
```

```
#
# Overlay four plots
#
# Gterm1
  plot(tm,Gterm1,xlab="t",
  ylab="Gterm1,Gterm2,Gterm3,dG/dt",
  xlim=c(0,5),ylim=c(-5,5),type="b",lty=1,pch="1",lwd=2,
  main="Gterm1,Gterm2,Gterm3,dG/dt vs t")
#
# Gterm2
  lines(tm,Gterm2,type="b",lty=1,pch="2",lwd=2)
#
# Gterm3
  lines(tm,Gterm3,type="b",lty=1,pch="3",lwd=2)
#
# dG/dt
  lines(tm,dG,type="b",lty=1,pch="4",lwd=2)
#
# Plot the terms of the P(t) ODE
#
# Single plot
  par(mfrow=c(1,1))
#
# Overlay four plots
#
# Pterm1
  plot(tm,Pterm1,xlab="t",
  ylab="Pterm1,Pterm2,Pterm3,dP/dt",
  xlim=c(0,5),ylim=c(-10,10),type="b",lty=1,pch="1",
     lwd=2,
  main="Pterm1,Pterm2,Pterm3,dP/dt vs t")
#
# Pterm2
  lines(tm,Pterm2,type="b",lty=1,pch="2",lwd=2)
#
# Pterm3
  lines(tm,Pterm3,type="b",lty=1,pch="3",lwd=2)
#
# dP/dt
  lines(tm,dP,type="b",lty=1,pch="4",lwd=2)
#
```

```
# Next case
 }
```

Listing 5.3 Additional programming to analyze the terms of eqs. (5.1).

We can note the following details of this programming.

- Six arrays are declared for the three RHS terms of eqs. (5.1).

```
#
# Declare (preallocate) additional arrays for ODE
#     analysis
  Gterm1=rep(0,nout);Gterm2=rep(0,nout);Gterm3=rep(0,
    nout);
  Pterm1=rep(0,nout);Pterm2=rep(0,nout);Pterm3=rep(0,
    nout);
```

- The RHS terms of eqs. (5.1) are computed through t with a for.

```
#
# Compute and save the RHS terms of the ODEs
  for(i in 1:nout){
  Gterm1[i]=a1*G[i]^n/(tha1^n+G[i]^n);
  Gterm2[i]=b1*thb1^m/(thb1^m+G[i]^m*P[i]^m);
  Gterm3[i]=-k1*G[i];
  Pterm1[i]=a2*P[i]^n/(tha2^n+P[i]^n);
  Pterm2[i]=b2*thb2^m/(thb2^m+G[i]^m*P[i]^m);
  Pterm3[i]=-k2*P[i];
  }
```

  The individual terms follow from the programming of eqs. (5.1) in stem_1 (Listing 5.2).
- With the six arrays Gterm1 to Pterm3 available, a graph is produced for each of eqs. (5.1) that indicates the RHS terms and the sum of these terms to give the LHS derivative. This graphical output is in Figs. 5.3 and 5.4 (for ncase=2).

Figure 5.3 indicates the following details.

- The first RHS term of eq. (5.1a) has a small transient initially but then has a nearly constant value at 5. For example (from

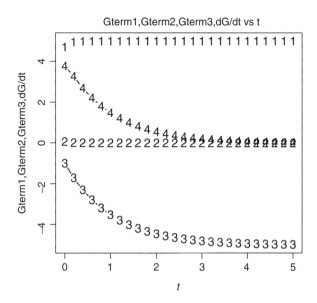

Figure 5.3   RHS terms and LHS derivative of eq. (5.1a) vs. t.

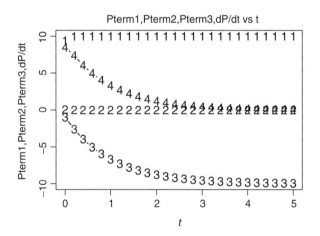

Figure 5.4   RHS terms and LHS derivative of eq. (5.1b) vs. t.

Table 5.1, ncase=2), at $t = 1$,

$$a_1 \frac{[G]^n /}{\theta_{a1}^n + [G]^n)} = (5)(3.521^4)/(0.5^4 + 3.521^4) = 4.9980$$

At $t = 5$, this term is

$$a_1 \frac{[G]^n}{(\theta_{a1}^n + [G]^n)} = (5)(4.974^4)/(0.5^4 + 4.974^4) = 4.9995$$

- The second RHS term of eq. (5.1a) is nearly constant at zero. For example (from Table 5.1, ncase=2), at $t = 0$,

$$+b_1 \frac{\theta_{b1}^m}{\theta_{b1}^m + [G]^m [P]^m} = (1)(0.07^1)/(0.07^1 + 1^1 1^1) = 0.0654$$

At $t = 5$, this term is

$$+b_1 \frac{\theta_{b1}^m}{\theta_{b1}^m + [G]^m [P]^m} = (1)(0.07^1)/(0.07^1 + 4.974^1 9.941^1)$$

$$= 0.0014$$

- The third RHS term of eq. (5.1a) varies with $G(t)$. For example (from Table 5.1, ncase=2), at $t = 0$,

$$-k_1[G] = -(1)(1) = -1$$

At $t = 5$, this term is

$$-k_1[G] = -(1)(4.974) = -4.974$$

- The net result of summing these terms according to eq. (5.1a) is that the derivative at $t = 0$ is

$$(5)(1^4)/(0.5^4 + 1^4) + 0.0654 - 1 = 3.7713$$

which agrees with Table 5.1.
At $t = 5$, the derivative is

$$(5)(4.974^4)/(0.5^4 + 4.974^4) + 0.0014 - 4.974 = 0.0269$$

which agrees with Table 5.1.

These numbers give a detailed picture of how the derivative $dG(t)/dt$ of eq. (5.1a) approaches zero at $t = 5$, that is, `Gterm1` = 5, `Gterm2` = 0, `Gterm3` = -4.974 so dG/dt at $t = 5$ is $dG/dt = 5 - 4.974 \approx 0$. Also, the second term `Gterm2` is a minor contributor to the derivative that calls into question whether this term should be included in the model, at least for the numerical parameters that were used; increasing b_1 by a factor of 100 could change this.

Thus, Fig. 5.3 gives a rather complete picture of the evolution of $G(t)$ according to eq. (5.1a); similar conclusions follow for $P(t)$ from Fig. 5.4. If any RHS term is relatively complicated, the components of the term can be individually computed and plotted. This type of detailed analysis of the ODEs is particularly informative as multiple cases are executed with varying parameter sets (the changes in the RHS terms can be observed as the model parameters are changed).

5.3.5 Stable States

The preceding output in Table 5.1 for `ncase=1` indicates the ODE system remains at the stable equilibrium solution $G(t) = P(t) = 1$ [1, Fig. 7a]. We can now consider introducing differences in the ICs and/or parameters for eqs. (5.1a) and (5.1b) such as for `ncase=2` of Listing 5.1. An interesting aspect of this type of investigation is if the solutions proceed to a stable equilibrium other than $G(t) = P(t) = 1$, or do not reach a stable point, perhaps by going into a sustained oscillation. To identify these various possibilities, a phase-plane plot can be used in which $P(t)$ is plotted against $G(t)$, which is easily accomplished with the `plot` utility. A sustained oscillation would be manifest as a limit cycle as described in Chapter 4.

5.4 Summary

The basic 2×2 model of eqs. (5.1) has a variety of properties depending on the ICs and parameters, and this is only an introductory model for a complex situation (stem cell differentiation). If the model is extended by adding more equations and mathematical details, the variety of solutions would increase. However, the numerical approach illustrated in the preceding example can be extended to accommodate a model of essentially any complexity. This is an important distinction with an analytical approach to the ODE system, which becomes increasingly difficult as the complexity of the model increases.

To conclude, we again note that the stable equilibrium solutions corresponding to $dG(t)/dt = dP(t)/dt = 0$ are also a solution to a 2×2 nonlinear algebraic system. For example, in the case of eqs. (5.2), the algebraic system is

$$0 = a \frac{x^n}{\theta_1^n + x^n} + b \frac{\theta_2^m}{\theta_2^m + x^m y^m} - x \qquad (5.3a)$$

$$0 = a \frac{y^n}{\theta_1^n + y^n} + b \frac{\theta_2^m}{\theta_2^m + x^m y^m} - y \qquad (5.3b)$$

and the solution would be (x, y) that satisfies eqs. (5.3).

This idea can be reversed, that is, to solve a nonlinear algebraic system such as eqs. (5.3), first convert the algebraic equations to an ODE system and then integrate the ODEs until they reach a stable equilibrium solution. The key word here is *stable*. In other words, the algebraic equations must be converted to stable ODEs. This is not always an obvious step (even a difference in a sign when adding the derivatives can preclude a stable solution). A systematic procedure for adding the derivatives to produce a stable ODE system is available that involves using the ODE Jacobian matrix, in this case, a 2×2 matrix of first-order partial derivatives of the ODE RHSs with respect to the two dependent variables G, P. We will not go into this procedure here. A detailed example is given in [1, pp 177–193].

As a related point, a nonlinear solver such as Newton's method could be applied directly to eqs. (5.3), but this would also require the Jacobian matrix. Also, an initial estimate of the solution that generally is not obvious for nonlinear algebraic systems would be required. The differential approach (based on the use of ODEs), therefore, does not require anything beyond that of a conventional nonlinear algebraic solver such as Newton's method. The differential approach, however, has the advantage of using a readily available ODE solver that essentially takes care of the stepping required by a nonlinear algebraic solver. In other words, the ODE solver steps from the assumed ODE ICs and does not require something like the Newton step that might have to be adjusted to reach a stable solution to the algebraic system.

Reference

[1] C. Duff, K. Smith-Miles, L. Lopes, T. Tian (2012), Mathematical modelling of stem cell differentiation: the PU.1_GATA-1 interaction, *J. Math. Biol.*, **64**, 449–468

## CHAPTER 6

Acetylcholine Neurocycle[1]

6.1 Introduction

We consider in this chapter a kinetic model for two enzyme-catalyzed reactions that determine the concentration of a key neurotransmitter, acetylcholine. The model consists of eight ODEs with time as the independent variable. The details of the model are first considered followed by a discussion of the model numerical solution. The latter includes a detailed discussion of the R routines for the calculation of the numerical solution.

6.2 ODE Model

We start with an ODE model reported in [5, 6, 7, 8]. A basic assumption for the model structure is two completely mixed compartments so that the concentrations of the various chemical specifies are uniform throughout the compartments (spatial effects are not considered). Subsequently, an ODE/PDE model in which spatial variation because of an interconnecting membrane between the two compartments is included is considered.

The ODE model is diagrammed in Fig. 6.1.

[1]This chapter is based in part on the papers by Mustafa et al. cited in the references. The contributions and guidance of Dr. I. H. Mustafa and Dr. A. Elkamel, University of Waterloo, are gratefully acknowledged.

Differential Equation Analysis in Biomedical Science and Engineering: Ordinary Differential Equation Applications with R, First Edition. William E. Schiesser.
© 2014 John Wiley & Sons, Inc. Published 2014 by John Wiley & Sons, Inc.

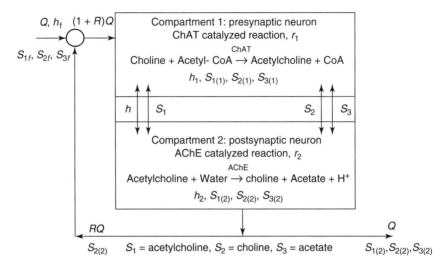

Figure 6.1   Diagram for the model of eqs. (6.1).

We can note the following details about Fig 6.1.

- The dependent variables of ODE for compartment 1 are h_1, $s_{1(1)}, s_{2(1)}$, and $s_{3(1)}$. Similarly, the dependent variables for compartment 2 are $h_2, s_{1(2)}, s_{2(2)}$, and $s_{3(2)}$. Thus, there are a total of eight dependent variables defined by eight ODEs discussed next.

- The principal difference between the two compartments is the reaction in compartment 1 catalyzed by an enzyme denoted as ChAT and the reaction in compartment 2 catalyzed by an enzyme denoted as AChE. The rates of these reactions are given by two algebraic equations that are added to the eight ODEs to complete the model.

- The eight dependent variables are chemical concentrations of four chemical species in each of the two compartments. As a result of differences in these concentrations between the two compartments, mass transfer takes place between the compartments through a separating membrane (note the double arrows in Fig. 6.1 depicting this membrane mass transfer).

- Compartment 1 has four feed concentrations h_{1f}, s_{1f}, s_{2f}, and s_{3f}. The effect of variation of these feed concentrations is a primary objective in using the model.

- Compartment 2 has an exit stream that is divided into two streams. One stream is the product stream with compositions $h_2, s_{1(2)}, s_{2(2)},$ and $s_{3(2)}$ (which are also the concentrations in compartment 2 because of the perfect mixing assumption). The second stream is a recycle that sends concentration $s_{2(2)}$ back to compartment 1 at flow rate R, which is a key parameter in the model.

- Solution of the model gives the eight dependent variable as a function of time, t. Of particular interest is whether the solution approaches a stable equilibrium solution for which there is no further variation with t.

The 8×8 ODE system (eight ODEs in eight dependent variables) follows. These equations are in dimensionless form; the dimensional and dimensionless equations are derived in [5].

$$\frac{dy_1}{dt} = y_{1f} - \gamma(1/y_{1f}) - \alpha_H(y_1 - y_2) + \alpha_{OH}\gamma(1/y_1 - 1/y_2) \quad (6.1a)$$

$$\frac{dy_2}{dt} = [\alpha_H(y_1 - y_2) - \alpha_{OH}\gamma(1/y_1 - 1/y_2) - (y_2 - \gamma/y_2)$$
$$+ B_2 r_2/k_{h1}]v_r \quad (6.1b)$$

$$\frac{dy_3}{dt} = y_{3f} - \alpha_{s1}(y_3 - y_4) + B_1 r_1/k_{s1} \quad (6.1c)$$

$$\frac{dy_4}{dt} = [\alpha_{s1}(y_3 - y_4) - y_4 - B_2 r_2/k_{s1}]v_r \quad (6.1d)$$

$$\frac{dy_5}{dt} = y_{5f} + Ry_6 - \alpha_{s2}(y_5 - y_6) - B_1 r_1/s_{2ref} \quad (6.1e)$$

$$\frac{dy_6}{dt} = [\alpha_{s2}(y_5 - y_6) - (1 + R)y_6 + B_2 r_2/s_{2ref}]v_r \quad (6.1f)$$

$$\frac{dy_7}{dt} = y_{7f} - \alpha_{s3}(y_7 - y_8) - B_1 r_1/s_{3ref} \quad (6.1g)$$

$$\frac{dy_8}{dt} = [\alpha_{s3}(y_7 - y_8) - y_8 + B_2 r_2/s_{3ref}]v_r \quad (6.1h)$$

The dependent variables, $y_1, \ldots, y_8$, and independent variable t of eqs. (6.1) are defined in Table 6.1 [8]. Also, the notation (variable symbols or names) in Table 1 of [5] are listed in Table 6.1.

TABLE 6.1 Variables of eqs. (6.1) and Table 1 of [5].

Eqs. (6.1)	Eqs. [5] Table 1	Interpretation
y_1	$h_{(1)}$	hydrogen protons (ions), compartment 1
y_2	$h_{(2)}$	hydrogen protons (ions), compartment 2
y_3	$s_{1(1)}$	acetylcholine, compartment 1
y_4	$s_{1(2)}$	acetylcholine, compartment 2
y_5	$s_{2(1)}$	choline, compartment 1
y_6	$s_{2(2)}$	choline, compartment 2
y_7	$s_{3(1)}$	acetate, compartment 1
y_8	$s_{3(2)}$	acetate, compartment 2
t	t	time

All of the other entities in eqs. (6.1) are parameters (constants) or reaction rates. For example, the parameters of eq. (6.1a) are y_{1f}, γ, α_H, and α_{OH}.

The reaction rates r_1 and r_2 in eqs. (6.1) are given by

$$r_1 = \frac{c_5 y_7 y_5}{c_1 c_2 (1 + y_1 + \delta y_1^2)/y_1 + c_4 y_7 + c_2 y_5 + c_3 y_5 y_7} \tag{6.2a}$$

$$r_2 = \frac{y_4}{y_4 + (1 + y_2 + \delta y_2^2)/y_2 + \alpha y_4^2} \tag{6.2b}$$

Each of the eqs. (6.1) requires an IC. One approach to defining the IC vector (eight components) is to set the LHS derivatives in t in eqs. (6.1) to zero. This produces an 8×8 system of nonlinear algebraic equations in the variables $y_1, \ldots, y_8$. This algebraic system can then be solved by a nonlinear solver, typically a variant of Newton's method. We consider an algorithm and its use for the solution of the nonlinear algebraic system in a later section.

The resulting IC vector corresponds to an equilibrium solution of eqs. (6.1) in which the eight components of the derivative vector $dy_1/dt, \ldots, dy_8/dt$ are zero. If this IC vector corresponds to a stable equilibrium point, the solution of eqs. (6.1) should remain at the IC values. This property is illustrated with the following IC vector reported in [8].

TABLE 6.2   Equilibrium condition vector for eqs. (6.1).

IC	Value
$y_1(t = 0)$	0.003796824
$y_2(t = 0)$	0.1405804
$y_3(t = 0)$	3.8971322
$y_4(t = 0)$	0.2801880941
$y_5(t = 0)$	3.233
$y_6(t = 0)$	1.1606
$y_7(t = 0)$	8.2517318
$y_8(t = 0)$	4.960605

The ICs of Table 6.2 correspond to particular values of the parameters (constants) in eqs. (6.1) that will be specified when the coding of eqs. (6.1) is discussed.

We can note two details about the ICs of Table 6.2.

- The particular value of t where the ICs are applied is inconsequential because the RHSs of eqs. (6.1) do not contain t explicitly. In other words, when the nonlinear equation solver is applied to the RHSs of eqs. (6.1) when set to zero, the resulting solution does not depend on a specific value of t. Thus, we will take $t = 0$ (but any other value of t can be specified because the IC vector is independent of the value of t).
- The ICs in Table 6.2 are reported with as many as 10 figures. This is a reflection of the fact that these values were calculated by a nonlinear equation solver. This does not imply that the

values are known in a realistic physical application of eqs. (6.1) to this many figures. Rather, within a physical system context, we would probably not have ICs to any more than three to four significant figures.

In the chapter appendix, the solution of the nonlinear algebraic equation system by a differential Levenberg Marquardt (DLM) method is discussed, including the analytical and numerical evaluations of the Jacobian matrix of eqs. (6.1). The R routines are included in this discussion, which reproduce the ICs of Table 6.2.

6.3 Numerical Solution of the Model

We now consider a set of R routines for the numerical integration (solution) of eqs. (6.1) subject to the IC vector of Table 6.2 for a particular set of parameters defined numerically in the programming.

6.3.1 ODE Routine

An ODE routine for eqs. (6.1)–(6.2) is in Listing 6.1.

```
  trans_1=function(t,y,parms) {
#
# Reaction rates
  r1=c5*y[7]*y[5]/(c1*c2*(1+y[1]+delta*y[1]^2)/y[1]+c4*
    y[7]+
    c2*y[5]+c3*y[5]*y[7]);
  r2=y[4]/(y[4]+(1+y[2]+delta*y[2]^2)/y[2]+alpha*y[4]^2);
#
# ODEs
  yt=rep(0,8);
  yt[1]=y1f-gamma*(1/y1f)-alphaH*(y[1]-y[2])+
      alphaOH*gamma*(1/y[1]-1/y[2]);
  yt[2]=(alphaH*(y[1]-y[2])-alphaOH*gamma*(1/y[1]-1/y[2])-
      (y[2]-gamma/y[2])+B2*r2/kh1)*vr;
  yt[3]= y3f-alphas1*(y[3]-y[4])+B1*r1/ks1;
  yt[4]=(alphas1*(y[3]-y[4])-y[4]-B2*r2/ks1)*vr;
  yt[5]=y5f+R*y[6]-alphas2*(y[5]-y[6])-B1*r1/s2ref;
  yt[6]=(alphas2*(y[5]-y[6])-(1+R)*y[6]+B2*r2/s2ref)*vr;
  yt[7]=y7f-alphas3*(y[7]-y[8])-B1*r1/s3ref;
```

```
  yt[8]=(alphas3*(y[7]-y[8])-y[8]+B2*r2/s3ref)*vr;
#
# Increment calls to trans_1
  ncall <<- ncall+1;
#
# Return derivative vector as list
  return(list(c(yt)));
}
```

Listing 6.1 ODE routine `trans_1` for eqs. (6.1).

We can note the following details about `ode_1`.

- The function is defined.

  ```
  trans_1=function(t,y,parms) {
  ```

  The dependent variable vector, y, is used in the programming of eqs. (6.1) and (6.2). The independent variable of ODE t and `parms` for parameters are not used in the programming.
- The reaction rates r_1 and r_2 of eqs. (6.2) are programmed.

  ```
  #
  # Reaction rates
    r1=c5*y[7]*y[5]/(c1*c2*(1+y[1]+delta*y[1]^2)/y[1]+
       c4*y[7]+
       c2*y[5]+c3*y[5]*y[7]);
    r2=y[4]/(y[4]+(1+y[2]+delta*y[2]^2)/y[2]+alpha*
       y[4]^2);
  ```

  This programming clearly demonstrates some of the nonlinearity of the model and how easily it can be accommodated by the numerical ODE integration.
- Equations (6.1) is programmed to give the eight ODE derivatives in t, y1t,...,y8t.

  ```
  #
  # ODEs
    yt=rep(0,8);
    yt[1]=y1f-gamma*(1/y1f)-alphaH*(y[1]-y[2])+
  ```

```
         alphaOH*gamma*(1/y[1]-1/y[2]);
  yt[2]=(alphaH*(y[1]-y[2])-alphaOH*gamma*(1/y[1]-1/
     y[2])-
        (y[2]-gamma/y[2])+B2*r2/kh1)*vr;
  yt[3]= y3f-alphas1*(y[3]-y[4])+B1*r1/ks1;
  yt[4]=(alphas1*(y[3]-y[4])-y[4]-B2*r2/ks1)*vr;
  yt[5]=y5f+R*y[6]-alphas2*(y[5]-y[6])-B1*r1/s2ref;
  yt[6]=(alphas2*(y[5]-y[6])-(1+R)*y[6]+B2*r2/s2ref)*
     vr;
  yt[7]=y7f-alphas3*(y[7]-y[8])-B1*r1/s3ref;
  yt[8]=(alphas3*(y[7]-y[8])-y[8]+B2*r2/s3ref)*vr;
```

Note that the vector yt is first declared (preallocated) (yt= rep(0,8)). The close correspondence of the programming with eqs. (6.1) again demonstrates the ease of numerically integrating systems of nonlinear ODEs (in contrast with analytical methods).

- The number of calls to trans_1 is incremented and returned to the main program with <<-.

```
#
# Increment calls to trans_1
  ncall <<- ncall+1;
```

- The derivative 8-vector yt is returned (to lsodes of deSolve) as a list.

```
#
# Return derivative vector as list
  return(list(c(yt)));
}
```

The final } concludes trans_1.

In summary, the ODE model of eqs. (6.1) and (6.2) is programmed in trans_1. The remaining details such as the IC vector of Table 6.2 and the numerical definition of the parameters passed to trans_1 are completed in Section 6.3.2.

6.3.2 Main Program

The main program is in Listing 6.2.

```
#
# Acetylcholine neurocycle
#
# Two cases are programmed for a variation in ODE
#    parameters.
#
# Access deSolve library (with lsodes)
  library("deSolve")
#
# ODE routine
  setwd("c:/R/bme_ode/chap6")
  source("trans_1.R")
#
# Select case
#
# ncase = 1 - equilibrium solution, y1f = 0.0062682
#
# ncase = 2 - nonequilibrum solution, y1f = 0.00600
#
  ncase=1;
#
# Parameters
  y1f=6.2682e-03; y3f=2.4;        y5f=1.15;      y7f=3.9;
  R=0.8;          gamma=0.01;     vr=1.2;        alpha=
                                                    0.5;
  delta=0.1;      kh1=1.0066e-06; alphaH=2.25;   alphaOH=
                                                    0.5;
  alphas1=1  ;    alphas2=1;      alphas3=1;     B1=5.033
                                                    e-05;
  B2=5.033e-05;   ks1=5.0033e-07; s2ref=1.0e-04; s3ref=1.0
                                                    e-06;
  c1=2.4;         c2=5;           c3=1;          c4=1000;
  c5=5.2;
#
# Initial conditions
  y0=rep(0,8);
  y0[1]=0.003796824;  y0[2]=0.1405804; y0[3]=3.8971322;
  y0[4]=0.2801880941; y0[5]=3.233;     y0[6]=1.1606;
```

```
  y0[7]=8.2517318;      y0[8]=4.960605;
  tf=20;nout=41;ncall=0;
  tm=seq(from=0,to=tf,by=tf/(nout-1));
#
# Changes from equilibrium solution
  if(ncase==2){ y1f=0.00600};
#
# Write heading
  cat(sprintf("\n ncase = %2d    y1f = %10.6e\n\n",ncase,
     y1f));
  cat(sprintf("    t            y[1]          y[2]          y[3]
     y[4]"));
  cat(sprintf("                 y[5]          y[6]          y[7]
     y[8]"));
#
# lsodes ODE integration
  parms=c(rtol=1e-8,atol=1e-8)
  out=lsodes(times=tm,y=y0,func=trans_1,parms=parms)
#
# Numerical output
  yn=matrix(0,nrow=nout,ncol=8);
  for(it in 1:nout){
    if(it==1){yn[1,]=y0;
    }else{
    yn[it,]=out[it,-1];}
    cat(sprintf("%5.2f%12.5f%12.5f%12.5f%12.5f\n",
                tm[it],yn[it,1],yn[it,2],yn[it,3],yn[it,
                4]));
    cat(sprintf("%17.5f%12.5f%12.5f%12.5f\n\n",
                yn[it,5],yn[it,6],yn[it,7],yn[it,8]));
  }
#
# Calls to trans_1
  cat(sprintf("\n ncall = %5d\n\n",ncall))
#
# Eight plots for y1(t) to y8(t) vs t
#
# y1(t)
  par(mfrow=c(4,2))
  plot(tm,yn[,1],xlab="t",ylab="H+, comp 1",xlim=c(0,20),
  type="l",lwd=2,main="H+, comp 1")
```

```
#
# y2(t)
  plot(tm,yn[,2],xlab="t",ylab="H+, comp 2",xlim=c(0,20),
  type="l",lwd=2,main="H+, comp 2")
#
# y3(t)
  plot(tm,yn[,3],xlab="t",ylab="acetylcholine",
      xlim=c(0,20),
  type="l",lwd=2,main="acetylcholine, comp 1")
#
# y4(t)
  plot(tm,yn[,4],xlab="t",ylab="acetylcholine",
      xlim=c(0,20),
  type="l",lwd=2,main="acetylcholine, comp 2")
#
# y5(t)
  plot(tm,yn[,5],xlab="t",ylab="choline",xlim=c(0,20),
  type="l",lwd=2,main="choline, comp 1")
#
# y6(t)
  plot(tm,yn[,6],xlab="t",ylab="choline",xlim=c(0,20),
  type="l",lwd=2,main="choline, comp 2")
#
# y7(t)
  plot(tm,yn[,7],xlab="t",ylab="acetate",xlim=c(0,20),
  type="l",lwd=2,main="acetate, comp 1")
#
# y8(t)
  plot(tm,yn[,8],xlab="t",ylab="acetate",xlim=c(0,20),
  type="l",lwd=2,main="acetate, comp 2")
#
# Four plots for compartments 1,2
#
# y1(t), y2(t) vs t
  par(mfrow=c(1,1))
  plot(tm,yn[,1],xlab="t",ylab="H+",xlim=c(0,20),
  ylim=c(0,0.6),type="b",lty=1,pch="1",lwd=2,main="H+",)
  lines(tm,yn[,2],type="b",lty=1,pch="2",lwd=2)
#
# y3(t), y4(t) vs t
  par(mfrow=c(1,1))
```

```
    plot(tm,yn[,3],xlab="t",ylab="acetylcholine",
      xlim=c(0,20),
    ylim=c(0,5),type="b",lty=1,pch="1",lwd=2,
      main="acetylcholine",)
    lines(tm,yn[,4],type="b",lty=1,pch="2",lwd=2)
#
# y5(t), y6(t) vs t
    par(mfrow=c(1,1))
    plot(tm,yn[,5],xlab="t",ylab="choline",xlim=c(0,20),
    ylim=c(0,4),type="b",lty=1,pch="1",lwd=2,
      main="choline",)
    lines(tm,yn[,6],type="b",lty=1,pch="2",lwd=2)
#
# y7(t), y8(t) vs t
    par(mfrow=c(1,1))
    plot(tm,yn[,7],xlab="t",ylab="acetate",xlim=c(0,20),
    ylim=c(4,10),type="b",lty=1,pch="1",lwd=2,
      main="acetate",)
    lines(tm,yn[,8],type="b",lty=1,pch="2",lwd=2)
```

Listing 6.2 Main program for eqs. (6.1) and (6.2).

We can note the following details.

- The library deSolve (with lsodes) and the ODE routine of Listing 6.1, trans_1, are accessed.

```
    #
    # Acetylcholine neurocycle
    #
    # Two cases are programmed for a variation in ODE
    #    parameters.
    #
    # Access deSolve library (with lsodes)
      library("deSolve")
    #
    # ODE routine
      setwd("c:/R/bme_ode/chap6")
      source("trans_1.R")
```

- One of two cases is selected.

```
#
# Select case
#
# ncase = 1 - equilibrium solution, y1f = 0.0062682
#
# ncase = 2 - nonequilibrum solution, y1f = 0.00600
#
  ncase=1;
```

These cases correspond to a variation in the entering hydrogen ion concentration, y1f. This variation is small, but the changes have a major effect on the solutions of eqs. (6.1) as discussed later.

• The parameters in eqs. (6.1) are defined numerically [8].

```
#
# Parameters
  y1f=6.2682e-03; y3f=2.4;          y5f=1.15;
                                    y7f=3.9;
  R=0.8;          gamma=0.01;       vr=1.2;
                                    alpha=0.5;
  delta=0.1;      kh1=1.0066e-06;   alphaH=2.25;
                                    alphaOH=0.5;
  alphas1=1   ;   alphas2=1;        alphas3=1;
                                    B1=5.033e-05;
  B2=5.033e-05;   ks1=5.0033e-07;   s2ref=1.0e-04;
                                    s3ref=1.0e-06;
  c1=2.4;         c2=5;             c3=1;
                                    c4=1000;
  c5=5.2;
```

These parameters are global so that they are available in trans _1 (see Listing 6.1). Note in particular y1f=6.2682e-03;, corresponding to the entering hydrogen ion concentration for ncase=1. This value is reset below for ncase=2.

• The ICs of Table 6.2 are set numerically.

```
#
# Initial conditions
  y0=rep(0,8);
```

```
y0[1]=0.003796824;  y0[2]=0.1405804;  y0[3]=3.8971322;
y0[4]=0.2801880941; y0[5]=3.233;      y0[6]=1.1606;
y0[7]=8.2517318;    y0[8]=4.960605;
tf=20;nout=41;ncall=0;
tm=seq(from=0,to=tf,by=tf/(nout-1));
```

The IC 8-vector y0 is declared (preallocated) as y0=rep (0,8). The ICs correspond to an equilibrium solution of eqs. (6.1) for which the LHS vector of derivatives $dy_1/dt,\ldots,$ dy_8/dt is effectively a zero vector. Again, for ncase=1, y1f=6.2682e-03 is set previously as the first parameter. The length of y0 informs lsodes of the number of ODEs to be integrated (eight for eqs. (6.1)).

The independent variable of ODE t is defined for $0 \le t \le 20$ with 41 output points (including $t = 0$). The counter for the calls to trans_1 is initialized.

- For ncase=2, y1f is changed. All other parameters remain unchanged.

```
#
# Changes from equilibrium solution
  if(ncase==2){ y1f=0.00600};
```

- A heading for the numerical solution is displayed.

```
#
# Write heading
  cat(sprintf("\n ncase = %2d   y1f = %10.6e\n\n",
    ncase,y1f));
  cat(sprintf("    t           y[1]            y[2]
    y[3]          y[4]"));
  cat(sprintf("                y[5]            y[6]
    y[7]          y[8]"));
```

- Equations (6.1) is integrated by lsodes in deSolve.

```
#
# lsodes ODE integration
  parms=c(rtol=1e-8,atol=1e-8)
  out=lsodes(times=tm,y=y0,func=trans_1,parms=parms)
```

Relative and absolute error tolerances for `lsodes` are set in `parms`. The numerical solution is returned by `lsodes` as the 2D array `out`. Note in the call to `lsodes`, the use of (i) the vector of output values of t, `tm`; (ii) the IC vector, `y0`; and (iii) the ODE routine, `trans_1` of Listing 6.1; and (iv) the parameter argument `parms`. `times,y,func,parms` are reserved names required by `lsodes`.

- The numerical solution is transferred from `out` to a 2D array, `yn`, for subsequent output.

```
#
# Numerical output
  yn=matrix(0,nrow=nout,ncol=8);
  for(it in 1:nout){
    if(it==1){yn[1,]=y0;
    }else{
    yn[it,]=out[it,-1];}
    cat(sprintf("%5.2f%12.5f%12.5f%12.5f%12.5f\n",
                tm[it],yn[it,1],yn[it,2],yn[it,3],
                  yn[it,4]));
    cat(sprintf("%17.5f%12.5f%12.5f%12.5f\n\n",
                yn[it,5],yn[it,6],yn[it,7],yn[it,8]));
  }
```

We can note the following details.

- A 2D array, `yn`, is defined for the numerical solution.

    `yn=matrix(0,nrow=nout,ncol=8);`

- The variation in t over $0 \le t \le 20$ is programmed as a `for`.

    `for(it in 1:nout){`

- For `it=1` corresponding to $t = 0$, the IC `y0` is placed in `yn`.

    `if(it==1){yn[1,]=y0;`

    The comma subscript , specifies all eight values of `y0`.

- `it=2,...,nout` correspond to the 40 values of t, $t = 0.5, 1, \ldots, 20$.

```
    }else{
    yn[it,]=out[it,-1];}
```

The subscript -1 specifies the index not 1, that is, 2,3,...,9. Thus, the eight dependent variables (from the integration of eqs. (6.1)) have been placed in yn for the 41 values of t.

- The independent variable t and the eight dependent variables, $y_1(t),...,y_8(t)$ from eqs. (6.1), are displayed numerically.

```
    cat(sprintf("%5.2f%12.5f%12.5f%12.5f%12.5f\n",
               tm[it],yn[it,1],yn[it,2],yn[it,3],
                 yn[it,4]));
    cat(sprintf("%17.5f%12.5f%12.5f%12.5f\n\n",
               yn[it,5],yn[it,6],yn[it,7],yn[it,
                 8]));
    }
```

The final } concludes the for in it.

- The number of calls to trans_1 at the end of the solution is displayed as

```
#
# Calls to trans_1
  cat(sprintf("\n ncall = %5d\n\n",ncall))
```

This final value of ncall gives a measure of the computational effort required to produce the numerical solution to eqs. (6.1).

- A composite (one page) of eight plots for $y_1(t),...,y_8(t)$ is produced from yn.

```
#
# Eight plots for y1(t) to y8(t) vs t
#
# y1(t)
  par(mfrow=c(4,2))
  plot(tm,yn[,1],xlab="t",ylab="H+, comp 1",
      xlim=c(0,20),
  type="l",lwd=2,main="H+, comp 1")
#
# y2(t)
```

```
  plot(tm,yn[,2],xlab="t",ylab="H+, comp 2",
      xlim=c(0,20),
  type="l",lwd=2,main="H+, comp 2")
#
# y3(t)
  plot(tm,yn[,3],xlab="t",ylab="acetylcholine",
      xlim=c(0,20),
  type="l",lwd=2,main="acetylcholine, comp 1")
#
# y4(t)
  plot(tm,yn[,4],xlab="t",ylab="acetylcholine",
      xlim=c(0,20),
  type="l",lwd=2,main="acetylcholine, comp 2")
#
# y5(t)
  plot(tm,yn[,5],xlab="t",ylab="choline",xlim=c(0,20),
  type="l",lwd=2,main="choline, comp 1")
#
# y6(t)
  plot(tm,yn[,6],xlab="t",ylab="choline",xlim=c(0,20),
  type="l",lwd=2,main="choline, comp 2")
#
# y7(t)
  plot(tm,yn[,7],xlab="t",ylab="acetate",xlim=c(0,20),
  type="l",lwd=2,main="acetate, comp 1")
#
# y8(t)
  plot(tm,yn[,8],xlab="t",ylab="acetate",xlim=c(0,20),
  type="l",lwd=2,main="acetate, comp 2")
```

Note the specification of a 4×2 (four rows and two columns) array of plots, par(mfrow=c(4,2)). The successive solutions yn[,1] to yn[,8] are used in the eight plots. The scaling of the abscissa (horizontal) axes is with xlim=c(0,20) corresponding to $0 \leq t \leq 20$. The ordinate (vertical) axes are scaled automatically by plots because the eight dependent variables have substantially different values. The eight plots in a single place (page) do not give a clear definition of the vertical axes (but the eight plots do give an indication of the simultaneous variation of y_1

to y_8). Therefore, the plotting is repeated next without so much graphical output in one place.

- Four separate plots are then produced, each with the same variable for the two compartments. In this way, the differences in the responses of the two compartments is apparent. Note in particular the use of pch=1 and pch=2 to number the solutions for compartments 1 and 2, respectively.

```
#
# Four plots for compartments 1,2
#
# y1(t), y2(t) vs t
  par(mfrow=c(1,1))
  plot(tm,yn[,1],xlab="t",ylab="H+",xlim=c(0,20),
  ylim=c(0,0.6),type="b",lty=1,pch="1",lwd=2,
     main="H+",)
  lines(tm,yn[,2],type="b",lty=1,pch="2",lwd=2)
#
# y3(t), y4(t) vs t
  par(mfrow=c(1,1))
  plot(tm,yn[,3],xlab="t",ylab="acetylcholine",
     xlim=c(0,20),
  ylim=c(0,5),type="b",lty=1,pch="1",lwd=2,main=
     "acetylcholine",)
  lines(tm,yn[,4],type="b",lty=1,pch="2",lwd=2)
#
# y5(t), y6(t) vs t
  par(mfrow=c(1,1))
  plot(tm,yn[,5],xlab="t",ylab="choline",xlim=c(0,20),
  ylim=c(0,4),type="b",lty=1,pch="1",lwd=2,
     main="choline",)
  lines(tm,yn[,6],type="b",lty=1,pch="2",lwd=2)
#
# y7(t), y8(t) vs t
  par(mfrow=c(1,1))
  plot(tm,yn[,7],xlab="t",ylab="acetate",xlim=c(0,20),
  ylim=c(4,10),type="b",lty=1,pch="1",lwd=2,main=
     "acetate",)
  lines(tm,yn[,8],type="b",lty=1,pch="2",lwd=2)
```

6.4   Model Output

We now consider the output for the two cases ncase=1,2 of List-ing 6.2.

6.4.1   Equilibrium Solution

Abbreviated numerical output from Listing 6.2 for ncase=1 is given in Table 6.3

We can note the following details about this output.

- The ICs of Table 6.2 are reproduced to six figures at $t = 0$. Although this is expected, it is a worthwhile check in the sense that if the ICs are incorrect, the solution will not be correct.
- The solution remains constant throughout the solution (to $t = 20$).
- The computational effort is modest (ncall=61) as might be expected because the solution does not change with t.

The solution in Table 6.3 clearly starts from a stable equilibrium point because it is invariant with t. In other words, the LHS deriva-tives of eqs. (6.1) are zero, which is illustrated by the following calculation. The programming of eq. (6.1a) from Listing 6.1 is

```
yt[1]=y1f-gamma*(1/y1f)-alphaH*(y[1]-y[2])+
      alphaOH*gamma*(1/y[1]-1/y[2]);
```

With numerical values for the parameters from Listing 6.2 and the ICs from Table 6.2, the calculation of dy_1/dt of eq. (6.1a) is

```
yt[1]=6.2682e-03-0.01*(1/6.2682e-03)-2.25*(0.003796824-
   0.1405804)+
      0.5*0.01*(1/0.003796824-1/0.1405804)=1.986102e-07
```

(computed by entering this calculation into R). The small result of 1.986102e-07 is essentially a zero value for dy_1/dt. A similar con-clusion follows for dy_2/dt to dy_8/dt from eqs. (6.1b) to (6.1h). The plots from Listing 6.2 are not reproduced here because they simply demonstrate that the solution does not change with t.

TABLE 6.3   Abbreviated output from Listings 6.1 and 6.2 for ncase=1.

ncase = 1 y1f = 6.268200e-03			
t	y[1]	y[2]	y[3]	y[4]
	y[5]	y[6]	y[7]	y[8]
0.00	0.00380	0.14058	3.89713	0.28019
	3.23300	1.16060	8.25173	4.96061
0.50	0.00380	0.14058	3.89713	0.28019
	3.23300	1.16060	8.25173	4.96061
1.00	0.00380	0.14058	3.89713	0.28019
	3.23300	1.16060	8.25173	4.96061
.	.			.
.	.			.
.	.			.
	Output for t = 1.50 to 18.5 removed			
.	.			.
.	.			.
.	.			.
19.00	0.00380	0.14058	3.89713	0.28019
	3.23300	1.16061	8.25173	4.96061
19.50	0.00380	0.14058	3.89713	0.28019
	3.23300	1.16061	8.25173	4.96061
20.00	0.00380	0.14058	3.89713	0.28019
	3.23300	1.16061	8.25173	4.96061
ncall = 61			

We now consider the effect of introducing a change away from the equilibrium condition. For example, for ncase=2 in Listing 6.2, the entering hydrogen ion flow h1f is changed from

6.2682e-03 for ncase=1 to 0.00600 for ncase=2, a change of only
((0.0062682-0.00600)/0.0062682)(100) = 4.28 %.

6.4.2   Nonequilibrium Solutions

Abbreviated tabulated output from Listing 6.2 for ncase=2 is given
in Table 6.4.

We can note the following details about this output.

- The ICs of Table 6.2 are again reproduced to six figures at $t = 0$
  (only h1f, a parameter, has been changed in Listing 6.2). But
  the initial derivatives are no longer zero because of the departure
  from the equilibrium solution. This change in the derivatives is
  illustrated with the following calculation of $dy_1(t = 0)/dt$.

  ```
  yt[1]=6.000e-03-0.01*(1/6.000e-03)-2.25*(0.003796824-
      0.1405804)+
          0.5*0.01*(1/0.003796824-1/0.1405804)=-0.07158034
  ```

  $dy_1(t = 0)/dt = $ -0.07158034 indicates a significant transient
  (change) in the solution of eqs. (6.1) can be expected, which is
  confirmed by the changes in Table 6.4 and the graphical output
  that follows.

- The computational effort (ncall=1788) is greater than that for
  ncase=1 (ncall=61) as expected because of the variation of the
  solution with t but is still modest.

These properties are reflected in Figs. 6.2 to 6.6 that follow (produced by Listing 6.2 with ncase=2).

Figure 6.2 indicates that the solution to eqs. (6.1) has a sustained
oscillation. This oscillation is further elucidated in Figs. 6.3–6.6 with
the plotting of the concentrations of the four components H^+, acetylcholine, choline, and acetate, respectively. Note in particular (i) in
Fig. 6.3, the H^+ concentration in compartment 1 has little variation compared to compartment 2 and (ii) the choline concentration
in Fig. 6.5 has little variation in both compartments 1 and 2. These
properties indicate the complexity of the solutions of eqs. (6.1). In

TABLE 6.4 Abbreviated output from Listings 6.1 and 6.2 for ncase=2.

ncase = 2	y1f = 6.000000e-03		
t	y[1]	y[2]	y[3]	y[4]
	y[5]	y[6]	y[7]	y[8]

t	y[1]	y[2]	y[3]	y[4]
0.00	0.00380	0.14058	3.89713	0.28019
	3.23300	1.16060	8.25173	4.96061
0.50	0.00212	0.00706	3.91235	0.73619
	3.23276	1.15850	8.24412	4.73246
1.00	0.00228	0.00915	4.15508	1.30369
	3.23070	1.15634	8.12267	4.44852
.	.			.
.	.			.
.	.			.

Output for t = 1.50 to 18.5 removed

t	y[1]	y[2]	y[3]	y[4]
.	.			.
.	.			.
.	.			.
19.00	0.00615	0.38764	4.11515	0.14269
	3.23080	1.16064	8.14265	5.02940
19.50	0.00510	0.31370	4.02265	0.16012
	3.23147	1.16065	8.18893	5.02068
20.00	0.00440	0.24589	3.95694	0.18593
	3.23197	1.16062	8.22181	5.00777

ncall = 1788

summary, the small change in h1f from ncase=1 to ncase=2 causes a significant departure of the solution from the equilibrium condition with no change in t. The solution of Fig. 6.2 can be characterized as a sustained oscillation. If h1f is changed to other values (than h1f=0.00600 for ncase=2), the solution can change character

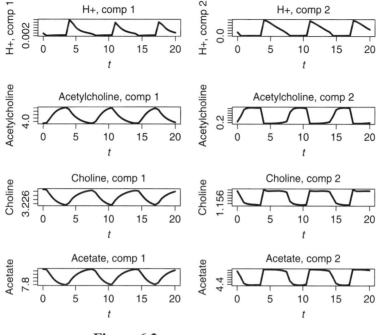

Figure 6.2 $y_1, \ldots, y_8$ versus t.

completely, such as a damped transient to an equilibrium point (rather than a sustained oscillation).

6.4.3   Analysis of the Terms in the ODEs

In order to have a more complete understanding of how parameter changes affect the model solution, we can consider the individual RHS terms in the ODEs. For example, we observed that a change in h1f from 0.0062682 to 0.006000 produced a change in the derivative $dy_1(t = 0)/dt$ from 1.986102e-07 (essentially zero) to -0.07158034 (a significant nonzero value). To understand how this happened, we can examine the individual RHS terms of eq. (6.1a) that are readily computed and displayed by using the numerical solution to eqs. (6.1). To illustrate this procedure, we add the following code to the end of Listing 6.2 (which also includes an analysis of $dy_2(t)/dt$ so that the pH in both compartments can be considered).

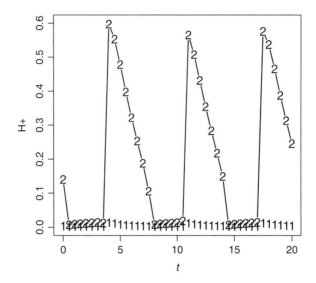

Figure 6.3 y_1, y_2 versus t.

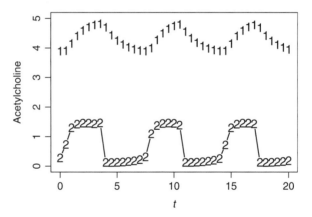

Figure 6.4 y_3, y_4 versus t.

```
#
# Analysis of dy1/dt, dy2/dt, reaction rates, pH
#
# Declare (preallocate) arrays
#
# Three RHS terms
  term11=rep(0,nout);
  term21=rep(0,nout);
```

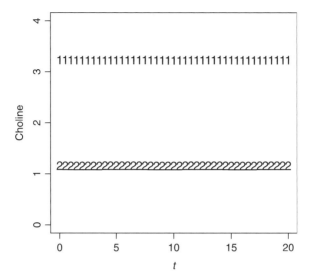

Figure 6.5 y_5, y_6 versus t.

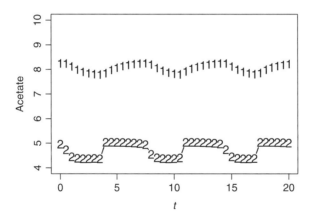

Figure 6.6 y_7, y_8 versus t.

```
term31=rep(0,nout);
dy1dt =rep(0,nout);
term12=rep(0,nout);
term22=rep(0,nout);
term32=rep(0,nout);
dy2dt =rep(0,nout);
#
```

```
# Reaction rates
  rate1=rep(0,nout);
  rate2=rep(0,nout);
#
# pH
  pH1=rep(0,nout);
  pH2=rep(0,nout);
#
# Step through the {\tt nout} values of t
  for(it in 1:nout){
#
#   r1,r2
    rate1[it]=c5*yn[it,7]*yn[it,5]/(c1*c2*(1+yn[it,1]+
        delta*yn[it,1]^2)/
               yn[it,1]+c4*yn[it,7]+c2*yn[it,5]+c3*yn[it,
                 5]*yn[it,7]);
    rate2[it]=yn[it,4]/(yn[it,4]+(1+yn[it,2]+delta*yn[it,
        2]^2)/yn[it,2]+
               alpha*yn[it,4]^2);
#
#   dy1/dt
    term11[it]=y1f-gamma*(1/y1f);
    term21[it]=-alphaH*(yn[it,1]-yn[it,2]);
    term31[it]=alphaOH*gamma*(1/yn[it,1]-1/yn[it,2]);
     dy1dt[it]=term11[it]+term21[it]+term31[it];
#
#   dy2/dt
    term12[it]=alphaH*(yn[it,1]-yn[it,2]);
    term22[it]=-alphaOH*gamma*(1/yn[it,1]-1/yn[it,2]);
    term32[it]=(yn[it,2]-gamma/yn[it,2])+B2*rate2[it]/kh1;
     dy2dt[it]=(term12[it]+term22[it]+term32[it])*vr;
#
#   pH
    pH1[it]=-log10(yn[it,1]*kh1);
    pH2[it]=-log10(yn[it,2]*kh1);
  }
#
# r1,r2
  par(mfrow=c(1,1))
  plot(tm,rate2,xlab="t",ylab="r1,r2",xlim=c(0,20),
  type="b",lty=1,pch="2",lwd=2,main="r1,r2",)
```

```
  lines(tm,rate1,type="b",lty=1,pch="1",lwd=2)
#
# dy1(t)/dt
#
# term1
  par(mfrow=c(2,2))
  plot(tm,term11,xlab="t",ylab="term1",xlim=c(0,20),
  type="l",lwd=2,main="dy1/dt, term1")
#
# term2
  plot(tm,term21,xlab="t",ylab="term2",xlim=c(0,20),
  type="l",lwd=2,main="dy1/dt, term2")
#
# term3
  plot(tm,term31,xlab="t",ylab="term3",xlim=c(0,20),
  type="l",lwd=2,main="dy1/dt, term3")
#
# dy1/dt
  plot(tm,dy1dt,xlab="t",ylab="dy1/dt",xlim=c(0,20),
  type="l",lwd=2,main="dy1/dt")
#
# dy2(t)/dt
#
# term1
  par(mfrow=c(2,2))
  plot(tm,term12,xlab="t",ylab="term1",xlim=c(0,20),
  type="l",lwd=2,main="dy2/dt, term1")
#
# term2
  plot(tm,term22,xlab="t",ylab="term2",xlim=c(0,20),
  type="l",lwd=2,main="dy2/dt, term2")
#
# term3
  plot(tm,term32,xlab="t",ylab="term3",xlim=c(0,20),
  type="l",lwd=2,main="dy2/dt, term3")
#
# dy1/dt
  plot(tm,dy2dt,xlab="t",ylab="dy2/dt",xlim=c(0,20),
  type="l",lwd=2,main="dy2/dt")
#
# pH1,pH2
```

```
par(mfrow=c(1,1))
plot(tm,pH2,xlab="t",ylab="pH1,pH2",xlim=c(0,20),
ylim=c(6,8.7),type="b",lty=1,pch="2",lwd=2,main="pH1,
   pH2",)
lines(tm,pH1,type="b",lty=1,pch="1",lwd=2)
```

Listing 6.3 Additional code added to the main program of
Listing 6.2.

We can note the following details of Listing 6.3.

• A series of rep statements are used to define arrays for the RHS
  terms of eqs. (6.1a) and (6.1b) (term11 to dy2/dt), the reaction
  rates of eqs. (6.2) (rate1 and rate2), and the *pH* corresponding
  to the hydrogen ion concentrations of the two compartments,
  y_1, y_2 (ph1,ph2).
• A for with index it is used to step through the 41 values of t. At
  each value of t, the various terms are calculated. For example, r_1
  and r_2 of eqs. (6.2) are calculated as rate1[it] and rate2[it],
  respectively. term11[it], term21[it], and term31[it] are calculated as the three RHS terms of eq. (6.1a) and these terms
  are then summed as dy1dt[it] according to eq. (6.1a). Note
  that the common factor vr in eq. (6.1b) is used in the calculation of dy2dt[it]. ph1[it] and ph2[it] are calculated from the
  equilibrium constant kh1 ([1]).
• After the various arrays are filled within the for, they are plotted
  against t, starting with rate1 and ending with ph2. rate2 is
  plotted first and then rate1 because the former has the larger
  range that is accommodated by automatic scaling of the vertical
  axis. Also, ph2 is plotted first with the scaling ylim=c(6,8.7)
  for the vertical axis followed by ph1 so that ph1 and ph2 appear
  in the composite plot with clear resolution.
• In all of the plots, pch=1 and pch=2 are used to identify compartments 1 and 2.

The plots that result from Listing 6.3 are in Figs. 6.7–6.10.

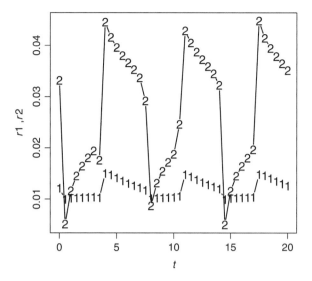

Figure 6.7 r_1, r_2 versus t.

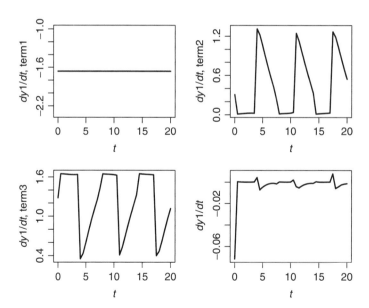

Figure 6.8   Components of dy_1/dt versus t from eq. (6.1a).

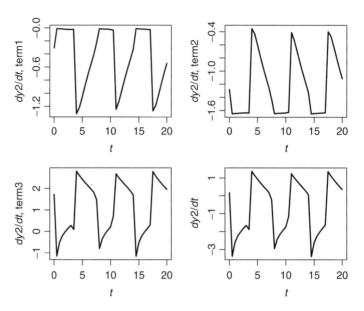

Figure 6.9   Components of dy_2/dt versus t from eq. (6.1b).

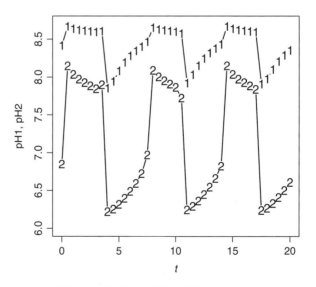

Figure 6.10   pH1, pH2 versus t.

The reaction rates of eqs. (6.2) have a sustained oscillation, with r_2 as the larger rate. `term1` in eq. (6.1a) is a constant. `term2` and `term3` have sustained oscillations. The three terms sum according to eq. (6.1a) to give a complicated dy_1/dt. For dy_2/dt of eq. (6.1b), `term1`,`term2`,`term3`, and `dy2/dt` all have sustained oscillations. `ph1` and `ph2` also have sustained oscillations, with `ph2` having a larger amplitude.

Clearly the solutions of eqs. (6.1a) and (6.1b) are complicated, but this type of graphical analysis can provide insight into the nature of the dynamics and how it changes with changes in the model ICs and parameters (and even changes in the RHS terms of eqs. (6.1)). Thus, experimentation with the model is facilitated, for example, in attempting to fit the solutions to experimental data.

In summary, the discussion of the model of eqs. (6.1) provides the following general conclusions:

- `h1f` is a sensitive parameter in the sense that the features of the solution to eqs. (6.1) change quite dramatically with small changes in `h1f`. This sensitivity illustrates a major benefit of mathematical modeling, that is, important parameters can be identified for further study. The values of `h1f` that are investigated in `ncase=1,2` are suggested in [5], which provides a detailed discussion of the model.

- The model of eqs. (6.1) has a set of parameters that could be investigated numerically (see the `Parameters` section of Listing 6.2). A parameter investigation and possibly a variation of the ODEs can, in principle, lead to a mathematical model that produces solutions that are consistent with experimental observations and thereby elucidate the essential features of the acetylcholine neurocycle.

- Ideally, this iterative process of model development will lead to improved insight into the causes of neurodegenerative diseases that can be used in the development of new therapies.

6.5 ODE/PDE Model

The ODE model of eqs. (6.1) could be extended in two ways.

- The mass transfer terms in eqs. (6.1) can be considered as approximations to the diffusion PDE as detailed in the following table.

Equation	Mass Transfer Term	Diffusion Term
(6.1a)	$-\alpha_H(y_1 - y_2)$	$-D_{12}\dfrac{y_1 - y_2}{z_m}$
(6.1b)	$-\alpha_H(y_2 - y_1)$	$-D_{12}\dfrac{y_2 - y_1}{z_m}$
(6.1c)	$-\alpha_{s1}(y_3 - y_4)$	$-D_{34}\dfrac{y_3 - y_4}{z_m}$
(6.1d)	$-\alpha_{s1}(y_4 - y_3)$	$-D_{34}\dfrac{y_4 - y_3}{z_m}$
(6.1e)	$-\alpha_{s2}(y_5 - y_6)$	$-D_{56}\dfrac{y_5 - y_6}{z_m}$
(6.1f)	$-\alpha_{s2}(y_6 - y_5)$	$-D_{56}\dfrac{y_6 - y_5}{z_m}$
(6.1g)	$-\alpha_{s3}(y_7 - y_8)$	$-D_{78}\dfrac{y_7 - y_8}{z_m}$
(6.1h)	$-\alpha_{s3}(y_8 - y_7)$	$-D_{78}\dfrac{y_8 - y_7}{z_m}$

Here, we have used a finite difference (FD) approximation of Fick's first law

$$j = -D\frac{\partial y}{\partial z} \approx -D\frac{\Delta y}{\Delta z}$$

where D is a diffusivity for the membrane and $\Delta z = z_m$ is the membrane thickness. This approach has the advantage that (i) the diffusivity may be more readily available than a mass transfer coefficient and (ii) the membrane is characterized in terms of its thickness, z_m.

Eqs. (6.1) can then be restated with the membrane diffusion terms as

$$\frac{dy_1}{dt} = y_{1f} - \gamma(1/y_{1f}) - D_{12}(y_1 - y_2)/z_m + \alpha_{OH}\gamma(1/y_1 - 1/y_2) \tag{6.3a}$$

$$\frac{dy_2}{dt} = [-D_{12}(y_2 - y_1)/z_m - \alpha_{OH}\gamma(1/y_1 - 1/y_2) - (y_2 - \gamma/y_2)$$
$$+ B_2 r_2/k_{h1}]v_r \tag{6.3b}$$

$$\frac{dy_3}{dt} = y_{3f} - D_{34}(y_3 - y_4)/z_m + B_1 r_1/k_{s1} \tag{6.3c}$$

$$\frac{dy_4}{dt} = [-D_{34}(y_4 - y_3)/z_m - y_4 - B_2 r_2/k_{s1}]v_r \tag{6.3d}$$

$$\frac{dy_5}{dt} = y_{5f} + Ry_6 - D_{56}(y_5 - y_6)/z_m - B_1 r_1/s_{2ref} \tag{6.3e}$$

$$\frac{dy_6}{dt} = [-D_{56}(y_6 - y_5)/z_m - (1 + R)y_6 + B_2 r_2/s_{2ref}]v_r \tag{6.3f}$$

$$\frac{dy_7}{dt} = y_{7f} - D_{78}(y_7 - y_8)/z_m - B_1 r_1/s_{3ref} \tag{6.3g}$$

$$\frac{dy_8}{dt} = [-D_{78}(y_8 - y_7)/z_m - y_8 + B_2 r_2/s_{3ref}]v_r \tag{6.3h}$$

- The membrane can be represented with a diffusion PDE, that is, Fick's second law, rather than in terms of a mass transfer coefficient or an FD approximation as detailed in the following table.

	Mass	
Equation	Transfer Term	Diffusion Term
(6.1a)	$-\alpha_H(y_1 - y_2)$	$j_{12}(z = 0, t) = -D_{12}\dfrac{\partial y_{12}(z = 0, t)}{\partial z}$
(6.1b)	$-\alpha_H(y_2 - y_1)$	$j_{12}(z = z_m, t) = -D_{12}\dfrac{\partial y_{12}(z = z_m, t)}{\partial z}$
(6.1c)	$-\alpha_{s1}(y_3 - y_4)$	$j_{34}(z = 0, t) = -D_{34}\dfrac{\partial y_{34}(z = 0, t)}{\partial z}$
(6.1d)	$-\alpha_{s1}(y_4 - y_3)$	$j_{34}(z = z_m, t) = -D_{34}\dfrac{\partial y_{34}(z = z_m, t)}{\partial z}$
(6.1e)	$-\alpha_{s2}(y_5 - y_6)$	$j_{56}(z = 0, t) = -D_{56}\dfrac{\partial y_{56}(z = 0, t)}{\partial z}$
(6.1f)	$-\alpha_{s2}(y_6 - y_5)$	$j_{56}(z = z_m, t) = -D_{56}\dfrac{\partial y_{56}(z = z_m, t)}{\partial z}$
(6.1g)	$-\alpha_{s3}(y_7 - y_8)$	$j_{78}(z = 0, t) = -D_{78}\dfrac{\partial y_{78}(z = 0, t)}{\partial z}$
(6.1h)	$-\alpha_{s3}(y_8 - y_7)$	$j_{78}(z = z_m, t) = -D_{78}\dfrac{\partial y_{78}(z = z_m, t)}{\partial z}$

where the spatial variable z represents position in the membrane, $0 \le z \le z_m$ and y_{12}, y_{34}, y_{56}, and y_{78} are concentrations within the membrane.

Eqs. (6.1) now become a system of ODEs/PDEs.

$$\frac{dy_1}{dt} = y_{1f} - \gamma(1/y_{1f}) - j_{12}(z = 0, t)$$
$$+ \alpha_{OH}\gamma(1/y_1 - 1/y_2) \tag{6.4a}$$

$$\frac{dy_2}{dt} = [j_{12}(z = z_m, t) - \alpha_{OH}\gamma(1/y_1 - 1/y_2)$$
$$- (y_2 - \gamma/y_2) + B_2 r_2/k_{h1}]v_r \tag{6.4b}$$

$$\frac{dy_3}{dt} = y_{3f} - j_{34}(z = 0, t) + B_1 r_1/k_{s1} \tag{6.4c}$$

$$\frac{dy_4}{dt} = [j_{34}(z = z_m, t) - y_4 - B_2 r_2/k_{s1}]v_r \qquad (6.4d)$$

$$\frac{dy_5}{dt} = y_{5f} + Ry_6 - j_{56}(z = 0, t) - B_1 r_1/s_{2ref} \qquad (6.4e)$$

$$\frac{dy_6}{dt} = [j_{56}(z = z_m, t) - (1 + R)y_6 + B_2 r_2/s_{2ref}]v_r$$
$$(6.4f)$$

$$\frac{dy_7}{dt} = y_{7f} - j_{78}(z = 0, t) - B_1 r_1/s_{3ref} \qquad (6.4g)$$

$$\frac{dy_8}{dt} = [j_{78}(z = z_m, t) - y_8 + B_2 r_2/s_{3ref}]v_r \qquad (6.4h)$$

$$\frac{\partial y_{12}}{\partial t} = D_{12}\frac{\partial^2 y_{12}}{\partial z^2}$$
$$y_{12}(z = 0, t) = y_1; \; y_{12}(z = z_m, t) = y_2; \; y_{12}(z, t = 0) = y_{12,0}$$
$$(6.5a,b,c,d)$$

$$\frac{\partial y_{34}}{\partial t} = D_{34}\frac{\partial^2 y_{34}}{\partial z^2}$$
$$y_{34}(z = 0, t) = y_3; \; y_{34}(z = z_m, t) = y_4; \; y_{34}(z, t = 0) = y_{34,0}$$
$$(6.6a,b,c,d)$$

$$\frac{\partial y_{34}}{\partial t} = D_{34}\frac{\partial^2 y_{34}}{\partial z^2}$$
$$y_{56}(z = 0, t) = y_5; \; y_{56}(z = z_m, t) = y_6; \; y_{56}(z, t = 0) = y_{56,0}$$
$$(6.7a,b,c,d)$$

$$\frac{\partial y_{78}}{\partial t} = D_{78}\frac{\partial^2 y_{78}}{\partial z^2}$$
$$y_{78}(z = 0, t) = y_7; \; y_{78}(z = z_m, t) = y_8; \; y_{78}(z, t = 0) = y_{78,0}$$
$$(6.8a,b,c,d)$$

This model is diagrammed in Fig. 6.11.

The ODE/PDE model of eqs. (6.4)–(6.8) might provide a more detailed representation of the membrane than that of eqs. (6.1), for

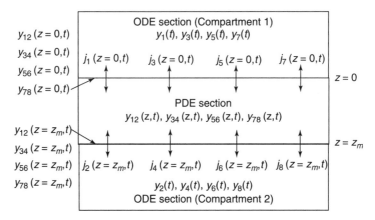

Figure 6.11   Diagram for the model of eqs. (6.4)–(6.8).

example, since the membrane thickness and diffusional resistance to mass transfer are explicitly included. Furthermore, the method of lines (MOL) is well suited for the implementation of the ODE/PDE model such as eqs. (6.4)–(6.8), so this extension is amenable to computer MOL analysis.

This chapter concludes with a discussion of a computational method, the DLM method, for the calculation of an equilibrium IC vector for eqs. (6.1), including the IC vector of Table 6.2. This discussion in Appendix A1 includes a set of R routines for the DLM method that can be applied to a system of nonlinear algebraic equations such as the 8×8 system from eqs. (6.1) with the LHS derivative vector set to zero.

Appendix A1: IC Vector by a Differential Levenberg Marquardt Method

The solution of the nonlinear algebraic equations resulting from setting the LHS derivatives of eqs. (6.1) to zero requires the use of a numerical nonlinear equation solver. Typically, this is some variant of Newton's method that requires the Jacobian matrix of the algebraic system.

A1.1   ODE Jacobian Matrix

To discuss these ideas, we consider the general $n \times n$ (n equations in n unknowns) ODE system[1]

$$\frac{d\mathbf{y}}{dt} = \mathbf{f}(\mathbf{y}, t) \tag{6.9}$$

where

$$\mathbf{y} = \begin{bmatrix} y_1 \\ y_2 \\ \vdots \\ y_n \end{bmatrix}$$

is the dependent variable vector,

$$\frac{d\mathbf{y}}{dt} = \begin{bmatrix} dy_1/dt \\ dy_2/dt \\ \vdots \\ dy_n/dt \end{bmatrix}$$

is the LHS derivative vector, and

$$\mathbf{f} = \begin{bmatrix} f_1(y_1, y_2, ..., y_n, t) \\ f_2(y_1, y_2, ..., y_n, t) \\ \vdots \\ f_n(y_1, y_2, ..., y_n, t) \end{bmatrix}$$

is the RHS function vector. For eqs. (6.1), $\mathbf{y} = [y_1, y_2, \ldots, y_8]^T$ (T denotes a transpose) and $\mathbf{f}$ is the vector of the eight RHS functions.

The Jacobian matrix of the ODE system of eq. (6.9) is

$$\mathbf{J} = \begin{bmatrix} \partial f_1/\partial y_1 & \partial f_1/\partial y_2 & \cdots & \partial f_1/\partial y_n \\ \partial f_2/\partial y_1 & \partial f_2/\partial y_2 & \cdots & \partial f_2/\partial y_n \\ & & \ddots & \\ \partial f_n/\partial y_1 & \partial f_n/\partial y_2 & \cdots & \partial f_n/\partial y_n \end{bmatrix} \tag{6.10}$$

---

[1]We use boldface notation for a vector or matrix.

We now proceed to the ODE Jacobian matrix consisting of the partial derivatives of the RHSs of eqs. (6.1) with respect to each of the dependent variables $y_1, \ldots, y_8$. The 8×8 Jacobian matrix has a typical element $\mathbf{J}(i,j)$ where i is the index for the ODE and j is the index for the dependent variable. Thus, $\mathbf{J}(1,1)$ pertains to eq. (6.1a) and y_1.

For eq. (6.1a) with the RHS function

$$y_{1f} - \gamma(1/y_{1f}) - \alpha_H(y_1 - y_2) + \alpha_{OH}\gamma(1/y_1 - 1/y_2)$$

the elements of the Jacobian matrix $\mathbf{J}(1,1), \ldots, \mathbf{J}(1,8)$ is as follows.

$$\mathbf{J}(1,1) = -\alpha_H + \alpha_{OH}\gamma(-1/y_1^2) \tag{6.11a}$$

$$\mathbf{J}(1,2) = \alpha_H + \alpha_{OH}\gamma(1/y_2^2) \tag{6.11b}$$

$$\mathbf{J}(1,3) = \mathbf{J}(1,4) = \mathbf{J}(1,5) = \mathbf{J}(1,6) = \mathbf{J}(1,7) = \mathbf{J}(1,8) = 0 \tag{6.11c}$$

A similar analysis of eqs. (6.1b)–(6.1h) gives the elements of the Jacobian matrix $\mathbf{J}(2,1), \mathbf{J}(2,2), \ldots, \mathbf{J}(8,7), \mathbf{J}(8,8)$, including the use of eqs. (6.3) and (6.4) where the reaction rates r_1 and r_2 are differentiated. The details are not given here because they appear in the Jacobian matrix routine `jacob_1` discussed subsequently. With this definition of the 8×8 ODE Jacobian matrix of eqs. (6.1), we can proceed with the calculation of an IC vector for eqs. (6.1).

A1.2 Newton's Method

The solution of the nonlinear algebraic system (from eqs. (6.1) with the LHSs set to zero) can be attempted by the classical Newton's method

$$\mathbf{J}(\mathbf{y})\Delta\mathbf{y} = -\mathbf{f}(\mathbf{y}) \tag{6.12a}$$

where $\Delta\mathbf{y}$ is a vector of Newton corrections. Equation (6.12a) is applied iteratively as

$$\mathbf{J}(\mathbf{y}^i)\Delta\mathbf{y}^{i+1} = -\mathbf{f}(\mathbf{y}^i) \tag{6.12b}$$

where i is an iteration counter, $i = 0, 1, 2, \ldots$ with $i = 0$ corresponding to an initial estimate of the solution. Equation (6.12b) is a linear algebraic system for the Newton corrections Δy^{i+1}. After this vector of corrections is computed, the solution vector is updated as

$$y^{i+1} = y^i + \Delta y^{i+1} \qquad (6.12c)$$

and eq. (6.12b) is repeated with the updated solution vector of eq. (6.12c) used as y^i.

Equation (6.12a) is quadratically convergent (the rate of convergence is proportional to the square of the distance from the final solution) and can be very effective, but it can also have some possible shortcomings.

- If J is singular, then Δy is undefined, that is, the problem is *singular*.
- If J is near singular (e.g., because of the finite word length of the computer), the problem is *ill-conditioned* and the calculation of Δy fails or is inaccurate.
- If J is not ill-conditioned, but Δy is large, the calculation of successive values of y may be unstable (some form of "damping" may be required to limit Δy).

The problems of ill-conditioning of J are emphasized through the alternate form of eq. (6.12a)

$$\Delta y = -J^{-1}(y)f(y) \qquad (6.12d)$$

In particular, note that J^{-1} precludes a solution if J is ill-conditioned. Newton's method is generally used in the form of eq. (6.12a) and not eq. (6.12d), that is, J^{-1} is not actually computed; the two forms are mathematically equivalent, but (6.12a) can be more efficient computationally.

We will not attempt the use of eq. (6.12a) for the solution of the nonlinear algebraic system but rather consider some extensions, finally arriving at the DLM method that is then used for the solution of the nonlinear 8×8 algebraic system stemming from eq. (6.1).

A1.3 Steepest Descent Method

The steepest descent method is (in analogy with eq. (6.12d))

$$\Delta \mathbf{y} = -\mathbf{J}^T(\mathbf{y})\mathbf{f}(\mathbf{y}) \tag{6.13a}$$

$-\mathbf{J}^T\mathbf{f}$ is a descent direction and is, in fact, the steepest descent direction.

Note that $\mathbf{J}^{-1}$ is not required in using eq. (6.13a), that is, steepest descent can get past points where $\mathbf{J}$ is singular or ill-conditioned. This is the principal advantage of steepest descent. The disadvantages are

- Slow convergence (relative to Newton's method);
- Convergence to a local minimum rather than a solution to the original nonlinear problem.

The second point will now be analyzed briefly.

The origin of eq. (6.13a) can be explained through a sum of squares of the equation residuals, ss [1]

$$ss(y_1, y_2, \ldots, y_n) = \sum_{i=1}^{n} r_i(y_1, y_2, \ldots, y_n)^2 = \sum_{i=1}^{n} \left[\frac{dy_i(y_1, y_2, \ldots, y_n)}{dt} \right]^2$$

$$= \sum_{i=1}^{n} f_i(y_1, y_2, \ldots, y_n)^2 \tag{6.13b}$$

where dy_i/dt and f_i refer to eq. (6.9). We then seek the dependent variable vector $y_1, y_2, \ldots, y_n$ that minimizes ss. Note that $ss = 0$ implies that the equations are satisfied exactly in the sense that all of the RHS functions $f_1, f_2, \ldots, f_n$ of eq. (6.9) are zero, and thus, all of the LHS derivatives $dy_1/dt, dy_2/dt, \ldots, dy_n/dt$ are zero. In other words, we seek to closely achieve the condition $ss = 0$.

To minimize ss, we impose the first-order (necessary) conditions

$$\frac{\partial ss(y_1, y_2, \ldots, y_n)}{\partial y_j} = \sum_{i=1}^{n} 2f_i \frac{\partial f_i}{\partial y_j} = 0, \; j = 1, 2, \ldots, n \tag{6.13c}$$

The second summation can be written in expanded form as

$$f_1 \frac{\partial f_1}{\partial y_1} + f_2 \frac{\partial f_2}{\partial y_1} + \cdots + f_n \frac{\partial f_n}{\partial y_1} = 0$$

$$f_1 \frac{\partial f_1}{\partial y_2} + f_2 \frac{\partial f_2}{\partial y_2} + \cdots + f_n \frac{\partial f_n}{\partial y_2} = 0$$

$$\vdots$$

$$f_1 \frac{\partial f_1}{\partial y_n} + f_2 \frac{\partial f_2}{\partial y_n} + \cdots + f_n \frac{\partial f_n}{\partial y_n} = 0 \tag{6.13d}$$

or in matrix form

$$\begin{bmatrix} \partial f_1/\partial y_1 & \partial f_2/\partial y_1 & \cdots & \partial f_n/\partial y_1 \\ \partial f_1/\partial y_2 & \partial f_2/\partial y_2 & \cdots & \partial f_n/\partial y_2 \\ & & \ddots & \\ \partial f_1/\partial y_n & \partial f_2/\partial y_n & \cdots & \partial f_n/\partial y_n \end{bmatrix} \begin{bmatrix} f_1 \\ f_2 \\ \vdots \\ f_n \end{bmatrix} = \begin{bmatrix} 0 \\ 0 \\ \vdots \\ 0 \end{bmatrix} \tag{6.13e}$$

or

$$\mathbf{J}^T \mathbf{f} = \mathbf{0} \tag{6.13f}$$

where T denotes a transpose (note the interchange of the rows and columns of $\mathbf{J}$ and $\mathbf{J}^T$ of eqs. (6.10) and (6.13e)). Thus, ss will be minimized if $\mathbf{J}^T \mathbf{f} = \mathbf{0}$ (a necessary condition). Away from the minimum point, we can use eq. (6.13a) as a discrete stepping algorithm to approach the minimum (the method of steepest descent). Note that this algorithm does not necessarily lead to the minimum point $dy_1/dt = dy_2/dt = \cdots = dy_n/dt = 0$, but rather, only to a point where ss is minimized (i.e., a local minimum).

A1.4   The Levenberg Marquardt Method

The Levenberg Marquardt [3, 4] method is an attempt to combine the advantages of Newton's and the steepest descent methods (rapid convergence with Newton's method, avoidance of a singular system with steepest descent).

$$[(1 - \mu)\mathbf{J}^T \mathbf{J} + \mu \mathbf{I}]\Delta \mathbf{y} = -\mathbf{J}^T \mathbf{f} \tag{6.14}$$

where $\mathbf{I}$ is the identity matrix.

The embedding of the parameter μ [1, 2] provides the following limiting cases.

- $\mu = 0$: Newton's method
- $\mu = 1$: Steepest descent

Intermediate values $(0 < \mu < 1)$ provide a linear combination of Newton's method and steepest descent. The value of μ can be determined by trial and error to arrive at an effective algorithm for the solution of the nonlinear equations.

A1.5 Differential Newton's Method

The steeping formulas for the three methods, Newton's, steepest descent, and Levenberg Marquardt, that is, eqs. (6.12d), (6.13a), and (6.14), respectively, define a vector of finite corrections, $\Delta \mathbf{y}$. These finite corrections might be too large (and, therefore, would require some attenuation or damping to maintain a stable calculation). We now consider how these finite changes can be replaced by differential changes that will better control the process of converging to a solution. For example, eq. (6.12a) can be changed to the differential equation

$$\mathbf{J}\frac{d\mathbf{y}}{dt} = -\mathbf{f} \tag{6.15a}$$

Equation (6.15a) is a system of implicit ODEs, usually termed the Davidenko ODE (it is implicit because the LHS is a linear combination of derivatives rather than just a single derivative in each ODE). Thus, eq. (6.15a) requires a numerical ODE integrator for implicit ODEs.

The alternate form

$$\frac{d\mathbf{y}}{dt} = -\mathbf{J}^{-1}\mathbf{f} \tag{6.15b}$$

can be used to avoid the coupling between the LHS derivatives. t can be considered as a continuation parameter. For $t = 0$, an IC vector is specified for eq. (6.15b). For large t, the condition $dy/dt \approx 0$ implies the solution $\mathbf{f} = \mathbf{0}$; the corresponding $\mathbf{y}$ is the solution of the problem of interest for a particular $\mathbf{f}$.

Equations (6.15a) and (6.15b) have the advantage that the ODE integrator now determines the changes in $\mathbf{y}$ rather than using a finite step that might have to be adjusted (damped, attenuated) to maintain a stable calculation. In other words, eqs. (6.15a) and (6.15b) have the advantage of using a library integrator for the ODEs with the attendant automatic adjustment of the integration interval in t.

Equations (6.15a) and (6.15b) has been used to good effect for the solution of a spectrum of nonlinear problems. The principal limitation is that $\mathbf{J}$ cannot become ill-conditioned as the solution proceeds (as with Newton's method, eq. (6.12d)).

A1.6   Differential Steepest Descent Method

Equation (6.13a) can also be put into differential form.

$$\frac{d\mathbf{y}}{dt} = -\mathbf{J}^T \mathbf{f} \tag{6.16}$$

An IC can be specified for eq. (6.16) and the integration in t carried out until $dy/dt \approx 0$, which (ideally) implies the solution $\mathbf{f} = \mathbf{0}$; the corresponding $\mathbf{y}$ is then the solution to the problem of interest for a particular $\mathbf{f}$. However, $dy/dt \approx 0$ can also come about from $\mathbf{J}^T \mathbf{f} = 0$ (from eq. (6.16)), which is the minimization condition (6.13f) that does not necessarily give $\mathbf{f} = \mathbf{0}$ (the nonuniqueness problem). We, therefore, proceed to a differential form of the Levenberg Marquardt method.

A1.7   Differential Levenberg Marquardt Method

The differential form of eq. (6.14) (the DLM [1, 2] method) is

$$[(1 - \mu)\mathbf{J}^T \mathbf{J} + \mu \mathbf{I}]\frac{d\mathbf{y}}{dt} = -\mathbf{J}^T \mathbf{f} \tag{6.17a}$$

or

$$\frac{d\mathbf{y}}{dt} = -[(1 - \mu)\mathbf{J}^T \mathbf{J} + \mu \mathbf{I}]^{-1}\mathbf{J}^T \mathbf{f} \tag{6.17b}$$

Equation (6.17b) can be integrated numerically, starting from an IC

$$y(t = 0) = y_0 \tag{6.17c}$$

Integration to $dy/dt \approx 0$ implies $f = 0$. The corresponding y is the solution of interest.

A1.8 Solution for the IC Vector of the 8 × 8 ODE System

We now consider the application of eqs. (6.17b) and (6.17c) to eqs. (6.1) to arrive at an IC vector for these ODEs (corresponding to the LHS derivatives equal to zero). The following discussion is in terms of a set of R routines that implement eqs. (6.17b) and (6.17c). In particular, eq. (6.17b) requires the Jacobian matrix of eqs. (6.1) which in turn requires the partial derivatives of r_1 and r_2 of eqs. (6.2) with respect to each of the dependent variables $y_1, \ldots, y_8$. From eq. (6.2a) with the RHS function

$$\frac{c_5 y_7 y_5}{c_1 c_2 (1 + y_1 + \delta y_1^2)/y_1 + c_4 y_7 + c_2 y_5 + c_3 y_5 y_7}$$

we have for the partial derivatives of r_1

$$\frac{\partial r_1}{\partial y_1} = \frac{-(c_5 y_7 y_5)[c_1 c_2 (-1/y_1^2 + \delta)]}{[c_1 c_2 (1 + y_1 + \delta y_1^2)/y_1 + c_4 y_7 + c_2 y_5 + c_3 y_5 y_7]^2} \tag{6.18a}$$

$$\frac{\partial r_1}{\partial y_5} = \frac{(c_5 y_7)(c_1 c_2 (1 + y_1 + \delta y_1^2)/y_1 + c_4 y_7 + c_2 y_5 + c_3 y_5 y_7)}{[c_1 c_2 (1 + y_1 + \delta y_1^2)/y_1 + c_4 y_7 + c_2 y_5 + c_3 y_5 y_7]^2} \tag{6.18b}$$

$$\frac{\partial r_1}{\partial y_7} = \frac{(c_5 y_5)(c_1 c_2 (1 + y_1 + \delta y_1^2)/y_1 + c_4 y_7 + c_2 y_5 + c_3 y_5 y_7)}{[c_1 c_2 (1 + y_1 + \delta y_1^2)/y_1 + c_4 y_7 + c_2 y_5 + c_3 y_5 y_7]^2} \tag{6.18c}$$

Note that

$$\frac{\partial r_1}{\partial y_2} = \frac{\partial r_1}{\partial y_3} = \frac{\partial r_1}{\partial y_4} = \frac{\partial r_1}{\partial y_6} = \frac{\partial r_1}{\partial y_8} = 0 \tag{6.18d}$$

Similarly, from eq. (6.2b) with the RHS function

$$\frac{y_4}{y_4 + (1 + y_2 + \delta y_2^2)/y_2 + \alpha y_4^2}$$

we have for the partial derivatives of r_2

$$\frac{\partial r_2}{\partial y_2} = \frac{-y_4(-1/y_2^2 + \delta)}{[y_4 + (1 + y_2 + \delta y_2^2)/y_2 + \alpha y_4^2]^2} \qquad (6.19a)$$

$$\frac{\partial r_2}{\partial y_4} = \frac{(y_4 + (1 + y_2 + \delta y_2^2)/y_2 + \alpha y_4^2) - (y_4)(1 + 2\alpha y_4)}{[y_4 + (1 + y_2 + \delta y_2^2)/y_2 + \alpha y_4^2]^2}$$

$$(6.19b)$$

Note that

$$\frac{\partial r_2}{\partial y_1} = \frac{\partial r_2}{\partial y_3} = \frac{\partial r_2}{\partial y_5} = \frac{\partial r_2}{\partial y_6} = \frac{\partial r_2}{\partial y_7} = \frac{\partial r_2}{\partial y_8} = 0 \qquad (6.19c)$$

A1.8.1 *The Jacobian Matrix Routine* We can now proceed with the programming of the Jacobian matrix of eqs. (6.1) (recall again the discussion of the Jacobian matrix of eqs. (6.1) in Section A1.1). A routine, jacob_1.R, for the calculation of the 8×8 elements of the Jacobian matrix of the RHS vector of eqs. (6.1) is in Listing 6.4.

```
  jacob_1=function(t,y){
#
# Declare (preallocate) Jacobian matrix
  J=matrix(0,nrow=8,ncol=8);
#
# Reaction rates and partial derivatives
  r1=c5*y[7]*y[5]/(c1*c2*(1+y[1]+delta*y[1]^2)/y[1]+c4*
     y[7]+c2*y[5]+
     c3*y[5]*y[7]);
  r2=y[4]/(y[4]+(1+y[2]+delta*y[2]^2)/y[2]+alpha*y[4]^2);
#
# Partial derivatives of r1
  den1=(c1*c2*(1+y[1]+delta*y[1]^2)/y[1]+c4*y[7]+c2*y[5]+
     c3*y[5]*y[7])^2;
  dr1y1= -c5*y[7]*y[5]*(c1*c2*(-1/y[1]^2+delta))/den1;
```

```
    dr1y5=((c1*c2*(1+y[1]+delta*y[1]^2)/y[1]+c4*y[7]+c2*
       y[5]+c3*y[5]*y[7])*
          (c5*y[7])-(c5*y[7]*y[5])*(c2+c3*y[7]))/den1;
    dr1y7=((c1*c2*(1+y[1]+delta*y[1]^2)/y[1]+c4*y[7]+c2*
       y[5]+c3*y[5]*y[7])*
          (c5*y[5])-(c5*y[7]*y[5])*(c4+c3*y[5]))/den1;
#
# Partial derivatives of r2
    den2=(y[4]+(1+y[2]+delta*y[2]^2)/y[2]+alpha*y[4]^2)^2;
    dr2y2= -y[4]*(-1/y[2]^2+delta)/den2;
    dr2y4=((y[4]+(1+y[2]+delta*y[2]^2)/y[2]+alpha*y[4]^2)-
          y[4]*(1+2*alpha*y[4]))/den2;
#
# First row
# y1t=y1f-gamma*(1/y1f)-alphaH*(y1-y2)+alphaOH*gamma*(1/
#    y1-1/y2);
    J[1,1]=-alphaH+alphaOH*gamma*(-1/y[1]^2);
    J[1,2]= alphaH+alphaOH*gamma*( 1/y[2]^2);
    J[1,3]=0;
    J[1,4]=0;
    J[1,5]=0;
    J[1,6]=0;
    J[1,7]=0;
    J[1,8]=0;
#
# Second row
# y2t=(alphaH*(y1-y2)-alphaOH*gamma*(1/y1-1/y2)-
#     (y2-gamma/y2)+B2*r2/kh1)*vr;
    J[2,1]=(alphaH-alphaOH*gamma*(-1/y[1]^2))*vr;
    J[2,2]=(-alphaH+alphaOH*gamma*(1/y[2]^2)-
           (1+gamma/y[2]^2+B2*dr2y2/kh1))*vr;
    J[2,3]=0;
    J[2,4]=-(B2*dr2y4/kh1)*vr;
    J[2,5]=0;
    J[2,6]=0;
    J[2,7]=0;
    J[2,8]=0;
#
# Third row
# y3t= y3f-alphas1*(y3-y4)+B1*r1/ks1;
    J[3,1]=B1*dr1y1/ks1;
```

```
  J[3,2]=0;
  J[3,3]=-alphas1;
  J[3,4]= alphas1;
  J[3,5]=B1*dr1y5/ks1;
  J[3,6]=0;
  J[3,7]=B1*dr1y7/ks1;
  J[3,8]=0;
#
# Fourth row
# y4t=(alphas1*(y3-y4)-y4-B2*r2/ks1)*vr;
  J[4,1]=0;
  J[4,2]=-B2*dr2y2/ks1*vr;
  J[4,3]=alphas1*vr;
  J[4,4]=(-alphas1-1-B2*dr2y4/ks1)*vr;
  J[4,5]=0;
  J[4,6]=0;
  J[4,7]=0;
  J[4,8]=0;
#
# Fifth row
# y5t=y5f+R*y6-alphas2*(y5-y6)-B1*r1/s2ref;
  J[5,1]=-B1*dr1y1/s2ref;
  J[5,2]=0;
  J[5,3]=0;
  J[5,4]=0;
  J[5,5]=-alphas2-B1*dr1y5/s2ref;
  J[5,6]=R+alphas2;
  J[5,7]=-B1*dr1y7/s2ref;
  J[5,8]=0;
#
# Sixth row
# y6t=(alphas2*(y5-y6)-(1+R)*y6+B2*r2/s2ref)*vr;
  J[6,1]=0;
  J[6,2]=B2*dr2y2/s2ref*vr;
  J[6,3]=0;
  J[6,4]=B2*dr2y4/s2ref*vr;
  J[6,5]=alphas2*vr;
  J[6,6]=(-alphas2-(1+R))*vr;
  J[6,7]=0;
  J[6,8]=0;
#
```

```
# Seventh row
# y7t=y7f-alphas3*(y7-y8)-B1*r1/s3ref;
  J[7,1]=-B1*dr1y1/s3ref;
  J[7,2]=0;
  J[7,3]=0;
  J[7,4]=0;
  J[7,5]=-B1*dr1y5/s3ref;
  J[7,6]=0;
  J[7,7]=-alphas3-B1*dr1y7/s3ref;
  J[7,8]=alphas3;
#
# Eighth row
# y8t=(alphas3*(y7-y8)-y8+B2*r2/s3ref)*vr;
  J[8,1]=0;
  J[8,2]=B2*dr2y2/s3ref*vr;
  J[8,3]=0;
  J[8,4]=B2*dr2y4/s3ref*vr;
  J[8,5]=0;
  J[8,6]=0;
  J[8,7]=alphas3*vr;
  J[8,8]=(-alphas3-1)*vr;
#
# Return numerical Jacobian as a matrix
  J <<- J;
#
# End of jacob_1
  }
  }
```

Listing 6.4 jacob_1.R for the Jacobian matrix of eqs. (6.1).

We can note the following details about jacob_1.

- The function and array J for the computed Jacobian matrix are defined.

  ```
  jacob_1=function(t,y){
  #
  # Declare (preallocate) Jacobian matrix
    J=matrix(0,nrow=8,ncol=8);
  ```

- The reaction rates r_1 and r_2 of eqs. (6.2) are computed from the input vector y (second argument of jacob_1 with elements y[1],...,y[8] that are the dependent variables of eqs. (6.1)).

```
r1=c5*y[7]*y[5]/(c1*c2*(1+y[1]+delta*y[1]^2)/y[1]+
    c4*y[7]+c2*y[5]+
    c3*y[5]*y[7]);
r2=y[4]/(y[4]+(1+y[2]+delta*y[2]^2)/y[2]+alpha*
    y[4]^2);
```

Note that the various parameters, for example, c1,alpha, delta, are defined numerically in the ODE routine trans_2 discussed subsequently.

• The partial derivatives of r_1 are computed according to eq. (6.18).

```
#
# Partial derivatives of r1
    den1=(c1*c2*(1+y[1]+delta*y[1]^2)/y[1]+c4*y[7]+c2
        *y[5]+c3*y[5]*y[7])^2;
    dr1y1= -c5*y[7]*y[5]*(c1*c2*(-1/y[1]^2+delta))/den1;
    dr1y5=((c1*c2*(1+y[1]+delta*y[1]^2)/y[1]+c4*y[7]+
        c2*y[5]+c3*y[5]*y[7])*
            (c5*y[7])-(c5*y[7]*y[5])*(c2+c3*y[7]))/den1;
    dr1y7=((c1*c2*(1+y[1]+delta*y[1]^2)/y[1]+c4*y[7]+
        c2*y[5]+c3*y[5]*y[7])*
            (c5*y[5])-(c5*y[7]*y[5])*(c4+c3*y[5]))/den1;
```

• The partial derivatives of r_2 are computed according to eq. (6.19).

```
#
# Partial derivatives of r2
    den2=(y[4]+(1+y[2]+delta*y[2]^2)/y[2]+alpha*
        y[4]^2)^2;
    dr2y2= -y[4]*(-1/y[2]^2+delta)/den2;
    dr2y4=((y[4]+(1+y[2]+delta*y[2]^2)/y[2]+alpha*
        y[4]^2)-
            y[4]*(1+2*alpha*y[4]))/den2;
```

• The partial derivatives of the RHS of eq. (6.1a) are computed.

```
#
# First row
```

```
# y1t=y1f-gamma*(1/y1f)-alphaH*(y1-y2)+alphaOH*gamma
  *(1/y1-1/y2);
J[1,1]=-alphaH+alphaOH*gamma*(-1/y[1]^2);
J[1,2]= alphaH+alphaOH*gamma*( 1/y[2]^2);
J[1,3]=0;
J[1,4]=0;
J[1,5]=0;
J[1,6]=0;
J[1,7]=0;
J[1,8]=0;
```

Eq. (6.1a) is included as a comment to facilitate the programming of the eight partial derivatives

$$\partial(dy_1/dt)/\partial y_1 = J[1,1] = -\text{alpha H}$$
$$+\text{alpha OH} * \text{gamma} * (-1/y[1] \wedge 2)$$

to
$$\partial(dy_1/dt)/\partial y_8 = J[1,8] = 0$$

- Similarly, the partial derivatives for eqs. (6.1b)–(6.1h) are programmed, starting with the statement of the ODE as a comment, that is, J[2,1] to J[8,8].
- The numerical Jacobian matrix, J, is returned to the calling program; in this case, the ODE routine trans_2 discussed subsequently with <<-.

```
#
# Return numerical Jacobian as a matrix
  J <<- J;
```

- jacob_1 is completed with the final }.

```
#
# End of jacob_1
  }
```

J is now available for use in the ODE routine, trans_2, which is discussed next.

A1.8.2 *DLM ODE Routine* With the availability of the Jacobian matrix, the 8×8 ODE system of the DLM method of eq. (6.17b) can now be integrated. The ODE routine trans_2 is in Listing 6.5.

```
  trans_2=function(t,y,parms) {
#
# Access jacob_1.R
  setwd("c:/R/bme_ode/chap6");
  source("jacob_1.R");
#
# Parameters
  y1f=6.2682e-03;  y3f=2.4;        y5f=1.15;        y7f=3.9;
  R=0.8;           gamma=0.01;     vr=1.2;          alpha=
                                                     0.5;
  delta=0.1;       kh1=1.0066e-06; alphaH=2.25;     alphaOH=
                                                     0.5;
  alphas1=1   ;    alphas2=1;      alphas3=1;       B1=5.033
                                                     e-05;
  B2=5.033e-05;    ks1=5.0033e-07; s2ref=1.0e-04;   s3ref=1.0
                                                     e-06;
  c1=2.4;          c2=5;           c3=1;            c4=1000;
  c5=5.2;
#
# Reaction rates
  r1=c5*y[7]*y[5]/(c1*c2*(1+y[1]+delta*y[1]^2)/y[1]+c4*
     y[7]+
     c2*y[5]+c3*y[5]*y[7]);
  r2=y[4]/(y[4]+(1+y[2]+delta*y[2]^2)/y[2]+alpha*y[4]^2);
#
# ODEs
  yt=rep(0,8);
  yt[1]=y1f-gamma*(1/y1f)-alphaH*(y[1]-y[2])+
        alphaOH*gamma*(1/y[1]-1/y[2]);
  yt[2]=(alphaH*(y[1]-y[2])-alphaOH*gamma*(1/y[1]-1/y[2])-
        (y[2]-gamma/y[2])+B2*r2/kh1)*vr;
  yt[3]= y3f-alphas1*(y[3]-y[4])+B1*r1/ks1;
  yt[4]=(alphas1*(y[3]-y[4])-y[4]-B2*r2/ks1)*vr;
  yt[5]=y5f+R*y[6]-alphas2*(y[5]-y[6])-B1*r1/s2ref;
  yt[6]=(alphas2*(y[5]-y[6])-(1+R)*y[6]+B2*r2/s2ref)*vr;
  yt[7]=y7f-alphas3*(y[7]-y[8])-B1*r1/s3ref;
  yt[8]=(alphas3*(y[7]-y[8])-y[8]+B2*r2/s3ref)*vr;
```

```
#
# Jacobian matrix
  jacob_1(t,y);
#
# DLM ODE
  cm=(1-mu)*t(J)%*%J+mu*diag(8);
  yt=-solve(cm)%*%t(J)%*%yt;
#
# Increment calls to trans_2
  ncall <<- ncall+1;
#
# Return numerical derivative vector
  dydt <<- yt
#
# Return derivative vector as list
  return(list(c(yt)));
}
```

Listing 6.5 trans_2 for the DLM eq. (6.17b).

We can note the following details about trans_2.

- The function is defined and the Jacobian matrix routine jacob_1 of Listing 6.4 is accessed.

```
    trans_2=function(t,y,parms) {
#
# Access jacob_1.R
    setwd("c:/R/bme_ode/chap6");
    source("jacob_1.R");
```

- The model parameters are defined numerically (and they are available as global variables one level down for use in jacob_1 in Listing 6.4).
- The reaction rates r_1 and r_2 of eqs. (6.2) and the ODEs, eqs. (6.1), are programmed in the same way as in trans_1 of Listing 6.1.
- jacob_1 (Listing 6.4) computes the Jacobian matrix from the dependent variable vector y, which is the second RHS (input) vector of trans_2.

```
#
# Jacobian matrix
  jacob_1(t,y);
```

Note also that if the Jacobian matrix is an explicit function of
t, it could be included in the call to `jacob_1` because it is the
first RHS (input) argument of `trans_2`. In the case of eqs. (6.1),
t does not appear explicitly so it is not used in the calculation
of the Jacobian matrix. The Jacobian matrix is returned from
`jacob_1` to `trans_2` as the 2D array `J` (see Listing 6.4).

• Equation (6.17b) is programmed with several R vector–matrix
utilities.

```
#
# DLM ODE
  cm=(1-mu)*t(J)%*%J+mu*diag(8);
  yt=-solve(cm)%*%t(J)%*%yt;
```

The individual steps are explained in somewhat more detail as
follows.

— μ in eq. (6.17b) is available numerically from the main program to be discussed.

— J^T (the transpose of J in eq. (6.17b)) is computed as `t(J)`
(`t` is the R transpose operator).

— The product $(1 - \mu)(J^T)J$ in eq. (6.17b) is programmed as

`(1-mu)*t(J)%*%J`

where the single `*` is a scalar–matrix product and `%*%` is a
matrix–matrix product.

— The entire LHS coefficient matrix of eq. (6.17a) is computed
as `cm`.

`cm=(1-mu)*t(J)%*%J+mu*diag(8);`

`diag` is the R utility for the identity matrix, in this case
of dimension 8×8. The close correspondence of this
programming with eq. (6.17a) is clear. This programming

demonstrates the facility of R vector–matrix operations, but equivalent programming would be straightforward in any standard language (e.g., C, C++, Fortran, Java).

— The RHS of eq. (6.17b) is programmed to give the LHS DLM derivative vector yt (not the derivative vector of eqs. (6.1)). solve is the R matrix inverse operator (applied to cm from eq. (6.17b)).

```
yt=-solve(cm)%*%t(J)%*%yt;
```

Note that the derivative vector yt from the preceding programming of the ODEs, denoted as **f** in eq. (6.17b) (for which **f** = **0** is the final desired result), is used in the RHS of this calculation to give a revised DLM yt in the LHS.

— The objective then is to integrate the DLM ODEs until the LHS vector yt essentially equals the zero vector that implies the RHS vector yt is also the zero vector (so that the RHS vector of eqs. (6.1) is the zero vector). Whatever y is at the point is the solution of interest, that is, the values of $y_1, y_2, \ldots, y_8$ that correspond to an equilibrium solution of eqs. (6.1), which can then be used as an IC for eqs. (6.1); in particular, the IC vector of Table 6.2 results from this integration as explained in the following.

• The counter for the calls to trans_2 is incremented.

```
#
# Increment calls to trans_2
  ncall <<- ncall+1;
```

This value is returned to the main program through the <<- where it is displayed at the end of the solution.

• The DLM derivative vector yt is returned to the main program as dydt with <<-. dydt is then available in the main program for numerical and graphical outputs.

```
#
# Return numerical derivative vector
  dydt <<- yt
```

- The DLM derivative vector yt is also returned as a list for use by the ODE integrator, in this case lsodes, in the main program.

```
#
# Return derivative vector as list
  return(list(c(yt)));
}
```

The use of a list (rather than a numerical vector) is generally required by the ODE integrators of deSolve. The final } terminates trans_2.

This completes the programming eq. (6.17b). The main program that uses trans_2 (and thus jacob_1) through lsodes is listed next.

A1.8.3 Main Program
Listing 6.6 is the main program that calls trans_2 of Listing 6.5.

```
#
# Access deSolve library (with lsodes)
  library("deSolve")
#
# ODE routine
  setwd("c:/R/bme_ode/chap6")
  source("trans_2.R")
#
# Select case
#
# ncase = 1 - equilibrium ICs
#
# ncase = 2 - nonequilibrum ICs
#
  ncase=1;
#
# Parameters
  y1f=6.2682e-03;  y3f=2.4;         y5f=1.15;      y7f=3.9;
  R=0.8;           gamma=0.01;      vr=1.2;        alpha=
                                                       0.5;
```

```
  delta=0.1;         kh1=1.0066e-06; alphaH=2.25;   alphaOH=
                                                      0.5;
  alphas1=1  ;       alphas2=1;      alphas3=1;      B1=5.033
                                                      e-05;
  B2=5.033e-05;      ks1=5.0033e-07; s2ref=1.0e-04; s3ref=1.0
                                                      e-06;
  c1=2.4;            c2=5;           c3=1;           c4=1000;
  c5=5.2;
#
# Initial conditions
  y0=rep(0,8);
  if(ncase==1){
  y0[1]=0.003796824;  y0[2]=0.1405804;  y0[3]=3.8971322;
  y0[4]=0.2801880941; y0[5]=3.233;       y0[6]=1.1606;
  y0[7]=8.2517318;    y0[8]=4.960605;
  }
  if(ncase==2){
  y0[1]=1; y0[2]=1; y0[3]=1;
  y0[4]=1; y0[5]=1; y0[6]=1;
  y0[7]=1; y0[8]=1;
  }
#
# Differential Newton's
  tf=20;mu=0;
#
# Differential steepest descent
# tf=20;mu=1;
#
# Differential steepest descent + Newton's
# tf=20;mu=0.5;
#
# Output sequence in t
  nout=41;ncall=0;
  tm=seq(from=0,to=tf,by=tf/(nout-1));
#
# Write heading for y1 to y8
  cat(sprintf("\n ncase = %2d\n\n",ncase));
  cat(sprintf("    t           y[1]          y[2]          y[3]
     y[4]"));
  cat(sprintf("                y[5]          y[6]          y[7]
     y[8]"));
```

```
#
# lsodes ODE integration
  parms=c(rtol=1e-8,atol=1e-8)
  out=lsodes(times=tm,y=y0,func=trans_2,parms=parms)
#
# Numerical output
  yn=matrix(0,nrow=nout,ncol=8);
  for(it in 1:nout){
    if(it==1){yn[1,]=y0;
    }else{
    yn[it,]=out[it,-1];}
    cat(sprintf("%5.2f%12.5f%12.5f%12.5f%12.5f\n",
                tm[it],yn[it,1],yn[it,2],yn[it,3],yn[it,
                  4]));
    cat(sprintf("%17.5f%12.5f%12.5f%12.5f\n\n",
                yn[it,5],yn[it,6],yn[it,7],yn[it,8]));
  }
#
# Calls to trans_2
  cat(sprintf("\n ncall = %5d\n\n",ncall))
#
# Eight plots for y1(t) to y8(t) vs t
#
# y1(t)
# par(mfrow=c(1,1))
  par(mfrow=c(4,2))
  plot(tm,yn[,1],xlab="t",ylab="H+, comp 1",xlim=c(0,tf),
  type="l",lwd=2,main="H+, comp 1")
#
# y2(t)
  plot(tm,yn[,2],xlab="t",ylab="H+, comp 2",xlim=c(0,tf),
  type="l",lwd=2,main="H+, comp 2")
#
# y3(t)
  plot(tm,yn[,3],xlab="t",ylab="acetylcholine",xlim=c(0,
      tf),
  type="l",lwd=2,main="acetylcholine, comp 1")
#
# y4(t)
  plot(tm,yn[,4],xlab="t",ylab="acetylcholine",xlim=c(0,
      tf),
```

```
    type="l",lwd=2,main="acetylcholine, comp 2")
#
# y5(t)
    plot(tm,yn[,5],xlab="t",ylab="choline",xlim=c(0,tf),
    type="l",lwd=2,main="choline, comp 1")
#
# y6(t)
    plot(tm,yn[,6],xlab="t",ylab="choline",xlim=c(0,tf),
    type="l",lwd=2,main="choline, comp 2")
#
# y7(t)
    plot(tm,yn[,7],xlab="t",ylab="acetate",xlim=c(0,tf),
    type="l",lwd=2,main="acetate, comp 1")
#
# y8(t)
    plot(tm,yn[,8],xlab="t",ylab="acetate",xlim=c(0,tf),
    type="l",lwd=2,main="acetate, comp 2")
#
# Analysis of dy1/dt to dy8/dt
#
# Write heading for dy1/dt to dy8/dt
    cat(sprintf("\n ncase = %2d\n\n",ncase));
    cat(sprintf("    t    dy/dt[1]    dy/dt[2]    dy/dt[3]
      dy/dt[4]"));
    cat(sprintf("           dy/dt[5]    dy/dt[6]    dy/dt[7]
      dy/dt[8]"));
#
# Step through the {\tt nout} values of t
    dydt=rep(0,8);
    dydt_plot=matrix(0,nrow=nout,ncol=8);
    for(it in 1:nout){
#
#   dy/dt returned by trans_2
    trans_2(tm[it],out[it,-1],parms);
    cat(sprintf("%5.2f%12.5f%12.5f%12.5f%12.5f\n",
                tm[it],dydt[1],dydt[2],dydt[3],dydt[4]));
    cat(sprintf("%17.5f%12.5f%12.5f%12.5f\n\n",
                dydt[5],dydt[6],dydt[7],dydt[8]));
    dydt_plot[it,]=dydt;
    }
#
```

```
# Eight plots for dy1(t)/dt to dy8(t)/dt vs t
#
# dy1(t)/dt
  par(mfrow=c(1,1))
# par(mfrow=c(4,2))
  plot(tm,dydt_plot[,1],xlab="t",ylab="dy1/dt, comp 1",
    xlim=c(0,tf),
  type="l",lwd=2,main="dy1/dt, comp 1")
#
# dy2(t)/dt
  plot(tm,dydt_plot[,2],xlab="t",ylab="dy2/dt, comp 2",
    xlim=c(0,tf),
  type="l",lwd=2,main="dy2/dt, comp 2")
#
# dy3(t)/dt
  plot(tm,dydt_plot[,3],xlab="t",ylab="dy3/dt",xlim=c(0,
    tf),
  type="l",lwd=2,main="dy3/dt, comp 1")
#
# dy4(t)/dt
  plot(tm,dydt_plot[,4],xlab="t",ylab="dy4/dt",xlim=c(0,
    tf),
  type="l",lwd=2,main="dy4/dt, comp 2")
#
# dy5(t)/dt
  plot(tm,dydt_plot[,5],xlab="t",ylab="dy5/dt",xlim=c(0,
    tf),
  type="l",lwd=2,main="dy5/dt, comp 1")
#
# dy6(t)/dt
  plot(tm,dydt_plot[,6],xlab="t",ylab="dy6/dt",xlim=c(0,
    tf),
  type="l",lwd=2,main="dy6/dt, comp 2")
#
# dy7(t)/dt
  plot(tm,dydt_plot[,7],xlab="t",ylab="dy7/dt",xlim=c(0,
    tf),
  type="l",lwd=2,main="dy7/dt, comp 1")
#
# dy8(t)/dt
```

```
plot(tm,dydt_plot[,8],xlab="t",ylab="dy8/dt",xlim=c(0,
   tf),
type="l",lwd=2,main="dy8/dt, comp 2")
```

Listing 6.6 Main program for the DLM eq. (6.17b) programmed in
trans_2 and jacob_1.

We can note the following details about Listing 6.6.

- The library deSolve (which includes lsodes) and the ODE routine trans_2 are accessed.

```
#
# Access deSolve library (with lsodes)
  library("deSolve")
#
# ODE routine
  setwd("c:/R/bme_ode/chap6")
  source("trans_2.R")
```

- Two cases are programmed, ncase=1 for the equilibrium IC case
  of Table 6.2 and ncase=2 for an IC that is selected arbitrarily
  to determine if the DLM algorithm converges to an equilibrium
  solution.

```
#
# Select case
#
# ncase = 1 - equilibrium ICs
#
# ncase = 2 - nonequilibrum ICs
#
  ncase=1;
```

- The parameters of eqs. (6.1) are defined numerically. They are
  global in the sense they are available one level down to trans_2.

```
#
# Parameters
  y1f=6.2682e-03; y3f=2.4;           y5f=1.15;
                                     y7f=3.9;
```

```
R=0.8;              gamma=0.01;      vr=1.2;
                                     alpha=0.5;
delta=0.1;          kh1=1.0066e-06; alphaH=2.25;
                                     alphaOH=0.5;
alphas1=1    ;      alphas2=1;       alphas3=1;
                                     B1=5.033e-05;
B2=5.033e-05;       ks1=5.0033e-07; s2ref=1.0e-04;
                                     s3ref=1.0e-06;
c1=2.4;             c2=5;            c3=1;
                                     c4=1000;
c5=5.2;
```

- The ICs for ncase=1,2 are defined numerically.

```
#
# Initial conditions
  y0=rep(0,8);
  if(ncase==1){
  y0[1]=0.003796824;  y0[2]=0.1405804; y0[3]=3.8971322;
  y0[4]=0.2801880941; y0[5]=3.233;     y0[6]=1.1606;
  y0[7]=8.2517318;    y0[8]=4.960605;
  }
  if(ncase==2){
  y0[1]=1; y0[2]=1; y0[3]=1;
  y0[4]=1; y0[5]=1; y0[6]=1;
  y0[7]=1; y0[8]=1;
  }
```

For ncase=2, all of the dependent variables, $y_1, \ldots, y_8$, are set to a unit value. The question of interest then is whether the DLM method will compute a solution corresponding to the IC for ncase=1, or possibly another equilibrium solution. In general, we should expect multiple equilibrium solutions because eqs. (6.1) are nonlinear.

- Three variations of the parameter mu in eq. (6.17) are programmed.

```
#
# Differential Newton's
  tf=20;mu=0;
```

```
#
# Differential steepest descent
# tf=20;mu=1;
#
# Differential steepest descent + Newton's
# tf=20;mu=0.5;
```

A particular value of mu is selected by activating (decommenting) the corresponding statement. The final value of t is also specified. This can vary depending on how far in t the numerical integration of eq. (6.17b) must go to reach an equilibrium solution (corresponding to the LHS vector of derivatives of eqs. (6.1) effectively equal to the zero vector).

- The total independent variable interval is $0 \le t \le 20$ (from the previous value of tf). In this case, t is not the independent variable of eqs. (6.1). In other words, for Listing 6.2, t is the independent variable of eqs. (6.1), but for Listing 6.6, t is the independent variable of eqs. (6.17), that is, the DLM ODEs (which are not the same as the model ODEs of eqs. (6.1)). The final value of $t = 20$ was selected so that the DLM ODEs reached an equilibrium solution (and there was essentially no further change in the solution with t).

```
#
# Output sequence in t
  nout=41;ncall=0;
  tm=seq(from=0,to=tf,by=tf/(nout-1));
```

In other words, t of eqs. (6.1) is physical time. t of eq. (6.17b) is not part of the original ODE model but rather is a parameter that is introduced to continue the solution from an arbitrarily selected IC (ncase=2) to an equilibrium solution; therefore, t in eq. (6.17b) is a continuation parameter.

- Selected parameters and a heading for the numerical solution are displayed.

```
#
# Write heading for y1 to y8
```

```
cat(sprintf("\n ncase = %2d\n\n",ncase));
cat(sprintf("     t          y[1]          y[2]
     y[3]          y[4]"));
cat(sprintf("                    y[5]          y[6]
     y[7]          y[8]"));
```

- The integration of the 8×8 DLM ODE system is by lsodes.

```
#
# lsodes ODE integration
  parms=c(rtol=1e-8,atol=1e-8)
  out=lsodes(times=tm,y=y0,func=trans_2,parms=parms)
```

times,y,func,parms are reserved names as explained for Listing 6.2. Note the use of trans_2 of Listing 6.5 as the ODE routine. The organization of the 2D array out with the numerical solution of eqs. (6.1) is explained for Listing 6.2.

- The numerical solution returned by lsodes, the 2D array out, is placed in the 2D array yn for subsequent numerical and graphical outputs by a for that steps through t.

```
#
# Numerical output
  yn=matrix(0,nrow=nout,ncol=8);
  for(it in 1:nout){
    if(it==1){yn[1,]=y0;
    }else{
    yn[it,]=out[it,-1];}
    cat(sprintf("%5.2f%12.5f%12.5f%12.5f%12.5f\n",
                tm[it],yn[it,1],yn[it,2],yn[it,3],
                yn[it,4]));
    cat(sprintf("%17.5f%12.5f%12.5f%12.5f\n\n",
                yn[it,5],yn[it,6],yn[it,7],yn[it,8]));
  }
```

The IC vector (for it=1) is placed in yn as yn[1,]=y0;. For subsequent t (it>1), the solution is placed in yn as yn[it,]=out[it,-1];. The numerical solution yn is then displayed numerically. The final } concludes the for in it.

- The number of calls to trans_2 at the end of the solution is displayed as a measure of the computational effort required to produce the solution in out.

```
#
# Calls to trans_2
  cat(sprintf("\n ncall = %5d\n\n",ncall))
```

- Eight plots for $y_1(t)$ to $y_8(t)$ are produced.

```
#
# Eight plots for y1(t) to y8(t) vs t
#
# y1(t)
# par(mfrow=c(1,1))
  par(mfrow=c(4,2))
  plot(tm,yn[,1],xlab="t",ylab="H+, comp 1",xlim=c(0,
    tf),
  type="l",lwd=2,main="H+, comp 1")
      .
      .
      .
#
# y8(t)
  plot(tm,yn[,8],xlab="t",ylab="acetate",xlim=c(0,tf),
  type="l",lwd=2,main="acetate, comp 2")
```

If plots on separate pages are to be produced, par(mfrow=c(1,1)) is used. If a composite matrix of 4 rows × 2 columns of plots is to be produced, par(mfrow=c(4,2)) is used. Note that the particular column of yn used in each plot and the use of tf, the final value of t, used to set the scale of the abscissa (horizontal) axis.

- The derivative vector, $dy_1/dt, \ldots, dy_8/dt$, is also computed to give an indication of the approach to an equilibrium solution, starting with a heading for the numerical derivative vector.

```
#
# Analysis of dy1/dt to dy8/dt
```

```
#
# Write heading for dy1/dt to dy8/dt
  cat(sprintf("\n ncase = %2d\n\n",ncase));
  cat(sprintf("    t    dy/dt[1]    dy/dt[2]
    dy/dt[3]    dy/dt[4]"));
  cat(sprintf("            dy/dt[5]    dy/dt[6]
    dy/dt[7]    dy/dt[8]"));
```

- The derivative vector is then computed as a function of t.
  To start, a 1D vector, dydt, and a 2D array, dydt_plot, are
  defined.

```
#
# Step through the {\tt nout} values of t
  dydt=rep(0,8);
  dydt_plot=matrix(0,nrow=nout,ncol=8);
  for(it in 1:nout){
#
#   dy/dt returned by trans_2
    trans_2(tm[it],out[it,-1],parms);
    cat(sprintf("%5.2f%12.5f%12.5f%12.5f%12.5f\n",
                tm[it],dydt[1],dydt[2],dydt[3],dydt
                  [4]));
    cat(sprintf("%17.5f%12.5f%12.5f%12.5f\n\n",
                dydt[5],dydt[6],dydt[7],dydt[8]));
    dydt_plot[it,]=dydt;
  }
```

A call to trans_2 (Listing 6.5) inside a for gives the derivative
vector dydt at each value of t (each it). Also, the derivative vector is placed in the 2D array dydt_plot for subsequent plotting.
The final } concludes the for in it.

- The derivative vector is then plotted to give an indication of
  the approach to an equilibrium solution (for which the eight
  components of the derivative vector approach zero).

```
#
# Eight plots for dy1(t)/dt to dy8(t)/dt vs t
#
# dy1(t)/dt
```

```
    par(mfrow=c(1,1))
  # par(mfrow=c(4,2))
    plot(tm,dydt_plot[,1],xlab="t",ylab="dy1/dt,
        comp 1",xlim=c(0,tf),
    type="l",lwd=2,main="dy1/dt, comp 1")
             .
             .
             .
             .

  #
  # dy8(t)/dt
    plot(tm,dydt_plot[,8],xlab="t",ylab="dy8/dt",xlim=
        c(0,tf),
    type="l",lwd=2,main="dy8/dt, comp 2")
```

The output from the main program of Listing 6.6 is now considered.

A1.8.4 *DLM Equilibrium Numerical Solution*   The numerical solution from Listings 6.4 (jacob_1), 6.5 (trans_2), and 6.6 (main program) is discussed next. Abbreviated numerical output from Listing 6.6 for ncase=1 is given in Tables 6.5.

We note that the solution of eq. (6.17b) does not change, that is, this is an equilibrium solution; the computational effort is modest (ncall=61) as might be expected because the solution does not change with t. This equilibrium solution is confirmed by the derivative vector output of Table 6.5b.

The derivative vector remains at zero to five figures. As the solution is invariant with t, the graphical output from Listing 6.6 is not considered here.

The preceding results in Tables 6.5 clearly indicate that the ICs of Table 6.2 correspond to an equilibrium solution. We now consider the effect of introducing a change in the ICs of the DLM ODEs for ncase=2 (set in Listing 6.6).

A1.8.5 *DLM nonequilibrium solutions*   Abbreviated tabulated output from Listing 6.6 for ncase=2 is given in Tables 6.6.

TABLE 6.5a   Abbreviated output for the solution of eq. (6.17b) from Listings 6.4–6.6 for ncase=1.

```
ncase =  1

     t           y[1]            y[2]            y[3]            y[4]
                 y[5]            y[6]            y[7]            y[8]

  0.00         0.00380         0.14058         3.89713         0.28019
               3.23300         1.16060         8.25173         4.96061

  0.50         0.00380         0.14058         3.89713         0.28019
               3.23300         1.16060         8.25173         4.96061

  1.00         0.00380         0.14058         3.89713         0.28019
               3.23300         1.16060         8.25173         4.96061
                                  .               .
                                  .               .
                                  .               .
            Output for t = 1.5,...,18.5 removed
                                  .               .
                                  .               .
                                  .               .

 19.00         0.00380         0.14058         3.89713         0.28019
               3.23300         1.16061         8.25173         4.96061

 19.50         0.00380         0.14058         3.89713         0.28019
               3.23300         1.16061         8.25173         4.96061

 20.00         0.00380         0.14058         3.89713         0.28019
               3.23300         1.16061         8.25173         4.96061

ncall =  61
```

We can note the following details about this output.

- The IC is an 8-vector of ones. Also, the derivatives are relatively large (compared to ncase=1) as expected because the IC departs from an equilibrium solution.

TABLE 6.5b Abbreviated output for the derivative vector of eq. (6.17b) from Listings 6.4–6.6 for ncase=1.

```
ncall =    61
ncase =  1
```

t	dy/dt[1] dy/dt[5]	dy/dt[2] dy/dt[6]	dy/dt[3] dy/dt[7]	dy/dt[4] dy/dt[8]
0.00	0.00000 0.00000	-0.00000 0.00001	0.00000 0.00000	0.00000 0.00000
0.50	0.00000 0.00000	-0.00000 0.00000	0.00000 0.00000	0.00000 0.00000
1.00	0.00000 0.00000	-0.00000 0.00000	0.00000 0.00000	0.00000 0.00000

```
                           .                  .
                           .                  .
                           .                  .
        Output for t = 1.5,...,18.5 removed
                           .                  .
                           .                  .
                           .                  .
```

t	dy/dt[1] dy/dt[5]	dy/dt[2] dy/dt[6]	dy/dt[3] dy/dt[7]	dy/dt[4] dy/dt[8]
19.00	0.00000 0.00000	0.00000 0.00000	-0.00000 0.00000	-0.00000 0.00000
19.50	0.00000 0.00000	0.00000 0.00000	-0.00000 0.00000	-0.00000 0.00000
20.00	0.00000 0.00000	0.00000 0.00000	-0.00000 0.00000	-0.00000 0.00000

- The solution varies with t because of the change in the IC. This variation is evident in Fig. 6.11 that follows, but at the end of the solution (at $t = 20$), the derivatives have approached small values as the solution approaches the ICs of Table 6.2 and Listing 6.2.

TABLE 6.6a Abbreviated output for the solution of eq. (6.17b) from Listings 6.4–6.6 for `ncase=2`, $\mu = 0$.

```
ncase =  2

    t        y[1]         y[2]         y[3]         y[4]
             y[5]         y[6]         y[7]         y[8]

 0.00     1.00000      1.00000      1.00000      1.00000
          1.00000      1.00000      1.00000      1.00000

 0.50     7.70460      7.98248      2.07396      0.46382
          1.87996      1.06446      3.88634      2.68494

 1.00     8.98291      9.42934      2.89007      0.30897
          2.41218      1.10270      5.55459      3.62167
                          .            .
                          .            .
                          .            .
          Output for t = 1.5,...,18.5 removed
                          .            .
                          .            .
                          .            .
19.00     0.00390      0.15414      3.88662      0.26084
          3.23313      1.16070      8.25699      4.97029

19.50     0.00389      0.15275      3.88755      0.26267
          3.23312      1.16069      8.25652      4.96937

20.00     0.00388      0.15152      3.88841      0.26433
          3.23311      1.16069      8.25610      4.96854

ncall =   338
```

```
Listing 6.2 (and Table 6.2):
#
# Initial conditions
  y0=rep(0,8);
  y0[1]=0.003796824;  y0[2]=0.1405804;  y0[3]=3.8971322;
```

TABLE 6.6b Abbreviated output for the derivative vector of eq. (6.17b) from Listings 6.4–6.6 for ncase=2, $\mu = 0$.

ncase = 2

t	dy/dt[1] dy/dt[5]	dy/dt[2] dy/dt[6]	dy/dt[3] dy/dt[7]	dy/dt[4] dy/dt[8]
0.00	17.26722 2.32361	17.97191 0.21298	-6.83756 12.12229	-11.18846 9.19838
0.50	6.62147 1.35224	7.04984 0.09698	2.11727 4.21824	-0.35034 2.35908
1.00	-0.43553 0.82058	-0.17572 0.05905	1.23883 2.58119	-0.25805 1.45364

Output for t = 1.5,...,18.5 removed

19.00	-0.00002 -0.00003	-0.00295 -0.00002	0.00195 -0.00097	0.00386 -0.00193
19.50	-0.00002 -0.00002	-0.00262 -0.00002	0.00179 -0.00089	0.00348 -0.00174
20.00	-0.00002 -0.00002	-0.00233 -0.00002	0.00163 -0.00082	0.00314 -0.00157

```
y0[4]=0.2801880941; y0[5]=3.233;   y0[6]=1.1606;
y0[7]=8.2517318;    y0[8]=4.960605;
tf=20;nout=41;ncall=0;
tm=seq(from=0,to=tf,by=tf/(nout-1));
```

Table 6.6a:

20.00	0.00388 3.23311	0.15152 1.16069	3.88841 8.25610	0.26433 4.96854

```
Table 6.6b:

20.00      -0.00002      -0.00233       0.00163       0.00314
           -0.00002      -0.00002      -0.00082      -0.00157
```

There are still differences in, for example, $y_2(t = 20)$ (0.1405804 and 0.15152) where the derivative is not close to zero (-0.00233). This suggests that the solution should be extended past $t = 20$. An execution of the main program in Listing 6.6 with tf=100 gives the following results.

```
y1,...,y8

100.00      0.00380       0.14058       3.89713       0.28019
            3.23300       1.16061       8.25173       4.96061


dy1/dt,...,dy8/dt

100.00      0.00000       0.00000      -0.00000      -0.00000
            0.00000       0.00000       0.00000       0.00000
```

At t=100, the DLM solution agrees with Table 6.2 and Listing 6.2 and the derivatives are zero to five figures.

- From Table 6.6b, the DLM ODEs have the largest derivatives at the beginning of the solution ($t = 0$). This is rather typical for ODE solutions with the largest derivatives at the beginning where the ICs (in this case $y_1(t = 0) = 1, \ldots, y_8(t = 0) = 1$) are relatively far from an equilibrium solution).

- The computational effort (ncall=338) is greater than that for ncase=1 (ncall=61) as expected because of the variation of the solution with t but is still modest.

These properties are reflected in Figs. 6.12–6.14. We can note the following details about Figs. 6.12–6.14.

- Figure 6.12 indicates a rapid departure from the unit ICs to a new solution that is the equilibrium solution of Table 6.2 and Listing 6.2 as reflected in the numerical output of Table 6.6.

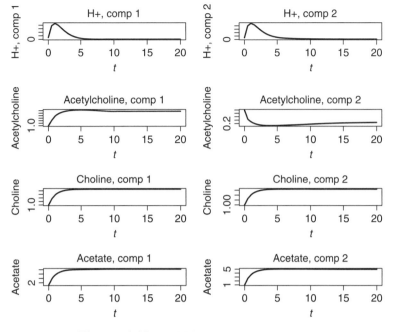

Figure 6.12 DLM $y_1, \ldots, y_4$ versus t.

- In Figs. 6.13 and 6.14, the derivatives dy_1/dt and dy_8/dt are nonzero as expected at $t = 0$ but they rapidly approach a near zero value corresponding to the equilibrium solution of Table 6.6 (as reflected in the numerical output at $t = 20$).

The preceding results indicate that the DLM of eq. (6.17b) worked well for the differential Newton's case with $\mu = 0$. We now consider the DLM performance with steepest descent that included $(0 < \mu \leq 1)$.

A1.8.6 *Variation in DLM Parameter μ* If the main program in Listing 6.6 is executed for the case mu=1

```
#
# Differential steepest descent
  tf=20;mu=1;
```

the numerical output is summarized in Tables 6.7.

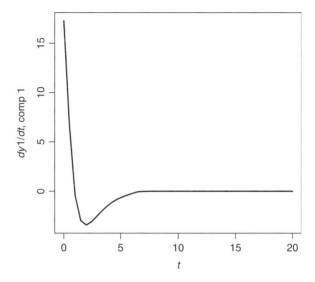

Figure 6.13   DLM dy_1/dt versus t.

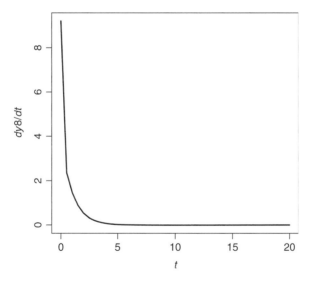

Figure 6.14   DLM dy_8/dt versus t.

We can note the following details about this output. The final solution at $t = 20$ for mu=0 (Tables 6.6) is different from that for mu=1 (Tables 6.7).

TABLE 6.7a   Abbreviated output for the solution of eq. (6.17b) from Listings 6.4–6.6 for ncase=2, $\mu = 1$.

ncase =   2

t	y[1] y[5]	y[2] y[6]	y[3] y[7]	y[4] y[8]
0.00	1.00000 1.00000	1.00000 1.00000	1.00000 1.00000	1.00000 1.00000
0.50	0.55178 1.24946	0.69157 0.36139	1.44093 1.86546	0.01481 0.59428
1.00	0.26912 1.24727	0.49694 0.35928	1.62962 2.28341	0.02534 0.87301

.
.
.

Output for t = 1.5,...,18.5 removed

.
.
.

19.00	0.00251 2.74821	0.01271 0.96235	4.65697 7.46076	1.43845 4.13950
19.50	0.00251 2.77045	0.01286 0.97136	4.67019 7.48577	1.43699 4.15881
20.00	0.00252 2.79183	0.01302 0.98002	4.68224 7.50894	1.43516 4.17689

ncall =   933

Table 6.6a (differential Newton's, mu=0)

| 20.00 | 0.00388
3.23311 | 0.15152
1.16069 | 3.88841
8.25610 | 0.26433
4.96854 |

ncall =   338

TABLE 6.7b   Abbreviated output for the derivative vector of eq. (6.17b) from Listings 6.4–6.6 for `ncase=2`, $\mu = 1$.

ncase =   2

t	dy/dt[1] dy/dt[5]	dy/dt[2] dy/dt[6]	dy/dt[3] dy/dt[7]	dy/dt[4] dy/dt[8]
0.00	-45.47436 3.79691	-227.85482 -10.19934	44.58470 -15.06174	-605.19172 33.73780
0.50	-0.60301 -0.02992	-0.42229 -0.01634	0.42818 0.90696	0.01611 0.48862
1.00	-0.52941 0.02058	-0.36609 0.00624	0.34484 0.80120	0.02489 0.56486

Output for t = 1.5,...,18.5 removed

19.00	-0.02316 0.04538	0.00071 0.01838	0.02766 0.05194	-0.00254 0.03993
19.50	0.00573 0.04362	0.00004 0.01766	0.02523 0.04813	-0.00330 0.03736
20.00	0.00459 0.04191	0.00065 0.01698	0.02300 0.04461	-0.00400 0.03499

Table 6.7a (differential steepest descent, mu=1)

| 20.00 | 0.00252
2.79183 | 0.01302
0.98002 | 4.68224
7.50894 | 1.43516
4.17689 |

ncall =   933

This difference in the solution is not totally unexpected because differential steepest descent (`mu=1`) is susceptible to ending at a local minimum.

Also, the derivative vector for steepest descent did not reach the zero vector equilibrium condition as closely as differential Newton's method by $t = 20$, even though the computational effort was substantially greater than that for Newton's method (ncall = 933 compared to ncall = 338). This is not unexpected because Newton's method is quadratically convergent (the approach to a solution is proportional to the square of the distance from the solution), whereas the rate of convergence of steepest descent is less than quadratic (less than second order).

Table 6.6b (differential Newton's, mu=0)

20.00	-0.00002	-0.00233	0.00163	0.00314
	-0.00002	-0.00002	-0.00082	-0.00157

Table 6.7b (differential steepest descent, mu=1)

20.00	0.00459	0.00065	0.02300	-0.00400
	0.04191	0.01698	0.04461	0.03499

Clearly, some of the derivatives at $t = 20$ are larger for mu=1 than for mu=0. This suggests that a solution beyond $t = 20$ might give a better approach to an equilibrium solution (but the solution might be different from that for mu=0 as reflected in the preceding comparison of the solutions for mu=0,1).

This result raises the basic question of why steepest descent would be used because it appears to be less effective in approaching a DLM equilibrium solution. The answer is that steepest descent will function when the Jacobian matrix J is singular or ill-conditioned (near singular) while the differential Newton's method will fail. The conclusion follows from eq. (6.17b). For $\mu = 1$, the inverse Jacobian matrix J^{-1} is not required (for steepest descent), whereas it is required for $\mu = 0$ (for Newton's method). In other words, steepest descent can move past a singular point for J.

This conclusion suggests that a combination of Newton's and steepest methods would be effective, that is, $0 < \mu < 1$, particularly if the Jacobian matrix becomes ill-conditioned along the solution in t. This variation in μ in eq. (6.17b) can easily be programmed (e.g., in List-ing 6.6). However, to keep this discussion to a reasonable length, we leave the study of the effect of variations in μ to the reader (also, because for $\mu = 0$, the differential Newton's method produced an accurate IC vector for eqs. (6.1), particularly for $0 \leq t \leq 100$).

Just to summarize, DLM can be used with a combination of New-ton's and steepest descent methods that ideally would combine the advantages of both the methods. Whether this turns out to be the case is generally determined by the characteristics of the problem system (i.e., the properties of the Jacobian matrix of the nonlinear algebraic system).

This conclusion also suggests that the linear combination in μ in eq. (6.17b) could be extended. For example, the condition number of J could be computed as the solution proceeds; specifically, in Jacob_1, μ could be adjusted according to the condition number. If the condition number is small, $\mu \approx 0$ would be used. If the condition number increases indicating J is becoming ill-conditioned (near sin-gular), μ could be increased until the solution is past the point where J is ill-conditioned.

As a final point, the DLM is basically a way of converting a non-linear algebraic system to an initial value ODE system that can then be integrated numerically by an ODE solver. A simpler approach would be to merely add a derivative to each of the nonlinear alge-braic equations. But this is not straightforward because adding the derivative to even one algebraic equation with the wrong sign could lead to an unstable ODE system. The advantage of the DLM is that the addition of the derivatives to the nonlinear algebraic equations is done in a systematic way that generally gives a stable ODE sys-tem, for example, the use of eq. (6.17b) with the coupling coefficient matrix cm.

A1.8.7 Conclusions We can conclude with the following points from the previous study of the DLM.

- The DLM method of eq. (6.17b) accurately produced the equi-librium solution of Table 6.2. More generally, the DLM method effectively solved an 8×8 nonlinear algebraic system. The principal requirement to use DLM in this way is the formulation of the algebraic system Jacobian matrix.

- Here, we have used an analytical Jacobian matrix (the 8×8 partial derivatives were programmed from the mathematical derivatives). As the number of algebraic equations, n, increases, the number of elements in the Jacobian matrix increases as n^2. Thus, the Jacobian matrix can quickly become too large for a feasible analytical evaluation and a numerical approximation may be required. For example, the partial derivatives can be approximated by FDs. This in turn usually requires some experimentation with the FDs such as the magnitudes of the changes in the dependent variables when calculating the FD approximations of the partial derivatives. Generally, the evaluation of the Jacobian matrix can be a substantial part of the total calculational effort in using a nonlinear equation solver such as the DLM method.

- One variant that may conserve computer time is to avoid the evaluation of the Jacobian matrix (e.g., through the call to `jacob_1`) at each point along the solution if the Jacobian matrix does not change significantly. In other words, the Jacobian matrix can often be used until it becomes outdated at which point a reevaluation may be required before taking the next step along the solution of the DLM ODEs.

- The topic of analytical versus numerical Jacobian matrices has been studied extensively. We do not consider this further but rather end by pointing out the utility of the DLM method and the need to evaluate a Jacobian matrix. As noted previously, an important feature of DLM is the facility to move past a singular point of the Jacobian matrix by including steepest descent ($0 < \mu \leq 1$ in eq. (6.17b)).

We generally have had success with DLM when Newton's method or steepest descent method has failed, particularly when using finite stepping versions of these methods (discussed previously). In other words, using a library ODE solver to move the solution forward in the continuation parameter t (e.g., in eq. (6.17b)) is an important feature of DLM. But again, some experimentation with DLM, for example, variation in μ, is generally required for a new application (system of nonlinear algebraic equations) and success in the use of DLM cannot be guaranteed in advance. Following the condition number of J may be a key step in implementing DLM.

References

[1] Anselmo, K.J. and W.E. Schiesser (1997), Some experiences with a differential Levenberg Marquardt method, presented at the SIAM Annual meeting, Stanford University, Stanford, CA, July 14–18, 1997.

[2] Belanger, P.W., private communication, 1997

[3] Levenberg K.A., (1944), A method for the solution of certain problems in least squares, *Quart. Appl. Math.*, **2**, 164–168.

[4] Marquardt, D.W. (1963), An algorithm for least-squares estimation of nonlinear parameters, *SIAM J. Appl. Math.*, **11**, 431–441.

[5] Mustafa, I.H., G. Ibrahim, A. Elkamel, S.S.E.H.Elnshaie, and P. Chen (2009a), Non-linear feedback modeling and bifurcation of the acetylcholine neurocycle and its relation to Alzheimer's and Parkinson's diseases, *Chem. Eng. Sci.*, **64**(1), 69–90.

[6] Mustafa, I.H., G. Ibrahim, A. Elkamel, S.S.E.H. Elnshaie, and P. Chen (2009b), Effect of choline and acetate substrates on bifurcation and chaotic behavior of acetycholine neurocycle and Alzheimer's and Parkinson's diseases, *Chem. Eng. Sci.*, **64**(9), 2096–2112.

[7] Mustafa, I.H., A. Elkamel, P. Chen, G. Ibrahim, S.S.E.H. Elnshaie (2012), Effect of cholineacetyltransferase activity and choline recycle tario on diffusion-reaction modeling, bifurcation and chaotic behavior of acetylcholine neurocycle and their relation to Alzheimer's and Parkinson's diseases, *Chem. Eng. Sci.*, **68**, 19–35.

[8] Mustafa, I.H. and A. Elkamel, private communications, 2012

## CHAPTER 7

Tuberculosis with Differential Infectivity[1]

7.1 Introduction

The model for tuberculosis is introduced by the following definitive statement from [2] (with slight editing).

> Tuberculosis (TB) is a disease caused by infection with myco-bacterium tuberculosis, which most frequently affects the lungs (pulmonary TB). It is one of the most common infectious diseases with about two billion people (one-third of the world's population) currently infected. About nine million new cases of active disease develop each year, resulting in two million deaths, mostly in developing countries. Despite intensive control efforts, recent data show that global incidence is increasing, largely due to an association with human immunodeficiency virus (HIV).

> Mathematical models have played a key role in the formulation of TB control strategies and the establishment of interim goals for intervention programs. Most of these models are of the SEIR class in which the host population is categorized by infection status as suscepti-ble (S), exposed (infected but not yet infectious) (E), infectious (I) and recovered (R). One of the principal attributes of these models is

[1]The contributions of Dr. Samuel Bowong, University of Douala, and Dr. Jean Jules Tewa, University of Yaounde, through their paper [2], are gratefully acknowledged.

Differential Equation Analysis in Biomedical Science and Engineering: Ordinary Differential Equation Applications with R, First Edition. William E. Schiesser.

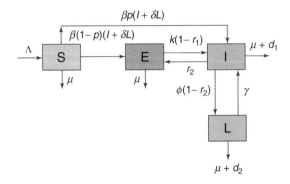

Figure 7.1   Diagram for the model of eqs. (7.1).

that the force of infection (the rate at which susceptible leaves the susceptible class and moves into an infected category, i.e., become infected) is a function of the number of infectious hosts in the population at any time t and is thus a nonlinear term. Other transitions, such as the recovery of infectious and death, are modeled as linear terms with constant coefficients. However, the enormous public health burden inflicted by tuberculosis necessitates the use of mathematical modeling to gain insights into the transmission dynamics and to determine effective control strategies.

These concepts are discussed in detail in [2]. Here, we only state the final mathematical model and illustrate its structure through the diagram in Fig. 7.1.

7.2 Mathematical Model

The ODE model illustrated in Fig. 7.1 follows.

$$\frac{dS}{dt} = \Lambda - \beta S(I + \delta L) - \mu S \tag{7.1a}$$

$$\frac{dE}{dt} = \beta(1-p)S(I + \delta L) + r_2 I - [\mu + k(1 - r_1)]E \tag{7.1b}$$

$$\frac{dI}{dt} = \beta p S(I + \delta L) + k(1 - r_1)E$$

$$+ \gamma L - [\mu + d_1 + \phi(1 - r_2) + r_2]I \tag{7.1c}$$

$$\frac{dL}{dt} = \phi(1 - r_2)I - (\mu + d_2 + \gamma)L \tag{7.1d}$$

where the dependent variable vector $[S(t)\ E(t)\ I(t)\ L(t)]^T$ is defined in Table 7.1.

TABLE 7.1   Dependent variables of eqs. (7.1).

Dependent variable	Interpretation
S	susceptible population
E	infected (exposed) population
I	infectious population
L	out of sight population

The relation between Fig. 7.1 and eqs. (7.1) is straightforward. For example, eq. (7.1a) has one input, Λ (a constant), and three outputs, μS, $\beta(1 - p)(I + \delta L)S$, and $\beta p(I + \delta L)S$. Note the sum $\beta(1 - p)(I + \delta L)S + \beta p(I + \delta L)S = \beta(I + \delta L)S$ as stated in the RHS of eq. (7.1a).

Also, the mathematical expressions in Fig. 7.1 next to the arrows from each block (box) are multiplying factors for the corresponding dependent variables. For example, E is multiplied by the two factors μ and $k(1 - r_1)$ as reflected in the third RHS term of eq. (7.1b), $-[\mu + k(1 - r_1)]E$, which has a negative sign because the corresponding arrows are directed from the E block (this term tends to decrease E with a negative effect on the derivative dE/dt of eq. (7.1b) through a mass balance). Terms corresponding to arrows directed toward the E block have a plus sign in the RHS of eq. (7.1b) (these terms tend to increase E with a positive effect on the derivative dE/dt). In this way, the diagram of Fig. 7.1 completely defines eq. (7.1b).

The parameters in eqs. (7.1) are explained and defined numerically in Table 7.2 ([2], p. 4011).

Eqs. (7.1) are first order in t, and therefore, each requires one IC. Two sets of ICs will subsequently be programmed. For the first set, we note that if $E = I = L = 0$, the RHSs of eqs. (7.1b)–(7.1d) are zero. Also, if $S = \Lambda/\mu$, the RHS of eq. (7.1a) is zero. This, if the IC vector is

$$[\Lambda/\mu\ 0\ 0\ 0]^T \tag{7.2a}$$

TABLE 7.2   Parameters of eqs. (7.1).

Parameter	Description	Estimated Value
Λ	recruitment rate of susceptible individuals in the community	2 (year)$^{-1}$
β	transmission coefficient	0.025
δ	fraction of loss of sight still infectious	1
p	proportion of newly infected who have fast progression to the infectious	0.3
μ	natural death rate	0.0101
k	rate of progression from infected to infectious	0.005
r_1	rate of effective chemoprophylaxis	0
r_2	rate of effective therapy	0.8182
ϕ	rate at which infectious become loss of sight	0.02
γ	rate at which loss of sight return to hospital	0.01
d_1	death rate of infectious	0.0227
d_2	death rate of loss of sight	0.20

the derivative vector (LHS) of eqs. (7.1) will be the zero vector and IC (7.2a) will correspond to an equilibrium solution of eqs. (7.1) for which there is no change with t. This case is the first programmed in the main program of Listing 7.1 considered next.

Then, to investigate the dynamics of eqs. (7.1), a change is made in the IC vector (7.2a) to

$$[\Lambda/\mu\ 1\ 0\ 0]^T \tag{7.2b}$$

As will be noted, the change in IC for E from 0 to 1 (a small perturbation in the infected or exposed population corresponding to the possible start of a tuberculosis epidemic) produces a substantial transient response in eqs. (7.1). IC (7.2b) is the second case programmed in the main program of Listing 7.1.

This completes the specification of the ODE model (eqs. (7.1) and (7.2) and the parameters of Table 7.2). We now consider the programming of this model.

7.3   R Routines for the ODE Model

We start with an ODE routine for eqs. (7.1). This routine is called by the ODE integrator lsodes in a main program that is discussed subsequently.

7.3.1   ODE Routine

The ODE routine tb_1.R is in Listing 7.1.

```
  tb_1=function(t,y,parms) {
#
# Definition of model dependent variables
  S=y[1];
  E=y[2];
  I=y[3];
  L=y[4];
#
# ODEs
  St=lambda-beta*S*(I+delta*L)-mu*S;
  Et=beta*(1-p)*S*(I+delta*L)+r2*I-(mu+k*(1-r1))*E;
  It=beta*p*S*(I+delta*L)+k*(1-r1)*E+gamma*L-
     (mu+d1+phi*(1-r2)+r2)*I;
  Lt=phi*(1-r2)*I-(mu+d2+gamma)*L;
#
# ODE derivative vector
  yt=rep(0,4);
  yt[1]=St;
  yt[2]=Et;
  yt[3]=It;
  yt[4]=Lt;
#
# Increment calls to tb_1
  ncall <<- ncall+1;
#
# Return derivative vector as list
```

```
  return(list(c(yt)));
}
```

Listing 7.1 ODE routine for eqs. (7.1).

We can note the following details about tb_1.R.

- The function is defined with the dependent variable 4-vector for eqs. (7.1) in the 1D array y.

```
  tb_1=function(t,y,parms) {
```

- y is transferred to four problem-oriented variables to facilitate the programming of eqs. (7.1).

```
#
# Definition of model dependent variables
  S=y[1];
  E=y[2];
  I=y[3];
  L=y[4];
```

- Eqs. (7.1) are programmed. The parameters in this coding, for example, lambda, beta, delta, and mu, are defined numerically in the main program discussed next; these values are available to tb_1 because it is a subordinate routine.

```
#
# ODEs
  St=lambda-beta*S*(I+delta*L)-mu*S;
  Et=beta*(1-p)*S*(I+delta*L)+r2*I-(mu+k*(1-r1))*E;
  It=beta*p*S*(I+delta*L)+k*(1-r1)*E+gamma*L-
     (mu+d1+phi*(1-r2)+r2)*I;
  Lt=phi*(1-r2)*I-(mu+d2+gamma)*L;
```

- A derivative 4-vector, yt, is declared and the derivatives from the ODEs are placed in this vector.

```
#
# ODE derivative vector
  yt=rep(0,4);
```

```
yt[1]=St;
yt[2]=Et;
yt[3]=It;
yt[4]=Lt;
```

- The number of calls to tb_1 is incremented and the value is returned to the main program through the <<-.

```
#
# Increment calls to tb_1
  ncall <<- ncall+1;
```

- The derivative vector yt is returned to lsodes as a list.

```
#
# Return derivative vector as list
  return(list(c(yt)));
}
```

The final } concludes tb_1.

The main program that calls tb_1 is listed in the following section.

7.3.2 Main Program

```
#
# Access deSolve library (with lsodes)
  library("deSolve")
#
# ODE routine
  setwd("c:/R/bme_ode/chap7")
  source("tb_1.R")
#
# Select case
#
# ncase = 1 - equilibrium, no disease
#
# ncase = 2 - endemic
#
  ncase=1;
```

```
#
# Parameters
  lambda=2; beta=0.01;  delta=1;       p=0.3;   mu=0.0101;
     k=0.005;
        r1=0; r2=0.8182; phi=0.02; gamma=0.01; d1=0.022722;
           d2=0.20;
#
# Modify parameters
  beta=0.025;
#
# Initial conditions
  y0=rep(0,4);
  if(ncase==1){ y0[1]=lambda/mu; y0[2]=0; y0[3]=0;
     y0[4]=0;}
  if(ncase==2){ y0[1]=lambda/mu; y0[2]=1; y0[3]=0;
     y0[4]=0;}
  tf=20;nout=41;ncall=0;
  tm=seq(from=0,to=tf,by=tf/(nout-1));
#
# Write heading
  cat(sprintf("\n ncase = %2d   beta = %6.3f\n\n",ncase,
     beta));
  cat(sprintf("    t          S             E            I
     L"));
#
# lsodes ODE integration
  parms=c(rtol=1e-8,atol=1e-8)
  out=lsodes(times=tm,y=y0,func=tb_1,parms=parms)
#
# Numerical output
  yn=matrix(0,nrow=nout,ncol=4);
  for(it in 1:nout){
    if(it==1){yn[1,]=y0;
    }else{
    yn[it,]=out[it,-1];}
    cat(sprintf("%5.2f%12.1f%12.2f%12.5f%12.5f\n",
                tm[it],yn[it,1],yn[it,2],yn[it,3],
                   yn[it,4]));
  }
#
# Calls to tb_1
```

```
  cat(sprintf("\n ncall = %5d\n\n",ncall))
#
# Four plots for y1(t) to y4(t) vs t
#
# S(t)
  par(mfrow=c(2,2))
  plot(tm,yn[,1],xlab="t",ylab="S(t)",xlim=c(0,20),
  type="l",lwd=2,main="S(t)")
#
# E(t)
  plot(tm,yn[,2],xlab="t",ylab="E(t)",xlim=c(0,20),
  type="l",lwd=2,main="E(t)")
#
# I(t)
  plot(tm,yn[,3],xlab="t",ylab="I(t)",xlim=c(0,20),
  type="l",lwd=2,main="I(t)")
#
# L(t)
  plot(tm,yn[,4],xlab="t",ylab="L(t)",xlim=c(0,20),
  type="l",lwd=2,main="L(t)")
```

Listing 7.2 Main program for eqs. (7.1) and (7.2).

We can note the following details about Listing 7.2.

- lsodes for the integration of eqs. (7.1) is accessed through the library deSolve. tb_1 is accessed through a setwd (set working directory) and source. Note the use of the forward slash (/) in setwd.

```
#
# Access deSolve library (with lsodes)
  library("deSolve")
#
# ODE routine
  setwd("c:/R/bme_ode/chap7")
  source("tb_1.R")
```

- Two cases are programmed corresponding to eqs. (7.2).

```
#
# Select case
```

```
#
# ncase = 1 - equilibrium, no disease
#
# ncase = 2 - endemic
#
  ncase=1;
```

- The parameters of Table 7.2 are defined numerically.

```
#
# Parameters
  lambda=2; beta=0.01;  delta=1;   p=0.3;    mu=0.0101;
    k=0.005;
    r1=0; r2=0.8182; phi=0.02; gamma=0.01; d1=0.022722;
      d2=0.20;
#
# Modify parameters
  beta=0.025;
```

These values were taken from [2], with a variation in beta to demonstrate some interesting features of the numerical solutions to eqs. (7.1).

- The ICs for eqs. (7.1) are specified for two cases. ncase=1,2 correspond to eqs. (7.2a) and (7.2b), respectively.

```
#
# Initial conditions
  y0=rep(0,4);
  if(ncase==1){ y0[1]=lambda/mu; y0[2]=0; y0[3]=0;
    y0[4]=0;}
  if(ncase==2){ y0[1]=lambda/mu; y0[2]=1; y0[3]=0;
    y0[4]=0;}
  tf=20;nout=41;ncall=0;
  tm=seq(from=0,to=tf,by=tf/(nout-1));
```

ncase=2 corresponds to a small increase in the E (exposed/infected) population initially. As Λ has the unit of year^{-1} (from Table 7.2), the range in t is taken as $0 \le t \le 20$ year, with 41 output points (counting $t = 0$), that is, outputs at $t = 0, 0.5, \ldots, 20$. Also, the counter for the calls to tb_1 is initialized (so that it is then available for use in the subordinate routine `tb_1` of Listing 7.1).

- A heading for the numerical solution is displayed.

```
#
# Write heading
  cat(sprintf("\n ncase = %2d    beta = %6.3f\n\n",
    ncase,beta));
  cat(sprintf("    t    S         E              I
    L"));
```

- Eqs. (7.1) are integrated with `lsodes`. Note the use of the vector of output values of t, `tm`, the IC vector `y0`, and the ODE routine `tb_1`. The argument `parms` is used to specify the error tolerances for the numerical ODE integration (the default tolerances produced the same numerical solution).

```
#
# lsodes ODE integration
  parms=c(rtol=1e-8,atol=1e-8)
  out=lsodes(times=tm,y=y0,func=tb_1,parms=parms)
```

The length of `y0` informs `lsodes` that four ODEs are to be integrated. The solution array `out` is dimensioned as `out(41,5)` as explained next.

- Array `yn` is defined for subsequent numerical and graphical display of the solution. A `for` (with index `it`) steps through the values $t = 0, 0.5, \ldots, 20$. With `it=1` corresponding to $t = 0$, the IC vector `y0` is placed in `yn[1,]` (note the use of , to include all four dependent variables of eqs. (7.1) at $t = 0$ corresponding to eqs. (7.2)). For `it>1`, the solution is placed in `yn` by using `-1` in `out` meaning the second subscript of `out` has the values `2,3,4,5` corresponding to the four dependent variables of eqs. (7.1)).

```
#
# Numerical output
  yn=matrix(0,nrow=nout,ncol=4);
  for(it in 1:nout){
    if(it==1){yn[1,]=y0;
    }else{
```

```
        yn[it,]=out[it,-1];}
        cat(sprintf("%5.2f%12.1f%12.2f%12.5f%12.5f\n",
                    tm[it],yn[it,1],yn[it,2],yn[it,3],
                    yn[it,4])));
    }
```

After the ODE solution is placed in yn, it is displayed as $S(t)$ = yn[it,1] to $L(t)$ = yn[it,4] versus t = tm[it]. The final } concludes the for.

- At the end of the solution ($t = 20$), the number of calls to tb_1 is displayed as an indication of the computational effort required to compute the solution.

```
#
# Calls to tb_1
    cat(sprintf("\n ncall = %5d\n\n",ncall))
```

- The four dependent variables of eqs. (7.1) are plotted as a 2×2 array.

```
#
# Four plots for y1(t) to y4(t) vs t
#
# S(t)
    par(mfrow=c(2,2))
    plot(tm,yn[,1],xlab="t",ylab="S(t)",xlim=c(0,20),
    type="l",lwd=2,main="S(t)")
#
# E(t)
    plot(tm,yn[,2],xlab="t",ylab="E(t)",xlim=c(0,20),
    type="l",lwd=2,main="E(t)")
#
# I(t)
    plot(tm,yn[,3],xlab="t",ylab="I(t)",xlim=c(0,20),
    type="l",lwd=2,main="I(t)")
#
# L(t)
    plot(tm,yn[,4],xlab="t",ylab="L(t)",xlim=c(0,20),
    type="l",lwd=2,main="L(t)")
```

Note the scaling of the abscissa (horizontal) axis as xlim=c(0, 20) for $0 \le t \le 20$ while automatic scaling by plot is used for the ordinate (vertical) axis.

This completes the programming of eqs. (7.1) and (7.2). The output from Listings 7.1 and 7.2 is considered next.

7.4 Model Output

Abbreviated numerical output for ncase=1 is given in Table 7.3.

TABLE 7.3   Abbreviated output from Listings 7.1 and 7.2, ncase=1.

```
ncase =  1   beta =    0.025

    t            S            E            I            L
 0.00         198.0         0.00      0.00000      0.00000
 0.50         198.0         0.00      0.00000      0.00000
 1.00         198.0         0.00      0.00000      0.00000
 1.50         198.0         0.00      0.00000      0.00000
 2.00         198.0         0.00      0.00000      0.00000
                 .                       .
                 .                       .
                 .                       .
        Output for t = 2.5 to 17.50 not included
                 .                       .
                 .                       .
                 .                       .
18.00         198.0         0.00      0.00000      0.00000
18.50         198.0         0.00      0.00000      0.00000
19.00         198.0         0.00      0.00000      0.00000
19.50         198.0         0.00      0.00000      0.00000
20.00         198.0         0.00      0.00000      0.00000

ncall =    53
```

The invariance of the equilibrium solution for IC (7.2a) is clear. Note that from Table 7.2, $S(t = 0) = \Lambda/\mu = 2/0.0101 = 198.0$.

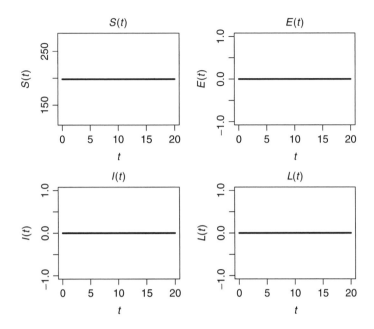

Figure 7.2   Solution of eqs. (7.1) for IC (7.2a) (ncase=1).

The computational effort is modest (ncall = 53) because the solution does not change. The graphical output in Fig. 7.2 also indicates the invariant solution.

Abbreviated numerical output from Listings 7.1 and 7.2 for ncase=2 is given in Table 7.4. We note that the loss in susceptibles, $S(t)$, is essentially equal to the gain in infected, $E(t)$. The infectious, $I(t)$, and out of sight, $L(t)$, increase and then go through a maximum; generally, the numbers for $I(t)$ and $L(t)$ are small. The computational effort for the solution in Table 7.4 is again modest with ncall = 133.

The overall variation of the solution is clear from the graphical output of Fig. 7.3.

The differential infectivity reflected in $E(t)$ and $L(t)$ indicates a substantial growth in $E(t)$ from a small initial value in eq. (7.2b). This can be interpreted as the onset of an epidemic. An explanation of these features of the solutions to eqs. (7.1) is available by examining the individual RHS terms of eqs. (7.1). This additional analysis is straightforward by using the numerical

TABLE 7.4   Abbreviated output from Listings 7.1 and 7.2, ncase=2.

```
ncase =   2   beta =   0.025
    t           S           E           I           L
  0.00       198.0        1.00      0.00000     0.00000
  0.50       198.0        1.00      0.00293     0.00000
  1.00       198.0        1.00      0.00695     0.00001
  1.50       198.0        1.01      0.01249     0.00003
  2.00       197.9        1.04      0.02016     0.00005
                 .                      .
                 .                      .
                 .                      .
         Output for t = 2.5 to 17.50 not included
                 .                      .
                 .                      .
                 .                      .
 18.00        57.2      137.01      3.27850     0.07702
 18.50        55.7      138.83      2.96727     0.07436
 19.00        54.4      140.33      2.70588     0.07148
 19.50        53.3      141.58      2.48841     0.06849
 20.00        52.5      142.63      2.30876     0.06548

ncall =     133
```

solution from lsodes and the ODE routine, tb_1, of Listing 7.1. An example of this additional analysis of the ODEs is given in Chapter 8.

7.5   Conclusions

The tuberculosis model of eqs. (7.1) and (7.2) is nonlinear (consider the RHSs of eqs. (7.1)), and therefore, an analytical approach to a solution is probably not feasible. However, the numerical approach as programmed in tb_1 of Listing 7.1 is quite straightforward. With the R routines in hand, experimentation with the parameters of Table 7.2 is easily accomplished, as well as changes in the structure of the model (variations in the programming of tb_1).

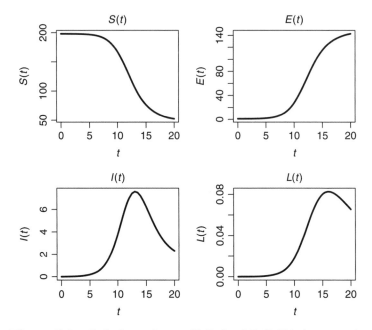

Figure 7.3   Solution of eqs. (7.1) for IC (7.2b) (ncase=2).

This model is offered as representative of a host of epidemic models that have been reported and discussed in the literature. These models include important conditions under which an epidemic might occur. For example, a tuberculosis model is reported in [1] that accounts for the effect of poverty.

References

[1] Bhunu, C.P., S. Mushayabasa, and R.J. Smith (2012), Assessing the effects of poverty in tuberculosis transmission dynamics, *Appl. Math. Model.*, **36**(9), 4173–4185.

[2] Bowong, S., and J.J. Tewa (2011), Mathematical analysis of a tuberculosis model with differential infectivity, *Commun. Nonlinear Sci. Numer. Simulat.*, **14**, 4010–4021.

## CHAPTER 8

Corneal Curvature

8.1   Introduction

The performance of the human cornea (the transparent, front part of the eye) is determined significantly by its curvature. In this case study, we analyze a boundary value ordinary differential equation (BVODE) model for the calculation of the cornea shape reported by Okrasiński and Płociniczak [1]. This study has a fivefold purpose:

1. A brief description of the BVODE model for the corneal shape.
2. A numerical procedure for the integration (solution) of the BVODE model.
3. Discussion of the R routines for the implementation of the numerical procedure.
4. Discussion of the numerical solution produced by the routines, including an assessment of the accuracy of the solution.
5. An introduction to initial values ordinary differential equations (IVODE), BVODE, and PDEs, all within a single application example.

8.2   Model Equations

The BVODE is derived by a static force balance on the cornea as detailed in [1]. Here, we have renumbered the original equations;

Differential Equation Analysis in Biomedical Science and Engineering: Ordinary Differential Equation Applications with R, First Edition. William E. Schiesser.
© 2014 John Wiley & Sons, Inc. Published 2014 by John Wiley & Sons, Inc.

and also, certain original equation numbers are repeated as a second number to facilitate reference to the original derivation and discussion, for example, (8.2; 4) with 8.2 as the new number and 4 as the original number in [1].

A force balance leads to the BVODE (see Fig. 1 in [1])

$$-T\frac{d^2h/dx^2}{\sqrt{1+(dh/dx)^2}} + kh = \frac{P}{\sqrt{1+(dh/dx)^2}} \qquad (8.1)$$

where

Variable Parameter	Interpretation
h	height of the corneal surface relative to the peripheral height; vertical coordinate y in a Cartesian (x,y) coordinate system
x	horizontal coordinate in a Cartesian (x,y) coordinate system
T	tension in the cornea
k	effective spring constant for the cornea
P	applied pressure

If dimensionless variables (based on the corneal radius R)

$$h^* = h/R, \; x^* = x/R \qquad (8.2a,b;4)$$

are introduced, eq. (8.1) becomes (with ($*$) dropped)

$$-T(R/R^2)\frac{d^2h/dx^2}{\sqrt{1+(dh/dx)^2}} + (R)kh = \frac{P}{\sqrt{1+(dh/dx)^2}}$$

or after multiplication by R/T,

$$-\frac{d^2h/dx^2}{\sqrt{1+(dh/dx)^2}} + (R^2/T)kh = (R/T)\frac{P}{\sqrt{1+(dh/dx)^2}} \qquad (8.3)$$

With $a = R^2 k/T$, $b = RT/P$, eq. (8.3) becomes

$$-\frac{d^2h/dx^2}{\sqrt{1 + (dh/dx)^2}} + ah = \frac{b}{\sqrt{1 + (dh/dx)^2}} \tag{8.4}$$

for the full nonlinear BVODE and

$$-\frac{d^2h}{dx^2} + ah = \frac{b}{\sqrt{1 + (dh/dx)^2}} \tag{8.5;5}$$

for an approximate nonlinear BVODE analyzed in [1]. Numerical solutions of eqs. (8.4) and (8.5) are calculated and compared subsequently.

For either nonlinear BVODE, eq. (8.4) or (8.5), the boundary conditions (BCs) are

$$h(1) = 0, \ dh(0)/dx = 0 \tag{8.6a,b;6}$$

Note that because of the nondimensional x of eq. (8.2b), with the corneal radius R the corneal periphery is at $x = 1$. BC (8.6a) specifies that the height of the corneal surface is zero on the periphery. BC (8.6b) specifies zero slope of the corneal surface at $x = 0$ (from symmetry about $x = 0$). Then, the solution to the BVODE, $h(x)$, gives the height of the cornea relative to the periphery.

The general numerical procedure for the solution of the BVODEs, eqs. (8.4) and (8.5), is to add a pseudo derivative in an initial value variable t, thereby producing a PDE in (x, t) that can be integrated by the method of lines (MOL) [2]. The solution is continued (integrated) until the derivative in t reaches an approximately zero value. The resulting solution in x is the required solution to the starting BVODE.

Specifically, eq. (8.4) can be converted to a PDE by adding a pseudo time derivative in t

$$\frac{\partial h}{\partial t} = \frac{1}{\sqrt{1 + (\partial h/\partial x)^2}} \frac{\partial^2 h}{\partial x^2} - ah + \frac{b}{\sqrt{1 + (\partial h/\partial x)^2}} \tag{8.7}$$

with the IC

$$h(x, t = 0) = h_0 \tag{8.8}$$

and BCs

$$h(x = 1, t) = 0, \quad \frac{\partial h(x = 0, t)}{\partial x} = 0 \qquad (8.9a,b)$$

h_0 is a pseudo IC (it is not part of the original model). For $a = b = 0$, $\partial h/\partial x \ll 1$, eq. (8.7) reduces to the 1D diffusion equation (Fick's second law). Eqs. (8.7)–(8.9) constitute the PDE system to be integrated numerically.

8.3   Method of Lines Solution

Here, we consider just a few basic ideas for the MOL solution of eqs. (8.7)–(8.9). A detailed discussion of the MOL is given in [2]. The basic idea in the MOL is to replace the partial derivatives in the spatial (boundary value) independent variables, in this case x, with algebraic approximations. We have selected finite difference (FD) for these algebraic approximations; other possibilities include finite elements, finite volumes, and radial basis functions.

The derivatives in x in eq. (8.7) can be approximated by second-order centered FDs.

$$\left(\frac{\partial h}{\partial x} \right)_i \approx \frac{h_{i+1} - h_{i+1}}{2\Delta x} + O(\Delta x^2) \qquad (8.10a)$$

$$\left(\frac{\partial^2 h}{\partial x^2} \right)_i \approx \frac{h_{i+1} - 2h_i + h_{i+1}}{\Delta x^2} + O(\Delta x^2) \qquad (8.10b)$$

where i is the index for a grid in x with spacing Δx and $1 \le i \le N$; the total number of grid points, N, is selected to give acceptable accuracy (resolution) in x. In the routines that follow, we take $N = 21$. Eqs. (8.10) are second order in x, as denoted by $O(\Delta x^2)$. In the programming that follows, we will actually use sixth-order FD approximations $(O(\Delta x^6))$; eqs. (8.10) are presented here just for the purpose of illustrating FD approximations.

If eqs. (8.10) are substituted in eq. (8.7), we have a system of N initial value ODEs in t ($1 \le i \le N$).

$$\left(\frac{dh}{dt} \right)_i = \frac{1}{\sqrt{1 + \left(\frac{h_{i+1} - h_{i+1}}{2\Delta x} \right)^2}} \left(\frac{h_{i+1} - 2h_i + h_{i+1}}{\Delta x^2} \right) - ah_i$$

$$+ \frac{b}{\sqrt{1 + \left(\frac{h_{i+1}-h_{i+1}}{2\Delta x}\right)^2}} \tag{8.11a}$$

$$h(t=0)_i = h_0 \tag{8.11b}$$

and BCs

$$h(t)_{i=N} = 0, \quad \left(\frac{\partial h(x=0,t)}{\partial x}\right)_{i=1} \approx \frac{h_2 - h_0}{2\Delta x} = 0 \tag{8.11c,d}$$

The IC, eq. (8.11b), and the BCs, eqs. (8.11c,d), follow from eqs. (8.8), (8.9a,b), and (8.10a). BC (8.11c) leads to the ODE at $x = 1$

$$\left(\frac{dh}{dt}\right)_i = 0 \tag{8.11e}$$

That is, eq. (8.11c) is used in place of eq. (8.11a) with $i = N$. Equation (8.11d) can be used to eliminate the fictitious value h_0 (which is beyond the left end of the grid at $i = 1$) from eq. (8.11a) (with $i = 1$). That is, from eq. (8.11d), $h_0 = h_2$ can be substituted in eq. (8.11a) with $i = 1$.

Equation (8.11a) is clearly nonlinear in h_{i-1}, h_i, h_{i+1}, $1 \le i \le N$. This is not an obstacle in the integration with respect to t (using a library initial value ODE integrator such as lsodes). This illustrates one of the essential features of MOL analysis, that is, nonlinearity can usually be easily accommodated. We now consider the programming of eqs. (8.11).

8.4   R Routines

A main program for eqs. (8.7)–(8.9) is in Section 8.4.1. Subordinate routines called by this main program are considered subsequently.

8.4.1   Main Program

A main program for eqs. (8.7)–(8.9) is in Listing 8.1.

```
#
# Access deSolve library (with lsodes)
```

```
  library("deSolve")
#
# ODE/PDE routines
  setwd("c:/R/bme_ode/chap8");
  source("corneal_1.R");
  source("corneal_2.R");
  source("dss006.R");
  source("dss046.R");
#
# Select case
#
#   ncase = 1 - nonlinear ODE
#
#   ncase = 2 - approximate nonlinear ODE
#
  ncase=1;
#
# Parameters
  R=1; k=1; P=1; T=1; a=R^2*k/T; b=R*P/T; nx=21; xl=1;
#
# Write selected parameters
  cat(sprintf('\n\n xl = %5.2f    a = %5.2f
     b = %5.2f\n\n',xl,a,b));
#
# x grid, initial condition
  xg=seq(from=0,to=xl,by=xl/(nx-1));
  u0=rep(0.25,nx);
#
# Output sequence in t
  tf=1;nout=6;ncall=0;
  tm=seq(from=0,to=tf,by=tf/(nout-1));
#
# lsodes ODE integration
  parms=c(rtol=1e-8,atol=1e-8)
  out=lsodes(times=tm,y=u0,func=corneal_1,parms=parms);
#
# Numerical output
  cat(sprintf("    t      u(0,t)  u(0.25xl,t)  u(0.50xl,t)
                      u(0.75xl,t)  u(xl,t)"));
```

```
  un=matrix(0,nrow=nout,ncol=nx);
  for(it in 1:nout){
    if(it==1){un[1,]=u0;
    }else{
    un[it,]=out[it,-1];
    un[it,nx]=0;}
    cat(sprintf("%5.2f%13.5f%13.5f%13.5f%13.5f%13.5f\n",
      tm[it],un[it,1],un[it,6],un[it,11],un[it,16],
        un[it,21])));
  }
#
# Calls to corneal_1
  cat(sprintf("\n ncall = %5d\n\n",ncall))
#
# ux, ut for plotting
  ux_plot=matrix(0,nrow=nout,ncol=nx);
  ut_plot=matrix(0,nrow=nout,ncol=nx);
  for(it in 1:nout){
    ux_plot[it,]=dss006(0,xl,nx,un[it,]);
    ut_plot[it,]=corneal_2(tm[it],un[it,],parms);
  }
#
# u(x,t) vs x
  matplot(x=xg,y=t(un),type="l",xlab="x",ylab="u(x,t)",
    xlim=c(0,xl),
         lty=1,main="u(x,t), t=0,0.2,...,1",lwd = 2)
#
# ux(x,t) vs x
  matplot(x=xg,y=t(ux_plot),type="l",xlab="x",
    ylab="ux(x,t)",
         xlim=c(0,xl),lty=1,main="ux(x,t), t=0,0.2,...,
           1",lwd = 2)
#
# ut(x,t) vs x
  matplot(x=xg,y=t(ut_plot[2:nout,]),type="l",xlab="x",
    ylab="ut(x,t)",
         xlim=c(0,xl),lty=1,main="ut(x,t), t=0.2,...,1",
           lwd = 2)
```

Listing 8.1 Main program for the solution of eqs. (8.7)–(8.9).

We can note the following details about Listing 8.1.

- Library deSolve with lsodes, two ODE routines, corneal_1 and corneal_2, and two PDE routines, dss006 and dss046, are accessed.

```
#
# Access deSolve library (with lsodes)
  library("deSolve")
#
# ODE/PDE routines
  setwd("c:/R/bme_ode/chap8");
  source("corneal_1.R");
  source("corneal_2.R");
  source("dss006.R");
  source("dss046.R");
```

- Two cases are programmed. For ncase=1, eq. (8.4) (the nonlinear BVODE) is programmed (in the ODE routine corneal_1 considered subsequently). For ncase=2, eq. (8.5) (the approximate nonlinear BVODE) is programmed in ODE routine corneal_2.

```
#
# Select case
#
#   ncase = 1 - nonlinear ODE
#
#   ncase = 2 - approximate nonlinear ODE
#
  ncase=1;
```

By executing the two cases and comparing the solutions, the effect of the nonlinear term

$$-\frac{d^2h/dx^2}{\sqrt{1+(dh/dx)^2}}$$

in eq. (8.4) can be assessed.

- The parameters in eqs. (8.7)–(8.9) are defined numerically or computed.

```
#
# Parameters
  R=1; k=1; P=1; T=1; a=R^2*k/T; b=R*P/T; nx=21; xl=1;
#
# Write selected parameters
  cat(sprintf('\n\n xl = %5.2f    a = %5.2f
    b = %5.2f\n\n',xl,a,b));
```

A subset of the parameters is then displayed.

- The grid in x and the IC are defined.

```
#
# x grid, initial condition
  xg=seq(from=0,to=xl,by=xl/(nx-1));
  u0=rep(0.25,nx);
```

In this case, 21 points in x are used (from nx=21). Later, this number will be increased to investigate the effect of the grid spacing on the spatial resolution of the solution. The IC is a constant (eq. (8.8) with $h_0 = 0.25$) that is selected arbitrarily but has no effect on the final solution as $t \to 0$. In particular, $h_0 = 0.25$ was selected as an intermediate value for h which generally is in the range $0 \le h \le 0.35$ as indicated in the subsequent discussion of the solution.

- The interval in t is defined as $0 \le t \le 1$ with six outputs displayed at $t = 0, 0.2, \ldots, 1$.

```
#
# Output sequence in t
  tf=1;nout=6;ncall=0;
  tm=seq(from=0,to=tf,by=tf/(nout-1));
```

The counter for the calls to corneal_1 is also initialzed.

- The solution to the nx=21 ODEs is computed by lsodes. Note the use of corneal_1, the ODE routine considered next.

```
#
# lsodes ODE integration
  parms=c(rtol=1e-8,atol=1e-8)
  out=lsodes(times=tm,y=u0,func=corneal_1,parms=parms);
```

The vector of output values of t in tm and the IC vector u0 defined previously are inputs to the integrator; the length of u0 informs lsodes how many ODEs are to be integrated (nx=21 in this case). The fourth argument, parms, defines the integration error tolerances for lsodes.

The computed solution is in the 2D array out with dimensions out(nout=6,nx+1=22) as discussed next.

- A heading for the solution is first displayed. Then, a 2D matrix for the solution, un, is defined (preallocated).

```
#
# Numerical output
  cat(sprintf("     t         u(0,t)   u(0.25xl,t)
                   u(0.50xl,t)  u(0.75xl,t)  u(xl,t)"));
  un=matrix(0,nrow=nout,ncol=nx);
  for(it in 1:nout){
    if(it==1){un[1,]=u0;
    }else{
    un[it,]=out[it,-1];
    un[it,nx]=0;}
    cat(sprintf("%5.2f%13.5f%13.5f%13.5f%13.5f%
        13.5f\n",
      tm[it],un[it,1],un[it,6],un[it,11],un[it,16],
        un[it,21])));
  }
```

The solution is then placed in un for subsequent plotting with a for in the t index it. The details of the for are, briefly, as follows:

— For it=1 corresponding to $t = 0$, the IC u0 is placed in un[1,]. Note the use of ,] as the second subscript of un to include all nx=21 ODE solutions.

```
      if(it==1){un[1,]=u0;
```

— For it>1 corresponding to $t = 0.2, 0.4, \ldots, 1$, the solution from lsodes in out is placed in un. Note the use of ,-1] to include all values of the second subscript except 1 (the latter is for t as out is formed by lsodes, that is, out[it,1] corresponds to $t = 0, 0.2, \ldots, 1$).

```
un[it,]=out[it,-1];
un[it,nx]=0;}
```

Also, un[it,nx]=0 implements BC (8.9a). This setting of $h(x = 1, t) = 0$ is required because lsodes does not return any ODE dependent variables that are not computed as the solution to an ODE. In other words, in corneal_1, un[it,nx]=0 is set algebraically as

```
#
# BC
  u[nx]=0;
```

and not by the integration of an ODE corresponding to ut[nx]. Without this statement for $h(x = 1, t) = 0$, the IC $h(x = 1, t = 0) = 0.25$ would be retained and displayed for $t > 0$. The final } concludes the if.

— The solution is displayed at $x = 0, 0.25, 0.5, 0.75, 1$.

```
cat(sprintf("%5.2f%13.5f%13.5f%13.5f%13.5f%
    13.5f\n",
    tm[it],un[it,1],un[it,6],un[it,11],un[it,16],
      un[it,21])));
  }
```

The final } concludes the for.

• At the end of the solution, the number of calls to corneal_1 is displayed.

```
#
# Calls to corneal_1
  cat(sprintf("\n ncall = %5d\n\n",ncall))
```

• The derivatives $\partial h(x, t)/\partial x$ and $\partial h(x, t)/\partial t$ are placed in two 2D matrices, ux_plot and ut_plot, respectively, within a for in it.

```
#
# ux, ut for plotting
  ux_plot=matrix(0,nrow=nout,ncol=nx);
  ut_plot=matrix(0,nrow=nout,ncol=nx);
  for(it in 1:nout){
    ux_plot[it,]=dss006(0,xl,nx,un[it,]);
    ut_plot[it,]=corneal_2(tm[it],un[it,],parms);
  }
```

$\partial h(x,t)/\partial x$ is computed by a call to a differentiation routine, dss006, (discussed subsequently). $\partial h(x,t)/\partial t$ is computed by a call to corneal_2 (not corneal_1 which returns the derivative vector as a list as required by lsodes while corneal_2 returns the derivative vector as a numerical vector that is used in subsequent plotting).

- The solution to eq. (8.7), $h(x,t)$, is plotted as a function of x with t as a parameter using the R utility matplot.

```
#
# u(x,t) vs x
  matplot(x=xg,y=t(un),type="l",xlab="x",ylab="u(x,t)",
    xlim=c(0,xl),
          lty=1,main="u(x,t), t=0,0.2,...,1",lwd = 2)
```

Note that the vertical (ordinate) variable is programmed as y=t(un) rather than y=un by using the R transpose operator t( ). This transpose is required so that y=t(un) has nx=21 rows in agreement with the dimension of the horizontal (abscissa) variable xg; in other words, un has nout=6 rows (and nx=21 columns) and is therefore not compatible with xg when using matplot.

- $\partial h/\partial x$ is plotted as a function of x. Note again the use of the transpose operator in y=t(ux_plot).

```
#
# ux(x,t) vs x
  matplot(x=xg,y=t(ux_plot),type="l",xlab="x",
    ylab="ux(x,t)",
```

```
        xlim=c(0,xl),lty=1,main="ux(x,t), t=0,0.2,
           ...,1",lwd = 2)
```

- $\partial h/\partial t$ is plotted as a function of x. Again, the transpose operator is used in y=t(ut_plot[2:nout,]).

```
#
# ut(x,t) vs x
  matplot(x=xg,y=t(ut_plot[2:nout,]),type="l",
     xlab="x",ylab="ut(x,t)",
           xlim=c(0,xl),lty=1,main="ut(x,t), t=0.2,...,
              1",lwd = 2)
```

Also, only the values of $\partial h/\partial t$ for $t = 0.2, 0.4, \ldots 1$ (corresponding to 2:nout) are used because at $t = 0$ the discontinuity between $h(x < 1, t = 0) = 0.25$ and $h(x = 1, t = 0) = 0$ produces a rather distorted curve for $t = 0$. This detail emphasizes an important feature of eq. (8.7), that is, it is a parabolic PDE which smoothes the discontinuity at $t = 0$ so that the solution for $t > 0$ does not display any adverse evidence of this discontinuity. This smoothing is in contrast with hyperbolic PDEs that generally propagate discontinuities (in x and t).

This completes the main program. An important point is the calculation of not only the solution $h(x, t)$ for eq. (8.7), but also the derivatives $\partial h(x, t)/\partial x$ and $\partial h(x, t)/\partial t$. More generally, all of the RHS terms of a PDE can be easily calculated and displayed to elucidate the properties of the solution.

The ODE routine called by lsodes, corneal_1, is considered next.

8.4.2 ODE Routine

The ODE routine corneal_1 is in Listing 8.2.

```
  corneal_1=function(t,u,parms) {
#
# Function corneal_1 computes the PDE t derivative
#
# Declare (preallocate) arrays
```

```
  sr =rep(0,nx);
  ux =rep(0,nx);
  uxx=rep(0,nx);
  ut =rep(0,nx);
#
# BC
  u[nx]=0;
#
# ux
  ux=dss006(0,xl,nx,u);
#
# BC
  ux[1]=0;
#
# uxx
  nl=2; nu=1;
  uxx=dss046(0,xl,nx,u,ux,nl,nu);
#
# PDE
  for(i in 1:nx){
    sr[i]=sqrt(1+ux[i]^2);
    if(ncase==1){ut[i]=uxx[i]/sr[i]-a*u[i]+b/sr[i];}
    if(ncase==2){ut[i]=uxx[i]      -a*u[i]+b/sr[i];}
  }
  ut[nx]=0;
#
# Increment calls to corneal_1
  ncall <<- ncall+1;
#
# Return derivative vector
  return(list(c(ut)))
  }
```

Listing 8.2 `corneal_1` for eqs. (8.7)–(8.9).

We can note the following details about `corneal_1`.

- The function is defined.

```
  corneal_1=function(t,u,parms) {
#
```

```
# Function corneal_1 computes the PDE t derivative
```

The vector of dependent variables is named u rather than the previous y. This choice of a variable name is in conformity with the usual practice of naming PDE dependent variables, for example, eq. (8.7), as u, whereas dependent variables of ODE are typically named y.

- Arrays used in corneal_1 are declared (preallocated).

```
#
# Declare (preallocate) arrays
  sr =rep(0,nx);
  ux =rep(0,nx);
  uxx=rep(0,nx);
  ut =rep(0,nx);
```

- BC (8.9a) (also eq. (8.11c)) is set.

```
#
# BC
  u[nx]=0;
```

Note the use of u, the second RHS (input) argument of corneal_1, and subscript nx for $x = 1$.

- The derivative $\partial h / \partial x$ of eq. (8.7) is computed by a library routine, dss006.

```
#
# ux
  ux=dss006(0,xl,nx,u);
```

The second-order FD approximations of eqs. (8.10a) and (8.11a) are not actually used. Rather, dss006 has seven-point sixth-order $(O(\Delta x^6))$ FDs 1.

- BC (8.9b) redefines ux(1) $= \partial h(x = 0, t)/\partial x$ from dss006.

```
#
# BC
  ux[1]=0;
```

Note the subscript 1 corresponding to $x = 0$.

- The second derivative in eq. (8.7), $\partial^2 h/\partial x^2 =$ uxx, is computed by the library differentiator dss046 [2] directly from u. nl=2 specifies the Neumann BC (8.9b) at $x = 0$, and nu=1 specifies the Dirichlet BC (8.9a) at $x = 1$. Briefly, the Neumann BC defines the first derivative in x (in this case, $\partial u(x = 0, t)/\partial x$), and the Dirichlet BC defines the dependent variable (in this case, $u(x = 1, t)$). The use of the sixth-order FD approximations in dss046 permits a small number of points in x, n=21. Whether this number of points achieves acceptable accuracy in the numerical solution will be investigated later by computing a second solution with a larger number of points and comparing the two solutions.

```
#
# uxx
  nl=2; nu=1;
  uxx=dss046(0,xl,nx,u,ux,nl,nu);
```

Note that the first derivative ux is an input to dss046 so that the BC at $x = 0$, eq. (8.9b), is included in the calculation of the second derivative uxx.

- All of the derivatives in the RHS of eq. (8.7) are now available, so the LHS can be programmed.

```
#
# PDE
  for(i in 1:nx){
    sr[i]=sqrt(1+ux[i]^2);
    if(ncase==1){ut[i]=uxx[i]/sr[i]-a*u[i]+b/sr[i];}
    if(ncase==2){ut[i]=uxx[i]      -a*u[i]+b/sr[i];}
  }
  ut[nx]=0;
```

The for steps through the grid in x. At each point in x, $\sqrt{1 + (\partial h/\partial x)^2} =$ sr is computed. Then this term is included in the nonlinear second-derivative term of eq. (8.7) for ncase=1

$$\frac{1}{\sqrt{1 + (\partial h/\partial x)^2}} \frac{\partial^2 h}{\partial x^2}$$

or is not included in the linear term for `ncase=2`

$$\frac{\partial^2 h}{\partial x^2}$$

In this way, the effect of $\sqrt{1 + (\partial h/\partial x)^2}$ can be ascertained by comparing the solutions for the two cases. For $\partial h/\partial x \ll 1$, the effect should be negligible, but as we will observe in the numerical and graphical outputs, this is not the case, so the nonlinear term should be included rather than neglected as in [1]. After the derivative $\partial h/\partial t = $ ut is computed at each x (each i), this derivative is set to zero at $x = 1$ in accordance with BC (8.9a) (or eq. (8.11c)), `ut(nx)=0;`. Note the subscript nx corresponding to $x = 1$. This completes the programming of eq. (8.7).

- The counter for the calls to `corneal_1` is incremented.

```
#
# Increment calls to corneal_1
  ncall <<- ncall+1;
```

ncall is returned to the main program of Listing 8.1 with the `<<-` so that it can be displayed at the end of the numerical solution.

- The derivative vector ut is returned to lsodes as a list.

```
#
# Return derivative vector
  return(list(c(ut)))
  }
```

The final } concludes `corneal_1`.

This completes the programming of eqs. (8.7)–(8.9). The numerical solution from Listings 8.1 and 8.2 is discussed in Section 8.5.

8.5 Numerical Solution

Abbreviated output for `ncase=1` (set in Listing 8.1) follows in Table 8.1.

TABLE 8.1   Selected output from Listings 8.1 and 8.2 for ncase=1.

```
xl =   1.00    a =   1.00    b =   1.00

    t        u(0,t)  u(0.25xl,t)  u(0.50xl,t)  u(0.75xl,t)
                                                u(xl,t)
  0.00       0.25000     0.25000      0.25000     0.25000
                                                  0.25000
  0.20       0.32839     0.31021      0.25354     0.15276
                                                  0.00000
  0.40       0.33946     0.31979      0.25965     0.15538
                                                  0.00000
  0.60       0.34437     0.32432      0.26310     0.15724
                                                  0.00000
  0.80       0.34681     0.32658      0.26483     0.15817
                                                  0.00000
  1.00       0.34803     0.32771      0.26570     0.15864
                                                  0.00000

ncall =    222
```

We note the following details about this output.

- The six values of t, $t = 0, 0.2, \ldots, 1$ appear in the output.
- The IC, u0(i)=0.25 in Listing 8.1, is displayed at $t = 0$. Checking the IC is a good procedure because if it is not correct due to a programming error, the remainder of the solution $(t > 0)$ will be incorrect.
- At the final value $t = 1$, the profile in h has the terminal values $h(x = 0, t = 1) = u(x = 0, t = 1) = 0.34803$, $h(x = 1, t = 1) = u(x = 1, t = 1) = 0$. The latter is in accordance with BC (8.9a). The value at $x = 1$ also indicates why $h(x = 1, t) = 0$ is programmed explicitly in Listing 8.1 because otherwise the IC would be indicated, that is, $h(x = 1, t = 0) = h(x = 1, t) = 0.25$.
- The computational effort is quite modest.

```
ncall =    222
```

The graphical output is in Figs. 8.1–8.3.

Figure 8.1 indicates the evolution of the solution of eq. (8.7) from the IC $h(x,t=0) = 0.25$ to an equilibrium solution at $t = 1$. This figure is in approximate agreement with the solution of eq. (8.5) in Fig. 2 of [1]. Differences between the two solutions (Fig. 2 of [1] and Fig. 8.2) could be due to the nonlinear factor $1/\sqrt{1+(\partial h/\partial x)^2}$ in eq. (8.7). This point is discussed further when the solution for ncase=2 is considered. Figure 8.2 indicates the evolution of $\partial h(x,t)/\partial x$ from the initial value $\partial h(x,t=0)/\partial x = 0$ to an equilibrium profile at $t = 1$. The initial derivative is zero because the derivative in x of the constant IC $h(x,t=0) = 0.25$ (see Fig. 8.1) is zero.

$\partial h(x,t)/\partial x =$ ux has negative values as expected because u decreases with x. Also, ux does not satisfy the condition $\partial h(x,t)/\partial x \ll 1$, which implies the nonlinear factor $1/\sqrt{1+(\partial h/\partial x)^2}$ in the second-derivative term of eq. (8.7) might significantly affect the solution. This will be considered when the solution for ncase=1 (with the nonlinear factor) is subsequently compared with the solution for ncase=2 (without the nonlinear factor).

Figure 8.3 indicates the evolution of $\partial h(x,t)/\partial t$ from the value $\partial h(x,t=0.2)/\partial t$ to an equilibrium profile at $t = 1$. Note that

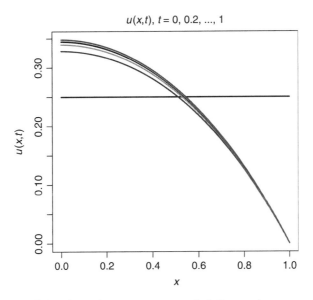

$u(x,t)$, $t = 0, 0.2, ..., 1$

Figure 8.1 $h(x,t)$ versus x, $t = 0, 0.2, \ldots, 1$, ncase=1.

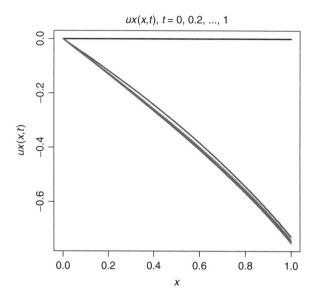

Figure 8.2 $\partial h(x,t)/\partial x$ versus x, $t = 0, 0.2, \ldots, 1$, ncase=1.

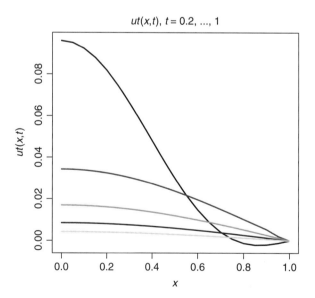

Figure 8.3 $\partial h(x,t)/\partial t$ versus x, $t = 0.2, \ldots, 1$, ncase=1.

$\partial h(x,t=0)/\partial x$ is not included because it has large values that distort the plot (recall again ut(1, :)=0 at $t=0$ in Listing 8.1 for the purpose of plotting). The reason for these large initial values can be explained by eq. (8.7) with $t=0$.

$$\frac{\partial h}{\partial t} = \frac{1}{\sqrt{1+(0)^2}}(0) - a(0.25) + \frac{b}{\sqrt{1+(0)^2}} = 0.75$$

with $a=b=1$. Here, we have used $\partial h(x,t=0)/\partial x = \partial^2 h(x,t=0)/\partial x^2 = 0$ because at $t=0$, the solution is constant, that is, $h(x,t=0)=0.25$. The value of the derivative, $\partial h(x,t=0)/\partial t=0.75$ is much larger than the values for $t>0$ in Fig. 8.3. Therefore, the $t=0$ derivative is not included in Fig. 8.3. In other words, the large initial derivative $\partial h(x,t=0)/\partial t$ quickly decays to the smaller values in Fig. 8.3 for $t>0$.

At the end of the solution ($t=1$), $\partial h(x,t)/\partial t=$ ut is small because the solution has reached an equilibrium (steady-state) condition.

The contribution of the nonlinear factor $1/\sqrt{1+(\partial h/\partial x)^2}$ in the second-derivative term of eq. (8.7) can be examined by executing Listing 8.1 with ncase=2. The output is discussed as previously (Table 8.1 and Figs. 8.1–8.3 which now become Table 8.2 and Figs. 8.4–8.6).

We note the following details about this output.

- The following comparison of the solutions for ncase=1,2 at $t=1$ (from Tables 8.1 and 8.2) gives an indication of the differences in the solutions.

```
ncase=1
1.00    0.34803    0.32771    0.26570    0.15864
        0.00000

ncase=2
1.00    0.33986    0.31928    0.25708    0.15167
        0.00000
```

The effect of the nonlinear term $1/\sqrt{1+(\partial h/\partial x)^2}$ in eq. (8.7) at $x=0$ is about $((0.34803-0.33986)/0.34803) \times 100 = 2.34\%$ so that neglecting the nonlinear has a small effect.

TABLE 8.2   Selected output from Listings 8.1 and 8.2 for ncase=2.

```
xl =  1.00   a =  1.00   b =  1.00
```

t	u(0,t)	u(0.25xl,t)	u(0.50xl,t)	u(0.75xl,t) u(xl,t)
0.00	0.25000	0.25000	0.25000	0.25000
				0.25000
0.20	0.32370	0.30496	0.24723	0.14697
				0.00000
0.40	0.33305	0.31305	0.25243	0.14925
				0.00000
0.60	0.33706	0.31672	0.25517	0.15067
				0.00000
0.80	0.33896	0.31846	0.25647	0.15135
				0.00000
1.00	0.33986	0.31928	0.25708	0.15167
				0.00000

```
ncall =    193
```

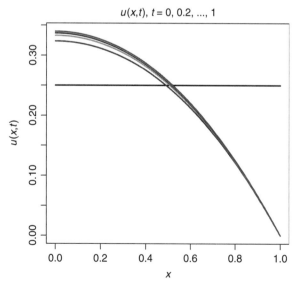

Figure 8.4 $h(x,t)$ vs. x, $t = 0, 0.2, \ldots, 1$, ncase=2.

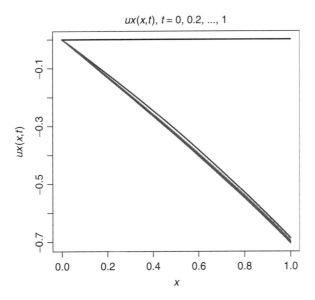

Figure 8.5 $\partial h(x,t)/\partial x$ versus x, $t = 0, 0.2, \ldots, 1$, ncase=2.

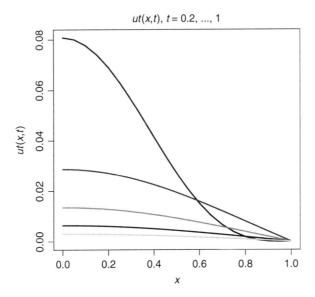

Figure 8.6 $\partial h(x,t)/\partial t$ versus x, $t = 0.2, \ldots, 1$, ncase=2.

- The computational effort for ncase=2 is quite modest.

```
ncall =   193
```

The graphical output for ncase=2, Figs. 8.4–8.6, is substantially different from that for ncase=1 in Figs. 8.1–8.3, but the final solution at t is approximately the same.

In summary, the inclusion of the nonlinear factor $1/\sqrt{1 + (\partial h/\partial x)^2}$ in the second-derivative term of eq. (8.7) has an observable but not large effect.

8.6 Error Analysis of the Numerical Solution

The solutions discussed previously were for a 21-point grid in x. We now consider the effect of increasing this number to 41, which requires only a change of nx=21 to nx=41 and the output statement in Listing 8.1 as follows.

```
cat(sprintf("%5.2f%13.5f%13.5f%13.5f%13.5f%13.5f\n",
    tm[it],un[it,1],un[it,11],un[it,21],un[it,31],
    un[it,41])));
```

Execution of the routines in Listings 8.1 and 8.2 with these changes gives the abbreviated output given in Table 8.3.

The following output indicates that the solution is essentially unchanged from nx=21.

```
ncase=1, nx=21 (Table 8.1)
1.00       0.34803     0.32771      0.26570      0.15864
    0.00000


ncase=1, nx=41 (Table 8.3)
1.00       0.34805     0.32772      0.26571      0.15865
    0.00000
```

This agreement implies that nx=21 achieved acceptable accuracy in the numerical solution. The computational effort for nx=41 is still quite modest with ncall=335 (however, additional computation is required in each execution of dss006 and dss046 as explained subsequently). As the solutions for nx=21,41 are essentially identical, the graphical output for the latter is not presented.

TABLE 8.3   Selected output from Listings 8.1 and 8.2 for nx=41, ncase=1.

x1 =	1.00	a =	1.00	b =	1.00

t	u(0,t)	u(0.25x1,t)	u(0.50x1,t)	u(0.75x1,t) u(x1,t)
0.00	0.25000	0.25000	0.25000	0.25000
				0.25000
0.20	0.32854	0.31036	0.25367	0.15284
				0.00000
0.40	0.33954	0.31987	0.25971	0.15541
				0.00000
0.60	0.34441	0.32436	0.26313	0.15725
				0.00000
0.80	0.34683	0.32660	0.26485	0.15818
				0.00000
1.00	0.34805	0.32772	0.26571	0.15865
				0.00000

ncall =   335

The change in nx results in a change in the grid spacing in x. As the grid spacing is often termed h in the literature, the change from 21 to 41 points is an example of h refinement to establish the accuracy of a numerical solution. An important point to note is that h refinement is a general procedure in the sense that it does not require an analytical solution to estimate the accuracy of the numerical solution (as is usually the case, an analytical solution to eq. (8.4) or (8.7) is not available).

Another possibility for the evaluation of the numerical solution is to change the order of the approximations used in the calculation of the solution. For example, the sixth-order FDs in dss006 and dss046 called in corneal_1 of Listing 8.2 can be replaced with eighth-order

FDs by calling `dss008` and `dss048`. This is easily done because the arguments for the differentiation routines are the same (only the names are different). The relevant statements in `corneal_1` become

```
#
# ux
   ux=dss008(0,xl,nx,u);
#
# BC
   ux[1]=0;
#
# uxx
   nl=2; nu=1;
   uxx=dss048(0,xl,nx,u,ux,nl,nu);
```

Abbreviated output for these changes is given in Table 8.4.

TABLE 8.4   Selected output from Listings 8.1 and 8.2 with `dss008`, `dss048`, `ncase=1`.

xl = 1.00	a = 1.00	b = 1.00		
t	u(0,t)	u(0.25xl,t)	u(0.50xl,t)	u(0.75xl,t) u(xl,t)
0.00	0.25000	0.25000	0.25000	0.25000
				0.25000
0.20	0.32839	0.31021	0.25354	0.15276
				0.00000
0.40	0.33946	0.31979	0.25965	0.15538
				0.00000
0.60	0.34436	0.32432	0.26310	0.15724
				0.00000
0.80	0.34681	0.32658	0.26483	0.15817
				0.00000
1.00	0.34803	0.32771	0.26570	0.15864
				0.00000

```
ncall =   242
```

The two solutions (in Tables 8.1 and 8.4) are identical. This is demonstrated in the following table.

```
ncase=1, nx=21, dss006, dss046 (Table 8.1)
1.00       0.34803    0.32771    0.26570    0.15864
   0.00000

ncase=1, nx=21, dss008, dss048 (Table 8.4)
1.00       0.34803    0.32771    0.26570    0.15864
   0.00000
```

This agreement implies that dss006, dss046 achieved acceptable accuracy in the numerical solution. The computational effort is still quite modest with ncall=242 (however, additional computation is required in each execution of dss008 and dss048 as explained subsequently). As the solutions for dss006, dss046 and dss008, dss048 are identical, the graphical output for the latter is not presented.

In this assessment of the accuracy of the numerical solution, the order of the FD approximations used to calculate the derivatives in x was changed. As in the literature, the order of an approximation is often denoted as p, the calculation and the comparison of the two solutions with FDs of different orders is termed as p refinement. The FD approximations in dss006, dss046 are $O(h^6)$ so $p = 6$, and the FD approximations in dss008, dss048 are $O(h^8)$ so $p = 8$.

In conclusion, nx=21 and dss006, dss046 appear to give numerical solutions of acceptable accuracy. This is inferred by a comparison of the solutions with different numbers of grid points and FD approximations. Of course, the integration in t could also introduce errors, so the error tolerances, rtol, atol, for lsodes could be changed and any differences in the numerical solutions are observed. As these tolerances are already stringent (1.0e-08), making these tolerances smaller is not expected to change the solution.

Also, lsodes is a sophisticated integrator in the sense that it automatically applies h and p refinement as the solution proceeds. This demonstrates a major advantage in using library routines, That is, they are usually written by experts and therefore have features and safeguards that would not be anticipated by less experienced analysts.

8.7 Library Routines for Differentiation in Space

The library differentiation routines dss006 and dss046 are listed in Listing 8.3.

```
  dss006=function(xl,xu,n,u) {
#
# Documentation comments removed to conserve space
#
# Preallocate arrays
  ux=rep(0,n);
#
# Grid spacing
  dx=(xu-xl)/(n-1);
#
# 1/(6!*dx) for subsequent use
  r6fdx=1/(720*dx);
#
# ux vector
#
# Boundaries (x=xl,x=xu)
  ux[1]=r6fdx*
    (-1764*u[  1]+4320*u[  2]-5400*u[  3]+4800*u[  4]-
      2700*u[  5] +864*u[  6] -120*u[  7]);
  ux[n]=r6fdx*
    ( 1764*u[  n]-4320*u[n-1]+5400*u[n-2]-4800*u[n-3]+
      2700*u[n-4] -864*u[n-5] +120*u[n-6]);
#
# dx in from boundaries (x=xl+dx,x=xu-dx)
  ux[  2]=r6fdx*
    (-120*u[  1]-924*u[  2]+1800*u[  3]-1200*u[  4]+
      600*u[  5]-180*u[  6] +24*u[  7]);
  ux[n-1]=r6fdx*
    ( 120*u[  n]+924*u[n-1]-1800*u[n-2]+1200*u[n-3]-
      600*u[n-4]+180*u[n-5]  -24*u[n-6]);
#
# 2*dx in from boundaries (x=xl+2*dx,x=xu-2*dx)
  ux[  3]=r6fdx*
    ( 24*u[  1]-288*u[  2]-420*u[  3]+960*u[  4]-
      360*u[  5] +96*u[  6] -12*u[  7]);
  ux[n-2]=r6fdx*
```

```
      (-24*u[   n]+288*u[n-1]+420*u[n-2]-960*u[n-3]+
        360*u[n-4] -96*u[n-5] +12*u[n-6]);
#
# Interior points (x=xl+3*dx,...,x=xu-3*dx)
  for(i in 4:(n-3))
  ux[i]=r6fdx*
    (-12*u[i-3]+108*u[i-2]-540*u[i-1]+
      12*u[i+3]-108*u[i+2]+540*u[i+1]);
#
# All points concluded (x=xl,...,x=xu)
  return(c(ux));
}
```

Listing 8.3 Differentiation routine dss006.

We can note the following details about dss006.

- The definition of the function is in accordance with its use in corneal_1 (i.e., the four input arguments). In particular, the 1D vector u is differentiated with respect to x using a grid of n points over the interval xl $\leq$ x $\leq$ xu.

  ```
      dss006=function(xl,xu,n,u) {
  ```

- The 1D array for the computed derivative, ux, is defined.

  ```
  #
  # Preallocate arrays
    ux=rep(0,n);
  #
  # Grid spacing
    dx=(xu-xl)/(n-1);
  #
  # 1/(6!*dx) for subsequent use
    r6fdx=1/(720*dx);
  ```

  The grid spacing dx and a multiplying factor r6fdx are computed.

- The elements of derivative vector ux are computed as weighted sums of the values of the elements in u. For example, at the left boundary x=xl,

```
ux[1]=r6fdx*
  (-1764*u[  1]+4320*u[  2]-5400*u[  3]+4800*u[  4]-
    2700*u[  5] +864*u[  6] -120*u[  7]);
```

We can note the following details about this calculation.

— The derivative at the left boundary, ux[1], is computed with only the interior points u[1], u[2], u[3], u[4], u[5], u[6], u[7]. In other words, the calculation of ux[1] does not require the use of fictitious points to the left of xl.

— The weighting coefficients -1764,...,-120 are derived from a Lagrange polynomial fitted to the seven values of u[1],...,u[7]. The details for deriving these coefficients are given in [2].

— R does not in general require special characters for continuing a line onto a second line. However, experience has indicated that the reliability of a continuation for a computation requires the first line end in an arithmetic operator. Therefore, for example, we use 4800*u[4]- to continue the first line rather than 4800*u[4] with the - placed at the beginning of the second line.

— The final line in the continuation should end with ;, for example, -120*u[7]);. In fact, ending each complete line in R with ; is recommended.

- ux is computed for all n grid points (ux[1] to ux[nx]) to produce the n-vector ux, which is then returned as a vector.

```
#
# All points concluded (x=xl,...,x=xu)
  return(c(ux));
}
```

The final } concludes dss006.

dss046 has a structure similar to dss004 (a weighted sum of the dependent variable), but it computes a second derivative in x rather than a first derivative, including the Neumann and the Dirichlet BCs (Listing 8.4).

```
dss046=function(xl,xu,n,u,ux,nl,nu) {
#
# Documentation comments removed to conserve space
#
# Preallocate arrays
  ux =rep(0,n);
  uxx=rep(0,n);
#
# Grid spacing
  dx=(xu-xl)/(n-1);
#
# 1/(dx**2) for subsequent use
  rdxs=1/dx^2;
#
# uxx vector
#
# Boundaries (x=xl,x=xu)
  if(nl==1)
    uxx[1]=rdxs*
    (  5.211111111111110*u[  1]-22.300000000000000*u[  2]+
      43.950000000000000*u[  3]-52.722222222222200*u[  4]+
      41.000000000000000*u[  5]-20.100000000000000*u[  6]+
       5.661111111111110*u[  7] -0.700000000000000*u[  8]);
  if(nu==1)
    uxx[n]=rdxs*
    (  5.211111111111110*u[n  ]-22.300000000000000*u[n-1]+
      43.950000000000000*u[n-2]-52.722222222222200*u[n-3]+
      41.000000000000000*u[n-4]-20.100000000000000*u[n-5]+
       5.661111111111110*u[n-6] -0.700000000000000*u[n-7]);
  if(nl==2)
    uxx[1]=rdxs*
    ( -7.493888888888860*u[  1]+12.000000000000000*u[  2]-
       7.499999999999940*u[  3] +4.444444444444570*u[  4]-
       1.874999999999960*u[  5] +0.479999999999979*u[  6]-
       0.055555555555568*u[  7] -4.900000000000000*ux[1]*
          dx);
```

```
if(nu==2)
  uxx[n]=rdxs*
  ( -7.493888888888860*u[n  ]+12.000000000000000*u[n-1]-
    7.499999999999940*u[n-2] +4.444444444444570*u[n-3]-
    1.874999999999960*u[n-4] +0.479999999999979*u[n-5]-
    0.055555555555568*u[n-6] +4.900000000000000*ux[n]*
      dx);
#
# dx in from boundaries (x=xl+dx,x=xu-dx)
  uxx[2]=rdxs*
  (  0.700000000000000*u[  1]-0.388888888888889*u[  2]-
    2.700000000000000*u[  3]+4.750000000000000*u[  4]-
    3.722222222222220*u[  5]+1.800000000000000*u[  6]-
    0.500000000000000*u[  7]+0.061111111111111*u[  8]);
  uxx[n-1]=rdxs*
  (  0.700000000000000*u[n  ]-0.388888888888889*u[n-1]-
    2.700000000000000*u[n-2]+4.750000000000000*u[n-3]-
    3.722222222222220*u[n-4]+1.800000000000000*u[n-5]-
    0.500000000000000*u[n-6]+0.061111111111111*u[n-7]);
#
# 2*dx in from boundaries (x=xl+2*dx,x=xu-2*dx)
  uxx[3]=rdxs*
  ( -0.061111111111111*u[  1]+1.188888888888890*u[  2]-
    2.100000000000000*u[  3]+0.722222222222223*u[  4]+
    0.472222222222222*u[  5]-0.300000000000000*u[  6]+
    0.088888888888889*u[  7]-0.011111111111111*u[  8]);
  uxx[n-2]=rdxs*
  ( -0.061111111111111*u[n  ]+1.188888888888890*u[n-1]-
    2.100000000000000*u[n-2]+0.722222222222223*u[n-3]+
    0.472222222222222*u[n-4]-0.300000000000000*u[n-5]+
    0.088888888888889*u[n-6]-0.011111111111111*u[n-7]);
#
# Remaining interior points (x=xl+3*dx,...,x=xu-3*dx)
  for(i in 4:(n-3))
    uxx[i]=rdxs*
    (  0.011111111111111*u[i-3]-0.150000000000000*u[i-2]+
      1.500000000000000*u[i-1]+0.011111111111111*u[i+3]-
      0.150000000000000*u[i+2]+1.500000000000000*u[i+1]-
      2.722222222222220*u[i  ]);
#
# All points concluded (x=xl,...,x=xu)
```

```
    return(c(uxx));
}
```

Listing 8.4 Differentiation routine `dss046`.

The similarity to `dss006` is clear. The following are essential differences.

- The second derivative is computed as `uxx` over the grid of `n` points.
- At the boundaries, points `1,n`, two forms of the calculation of `uxx` are programmed. For example, at point `1`, for a Dirichlet BC (`nl=1`), `uxx[1]` is given by

```
    if(nl==1)
      uxx[1]=rdxs*
      (   5.211111111111110*u[   1]-22.300000000000000*
           u[   2]+
          43.950000000000000*u[   3]-52.722222222222200*
           u[   4]+
          41.000000000000000*u[   5]-20.100000000000000*
           u[   6]+
           5.661111111111110*u[   7] -0.700000000000000*
           u[   8]);
```

For a Neumann BC, `nl=2`, `uxx[1]` is given by

```
    if(nl==2)
      uxx[1]=rdxs*
      (  -7.493888888888860*u[   1]+12.000000000000000*
           u[   2]-
           7.499999999999940*u[   3] +4.444444444444570*
           u[   4]-
           1.874999999999960*u[   5] +0.479999999999979*
           u[   6]-
           0.055555555555568*u[   7] -4.900000000000000*
           ux[1]*dx);
```

The important difference is that for the Neumann BC, a term involving the first derivative, `ux[1]`, is included in the calculation of `uxx[1]`.

```
-4.900000000000000*ux[1]*dx
```

`ux[1]` is an input to `dss046` through the fifth argument, that is, `ux` in

```
dss046=function(xl,xu,n,u,ux,nl,nu) {
```

Note also that `nl`, `nu` are input arguments to `dss046` for the Dirichlet and the Neumann BCs. Again, as in `dss006`, these differentiation formulas originate from a Lagrange interpolation polynomial [2].

The FD formulas in `dss006,dss046` are sixth-order correct. The `dss` series of differentiators has `ux` and `uxx` routines that are second- to tenth-order correct.

8.8 Summary

BVODEs are an important class of differential equations for applications. Several direct numerical methods are available for the solution of BVODEs. Here, we have used an indirect method in which the BVODE is converted to a PDE and then the PDE is integrated to an equilibrium solution that is also the solution of the BVODE. One way to view this is to consider that the PDE solution is *continued* to the BVODE solution. In other words, this approach can be considered as an example of a continuation method and t in eq. (8.7) is a continuation parameter.

Generally, continuation can be an effective approach to the solution of systems of nonlinear equations. This is illustrated by the preceding example. If eq. (8.4) is approximated directly by FDs, the result is eq. (8.11a) with $\left(\dfrac{dh}{dt}\right)_i = 0$.

$$0 = \frac{1}{\sqrt{1 + \left(\frac{h_{i+1}-h_{i+1}}{2\Delta x}\right)^2}} \left(\frac{h_{i+1}-2h_i+h_{i+1}}{\Delta x^2}\right) - ah_i$$

$$+ \frac{b}{\sqrt{1 + \left(\frac{h_{i+1}-h_{i+1}}{2\Delta x}\right)^2}} \tag{8.12}$$

Eqs. (8.12) constitute an $N \times N$ system of nonlinear algebraic equations for $h_1, h_2, \ldots, h_N$. The solution of this algebraic system would require an iterative method such as, for example, a variant of Newton's method that would be relatively difficult to derive (the $N \times N$ Jacobian matrix would be required for Newton's method) and program, and which might not converge. The success of this iterative approach would be dependent on the assumed initial estimate of the solution (which would have to be within the domain of convergence of the iterative algorithm).

By adding the derivative $(dh/dt)_i$ in eq. (8.11a), the solution of a system of nonlinear algebraic equations is replaced by the numerical integration of a system of ODEs, which is generally an easier problem because of the availability of quality library initial value ODE integrators (such as lsodes). This approach is discussed in terms of the differential Levenberg Marquardt method in the appendix of Chapter 6.

Also, the matter of selecting an initial estimate of the solution in an iterative algebraic method is replaced by the specification of an IC for the ODE system, for example, eq. (8.11b). Assuming that the ODE integration proceeds to a stable equilibrium solution for which $(dh/dt)_i \approx 0$, the final solution might not be the one of interest because systems of nonlinear ODEs can have multiple solutions. But this same problem (nonunique solutions) exists also for iterative algebraic methods. Therefore, some experimentation with the ODE IC, such as eq. (8.11b), may be required, but experience has demonstrated that this is usually not the case. Generally, the only significant complication is adding the pseudo t derivative to the BVODE system so that the resulting PDE has a stable equilibrium solution. In the present example, this step was guided to some extent by the knowledge that the diffusion equation, which is a special case of the PDE, is stable.

In other words, in going from eq. (8.4) to (8.7), the way in which the pseudo derivative in t is added is an important consideration. To direct this step, we can note for the special case $a = b = 0, \partial h / \partial x \ll 1$, eq. (8.7) reduces to the diffusion equation, which is known to have stable solutions. If the t derivative had been added with the opposite sign, the resulting PDE would probably be unstable (as is $\partial u / \partial t =$

$-\partial^2 u / \partial x^2$). Generally, the pseudo t derivative must be added with care to produce a PDE that will have a stable equilibrium solution.

The transformation of eq. (8.4) to (8.11a) is usually termed the *method of false transients*. Equation (8.11a) appears to give a transient solution, as in Fig. 8.1, but this solution is not for the original problem, eq. (8.4), except in the limiting case $t \to \infty$.

The preceding example illustrates three major classes of differential equations: (i) IVODEs, for example, eqs. (8.11a) and (8.11b) with solution by `lsodes`; (ii) BVODEs, for example, eq. (8.4); and (iii) PDEs (or more specifically, initial–boundary value PDEs), for example, eqs. (8.7)–(8.9). The numerical methods that were used are general purpose, but they require attention to the details of the particular problem including the coding.

In other words, these methods, as they are presented here, are not embedded in a software system that requires the analyst to merely specify the equations in some standard format with the expectation that a valid numerical solution will result. Rather, the coding is specific to the particular problem and generally requires an error analysis to provide confidence that the computed solution has an acceptable accuracy; for example, this might require some form of h and/or p refinement.

Also, the computation might be sensitive to the particular values of the problem parameters, particularly for nonlinear problems. For example, seemingly small changes in the parameter values might produce unexpectedly large changes in the solution, or the computation might fail altogether. Thus, each problem must be considered as a new problem, with no guarantee in advance of the successful calculation of a solution. For all of these reasons, the details of how a numerical solution is computed should be reported along with the solution so that analysts will understand the basis and possible limitations of the numerical methodology. An important part of this reporting of the numerical methods is the (documented) source code so that analysts can understand precisely how the calculations were performed and can verify the reported numerical results. After this verification, analysts can extend the methods with confidence to new cases, equation models, and applications.

In other words, this form of scientific computation should follow the usual standard for reporting the results of scientific research, that is, reporting the methodology in enough detail that other researchers can reproduce and verify the reported numerical results and then apply and extend the computational methods. Presenting a mathematical model as a system of equations followed by a computed solution, without giving the details of the intermediate steps and procedures used to compute the reported numerical solution, is not sufficient to meet the usual requirements and standards of scientific research.

References

[1] Okrasiński, W., and L. Płociniczak (2012), A nonlinear mathematical model of the corneal shape, *Nonlinear Anal. R. World Appl.*, **13**, 1498–1505.

[2] Schiesser, W.E., and G.W. Griffiths (2009), *A Compendium of Partial Differential Equation Models*, Cambridge University Press, Cambridge.

Stiff ODE Integration

A1.1   Introduction

The integrators implemented in `euler`, `meuler`, `rkc4`, and `rkf45` discussed previously can be used for a broad spectrum of applications. However, these explicit (nonstiff) integrators will require lengthy calculations for stiff ODE systems. This difficulty with stiff systems results from having to take small integration steps to maintain stability of the numerical integration (because of the stability constraints of explicit algorithms) while having to cover a large interval in the independent variable to compute a complete solution. This computational requirement will now be illustrated with the following 2×2 ODE system.

$$\begin{aligned} dy_1/dt &= f_1(y_1, y_2, t) & y_1(t = 0) &= y_{10} \\ dy_2/dt &= f_2(y_1, y_2, t) & y_2(t = 0) &= y_{20} \end{aligned} \tag{A1.1}$$

where f_1 and f_2 are arbitrary functions. As eqs. (A1.1) are first order, each equation requires one IC as stated in terms of arbitrary constants y_{10}, y_{20}.

We now consider the following special case of eqs. (A1.1) for which f_1 and f_2 are linear functions of y_1 and y_2, respectively.

$$\begin{aligned} \frac{dy_1}{dt} &= -ay_1 + by_2 & y_1(t = 0) &= y_{10} \\ \frac{dy_2}{dt} &= by_1 - ay_2 & y_2(t = 0) &= y_{20} \end{aligned} \tag{A1.2}$$

Differential Equation Analysis in Biomedical Science and Engineering: Ordinary Differential Equation Applications with R, First Edition. William E. Schiesser.

The constants a, b can be selected to make eqs. (A1.2) arbitrarily stiff (as explained subsequently).

A1.2   Analytical Solution of Second-Order ODE System

As eqs. (A1.2) are linear, they can be readily integrated by the well-known methods of linear algebra. We first derive the analytical solution to eqs. (A1.2) that can then be used as a test for selected numerical methods for stiff ODEs.

Generally, linear constant coefficient ODEs such as eqs. (A1.2) have exponential functions of the independent variable (t) as solutions, so as a starting point, we assume

$$y_1(t) = c_1 e^{\lambda t}$$
$$y_2(t) = c_2 e^{\lambda t} \tag{A1.3a}$$

where c_1, c_2, and λ are constants to be determined. Substitution of eqs. (A1.3a) in eqs. (A1.2) gives

$$c_1 \lambda e^{\lambda t} = a_{11} c_1 e^{\lambda t} + a_{12} c_2 e^{\lambda t}$$
$$c_2 \lambda e^{\lambda t} = a_{21} c_1 e^{\lambda t} + a_{22} c_2 e^{\lambda t} \tag{A1.3b}$$

Cancellation of $e^{\lambda t}$ gives a system of algebraic equations (this is the reason why assuming exponential solutions works in the case of linear constant coefficient ODEs—note that the exponential will in general not be zero, so this division is possible)

$$c_1 \lambda = a_{11} c_1 + a_{12} c_2$$
$$c_2 \lambda = a_{21} c_1 + a_{22} c_2$$

or

$$(a_{11} - \lambda) c_1 + a_{12} c_2 = 0$$
$$a_{21} c_1 + (a_{22} - \lambda) c_2 = 0 \tag{A1.3c}$$

Eqs. (A1.3c) are the 2×2 case of the linear algebraic eigenvalue problem. In other words, this discussion illustrates the relation between linear constant coefficient ODEs and linear algebraic equations.

Note that eqs. (A1.3c) are a linear homogeneous algebraic system (homogeneous means that the RHS is the zero vector). Therefore, eqs. (A1.3c) will have nontrivial solutions ($c_1 \neq 0$ and/or $c_2 \neq 0$) if and only if (iff) the determinant of the coefficient matrix is zero, that is,

$$\begin{vmatrix} a_{11} - \lambda & a_{12} \\ a_{21} & a_{22} - \lambda \end{vmatrix} = 0$$

or

$$(a_{11} - \lambda)(a_{22} - \lambda) - a_{21}a_{12} = 0$$

or

$$\lambda^2 - (a_{11} + a_{22})\lambda + a_{11}a_{22} - a_{21}a_{12} = 0 \qquad \text{(A1.4)}$$

Eqs. (A1.4) is the characteristic equation or characteristic polynomial for eqs. (A1.3c); note that because eqs. (A1.3c) constitute a 2×2 linear homogeneous algebraic system, the characteristic eq. (A1.4) is a second-order polynomial (in λ).

Eq. (A1.4) can be factored by the quadratic formula

$$\lambda_1, \lambda_2 = \frac{(a_{11} + a_{22}) \pm \sqrt{(a_{11} + a_{22})^2 - 4(a_{11}a_{22} - a_{21}a_{12})}}{2} \qquad \text{(A1.5)}$$

Thus, as expected, the 2×2 system of eqs. (A1.3c) has two eigenvalues (that may be real or complex conjugates, distinct or repeated).

As eqs. (A1.2) are linear constant coefficient ODEs, their general solution will be a linear combination of exponential functions, one for each eigenvalue.

$$y_1(t) = c_{11}e^{\lambda_1 t} + c_{12}e^{\lambda_2 t}$$
$$y_2(t) = c_{21}e^{\lambda_1 t} + c_{22}e^{\lambda_2 t} \qquad \text{(A1.6)}$$

This addition or superposition of solutions is a distinguishing feature of linear differential equations and follows from substituting eqs. (A1.6) in eqs. (A1.2).

$$\frac{dy_1}{dt} = c_{11}\lambda_1 e^{\lambda_1 t} + c_{12}\lambda_2 e^{\lambda_2 t}$$

$$= a_{11}[c_{11}e^{\lambda_1 t} + c_{12}e^{\lambda_2 t}] + a_{12}[c_{21}e^{\lambda_1 t} + c_{22}e^{\lambda_2 t}]$$

$$\frac{dy_2}{dt} = c_{21}\lambda_1 e^{\lambda_1 t} + c_{22}\lambda_2 e^{\lambda_2 t}$$

$$= a_{21}[c_{11}e^{\lambda_1 t} + c_{12}e^{\lambda_2 t}] + a_{22}[c_{21}e^{\lambda_1 t} + c_{22}e^{\lambda_2 t}]$$

or

$$[(a_{11} - \lambda_1)c_{11} + a_{12}c_{21}]e^{\lambda_1 t} + [(a_{11} - \lambda_2)c_{12} + a_{12}c_{22}]e^{\lambda_2 t} = 0$$

$$[(a_{22} - \lambda_1)c_{21} + a_{21}c_{11}]e^{\lambda_1 t} + [(a_{22} - \lambda_2)c_{22} + a_{21}c_{12}]e^{\lambda_2 t} = 0$$

Each of the terms in square brackets in this last result is zero from eqs. (A1.3c) for the two cases $\lambda = \lambda_1, \lambda_2$.

Eq. (A1.6) have four constants that occur in pairs, one pair for each eigenvalue. Thus, the pair $[c_{11} \ c_{21}]^T$ is the eigenvector for eigenvalue λ_1, whereas $[c_{12} \ c_{22}]^T$ is the eigenvector for eigenvalue λ_2. We can restate the two eigenvectors for eqs. (A1.6) as

$$\begin{bmatrix} c_{11} \\ c_{21} \end{bmatrix}_{\lambda_1}, \begin{bmatrix} c_{12} \\ c_{22} \end{bmatrix}_{\lambda_2} \tag{A1.7}$$

Finally, the four constants in eigenvectors (A1.7) are related through the ICs of eqs. (A1.2) and either of eqs. (A1.3c)

$$y_{10} = c_{11}e^{\lambda_1 0} + c_{12}e^{\lambda_2 0}$$
$$y_{20} = c_{21}e^{\lambda_1 0} + c_{22}e^{\lambda_2 0} \tag{A1.8}$$

We can simplify the analysis somewhat by considering the special case $a_{11} = a_{22} = -a, a_{21} = a_{12} = b$, where a and b are constants. Then, from eq. (A1.5), we have two real eigenvalues,

$$\lambda_1, \lambda_2 = \frac{-2a \pm \sqrt{(2a)^2 - 4(a^2 - b^2)}}{2}$$

$$= -a \pm b = -(a - b), -(a + b) \tag{A1.9}$$

The relationship of eq. (A1.9) between the eigenvalues λ_1, λ_2 and the constants a, b facilitates the subsequent analysis. From the first of eqs. (A1.3c) (the second equation could be used just as well), for $\lambda = \lambda_1$,

$$(a_{11} - \lambda_1)c_{11} + a_{12}c_{21} = 0$$

or

$$(-a + (a - b))c_{11} + bc_{21} = 0$$

$$c_{11} = c_{21}$$

Similarly, for $\lambda = \lambda_2$

$$(a_{11} - \lambda_2)c_{12} + a_{12}c_{22} = 0$$

or

$$(-a + (a + b))c_{12} + bc_{22} = 0$$

$$c_{12} = -c_{22}$$

Substitution of these results in eqs. (A1.8) gives

$$y_{10} = c_{11} - c_{22}$$

$$y_{20} = c_{11} + c_{22}$$

or

$$c_{11} = \frac{y_{10} + y_{20}}{2} = c_{21}$$

$$c_{22} = \frac{y_{20} - y_{10}}{2} = -c_{12}$$

Finally, the solution from eqs. (A1.6) is

$$y_1(t) = \frac{y_{10} + y_{20}}{2}e^{\lambda_1 t} - \frac{y_{20} - y_{10}}{2}e^{\lambda_2 t}$$

$$y_2(t) = \frac{y_{10} + y_{20}}{2}e^{\lambda_1 t} + \frac{y_{20} - y_{10}}{2}e^{\lambda_2 t}$$

(A1.10)

Eqs. (A1.10) can easily be checked by substitution in eqs. (A1.2) (with $a_{11} = a_{22} = -a, a_{21} = a_{12} = b$) and application of the ICs at $t = 0$

First of eqs. (A1.2)   First of eqs. (A1.10)

$$\frac{dy_1}{dt} \qquad \lambda_1 \frac{y_{10} + y_{20}}{2} e^{\lambda_1 t} - \lambda_2 \frac{y_{20} - y_{10}}{2} e^{\lambda_2 t}$$

$$= -(a - b)\frac{y_{10} + y_{20}}{2} e^{\lambda_1 t} + (a + b)\frac{y_{20} - y_{10}}{2} e^{\lambda_2 t}$$

$$+ay_1 \qquad + a\left(\frac{y_{10} + y_{20}}{2} e^{\lambda_1 t} - \frac{y_{20} - y_{10}}{2} e^{\lambda_2 t} \right)$$

$$-by_2 \qquad - b\left(\frac{y_{10} + y_{20}}{2} e^{\lambda_1 t} + \frac{y_{20} - y_{10}}{2} e^{\lambda_2 t} \right)$$

$$= \qquad\qquad =$$
$$0 \qquad\qquad 0$$

Second of eqs. (A1.2)   Second of eqs. (A1.10)

$$\frac{dy_2}{dt} \qquad \lambda_1 \frac{y_{10} + y_{20}}{2} e^{\lambda_1 t} + \lambda_2 \frac{y_{20} - y_{10}}{2} e^{\lambda_2 t}$$

$$= -(a - b)\frac{y_{10} + y_{20}}{2} e^{\lambda_1 t} - (a + b)\frac{y_{20} - y_{10}}{2} e^{\lambda_2 t}$$

$$+ay_2 \qquad + a\left(\frac{y_{10} + y_{20}}{2} e^{\lambda_1 t} + \frac{y_{20} - y_{10}}{2} e^{\lambda_2 t} \right)$$

$$-by_1 \qquad - b\left(\frac{y_{10} + y_{20}}{2} e^{\lambda_1 t} - \frac{y_{20} - y_{10}}{2} e^{\lambda_2 t} \right)$$

$$= \qquad\qquad =$$
$$0 \qquad\qquad 0$$

For the ICs of eqs. (A1.2),

$$y_{10} = \frac{y_{10} + y_{20}}{2} e^{\lambda_1 0} - \frac{y_{20} - y_{10}}{2} e^{\lambda_2 0} = y_{10}$$

$$y_{20} = \frac{y_{10} + y_{20}}{2} e^{\lambda_1 0} + \frac{y_{20} - y_{10}}{2} e^{\lambda_2 0} = y_{20}$$

as required.

For $y_{10} = 0, y_{20} = 2$, eqs. (A1.10) is

$$y_1(t) = e^{\lambda_1 t} - e^{\lambda_2 t}$$
$$y_2(t) = e^{\lambda_1 t} + e^{\lambda_2 t} \qquad \text{(A1.11)}$$

Eqs. (A1.11) are subsequently investigated numerically for various values of the stiffness ratio $\dfrac{\lambda_2}{\lambda_1}$.

To conclude this section on analytical solutions, the preceding analysis can be easily extended to the case of n linear constant coefficient ODEs (rather than just the 2 ODEs of eqs. (1.2)). The essential features of this more general case are (i) a characteristic equation that is an nth-order polynomial, (ii) n eigenvalues that are the roots of the nth-order characteristic equation, (iii) n eigenvectors corresponding to the n eigenvectors, and (iv) analytical solutions to the n ODEs that are a linear combination of n exponentials in t. The extension to n first-order, linear, constant coefficient ODEs is a standard part of linear algebra and therefore will not be considered further.

A1.3 Eigenvalue Stability Analysis

We now consider some particular values for a and b with $a_{11} = a_{22} = -a, a_{21} = a_{12} = b$ in eqs. (A1.2). Also, recall from eq. (A1.9) that $\lambda_1, \lambda_2 = -(a - b), -(a + b)$

Consider the maximum integration step h for the explicit Euler method (e.g., in function euler) for the stiff case of Table (A1.1). If $\lambda_2 = -1,000,000$, the maximum stable step for the explicit Euler method is given by $|\lambda h| = 2$ or $h = 2/1,000,000 = 0.000002$. However, to compute a complete solution, we require a final t given approximately by $\lambda_1 t \approx -10$ (or $t = 10$ so that $\exp(\lambda_1 t)$ $= \exp(-10)$ has decayed to insignificance compared to the IC $y_2(0) = 2$). Thus, we must take $10/0.000002 = 5 \times 10^6$ steps! If this does not seem like a large number of steps, consider $a = 500,000,000.5$, $b = 499,999,999.5$ for which the ratio $\dfrac{|\text{largest eigenvalue}|}{|\text{smallest eigenvalue}|} = \dfrac{|\lambda_{\max}|}{|\lambda_{\min}|} = \dfrac{|\lambda_2|}{|\lambda_1|} = 10^9$ and 5×10^9 steps would be required to compute a complete solution (physical problems in which the stiffness ratio $= \dfrac{|\lambda_{\max}|}{|\lambda_{\min}|} = 10^{12}$ to 10^{15} are not unusual).

TABLE A1.1 Degrees of stiffness of eqs. (A1.2).

Values of a,b	Values of λ_1, λ_2	$\dfrac{\|\lambda_2\|}{\|\lambda_1\|}$ and Description
Case 1		
$a = 50.5$	$\lambda_2 = -100$	$\dfrac{\|\lambda_2\|}{\|\lambda_1\|} = 100$
$b = 49.5$	$\lambda_1 = -1$	nonstiff
Case 2		
$a = 500.5$	$\lambda_2 = -1000$	$\dfrac{\|\lambda_2\|}{\|\lambda_1\|} = 1000$
$b = 499.5$	$\lambda_1 = -1$	moderately stiff
Case 3		
$a = 500,000.5$	$\lambda_2 = -1,000,000$	$\dfrac{\|\lambda_2\|}{\|\lambda_1\|} = 1,000,000$
$b = 499,999.5$	$\lambda_1 = -1$	stiff

In summary, numerical solutions of eqs. (A1.2) by the explicit Euler method for the stiff case of Table A1.1 require a large calculation. The same conclusion is true for the modified Euler method (meuler), classical Runge–Kutta method (rkc4), and the RKF45 method (rkf45). This is so because of the stability limit of explicit methods is approximately $|\lambda h| < 3$. To circumvent this stability of explicit methods, we turn to implicit methods, and in particular, the BDF (backward differentiation formula) methods.

Before considering BDF methods, we mention as an incidental point that the calculation of λ_1 requires a subtraction, $\lambda_1 = -(a - b)$. If a and b are nearly equal, for example, $a = 500,000.5, b = 499,999.5$, then this subtraction might be done with substantial error. For example, if the machine precision (often termed the *machine epsilon* or *unit roundoff*) is 10^{-7} (one part in 10^7) corresponding to 32-bit arithmetic, this stiff ODE system could not be integrated numerically because the calculation of $(a - b)$ requires a precision better than one part in 10^7. Although this is a heuristic argument, generally the conclusion is correct, that is, stiff systems require a precision that is substantially better than that set by $\dfrac{|\lambda_{\max}|}{|\lambda_{\min}|}$ ($1,000,000$

in the preceding stiff case of Table A1.1). As an example of available precision, the machine epsilon for R, Java, and double precision Fortran is approximately 10^{-15} so that an ODE system with a stiffness ratio approaching 10^{15} can be accommodated with these systems.

A1.4 BDF Methods for Stiff ODEs

The BDF method is first applied to the general (possibly nonlinear) 2×2 ODE system of eqs. (A1.1). The BDF equations to step forward in t are

$$\alpha_0 y_{i+1,1} + \alpha_1 y_{i,1} + \cdots + \alpha_v y_{i-v+1,1} = hf_1(y_{i+1,1}, y_{i+1,2}, t_{i+1})$$
$$\alpha_0 y_{i+1,2} + \alpha_1 y_{i,2} + \cdots + \alpha_v y_{i-v+1,2} = hf_2(y_{i+1,1}, y_{i+1,2}, t_{i+1})$$

or

$$hf_1(y_{i+1,1}, y_{i+1,2}, t_{i+1}) - [\alpha_0 y_{i+1,1} + \alpha_1 y_{i,1} + \cdots + \alpha_v y_{i-v+1,1}]$$
$$= g_1(y_{i+1,1}, y_{i+1,2} t_{i+1}) = 0$$
$$hf_2(y_{i+1,1}, y_{i+1,2}, t_{i+1}) - [\alpha_0 y_{i+1,2} + \alpha_1 y_{i,2} + \cdots + \alpha_v y_{i-v+1,2}]$$
$$= g_2(y_{i+1,1}, y_{i+1,2}, t_{i+1}) = 0$$

$$(A1.12)$$

Eqs. (A1.12) is a 2×2 nonlinear system (nonlinear if the original ODE system, eqs. (A1.1), is nonlinear), for the two unknowns $y_{i+1,1}, y_{i+1,2}$ (the ODE solution at the advanced point $i + 1$). We need to apply a nonlinear solver to eqs. (A1.12) such as Newton's method to compute the two unknowns, $y_{i+1,1}, y_{i+1,2}$.

$$\mathbf{J}\delta\mathbf{y} = -\mathbf{g}(\mathbf{y})$$
$$(A1.13a)$$

where for the $n \times n$ problem,

$$\mathbf{y} = \begin{bmatrix} y_1 \\ y_2 \\ \vdots \\ y_n \end{bmatrix}, \quad \delta\mathbf{y} = \begin{bmatrix} \delta y_1 \\ \delta y_2 \\ \vdots \\ \delta y_n \end{bmatrix} \qquad \text{(A1.13b)(A1.13c)}$$

$$\mathbf{g} = \begin{bmatrix} g_1 \\ g_2 \\ \vdots \\ g_n \end{bmatrix} = \begin{bmatrix} g_1(y_1, y_2, \cdots y_n, t) \\ g_2(y_1, y_2, \cdots y_n, t) \\ \vdots \\ g_n(y_1, y_2, \cdots y_n, t) \end{bmatrix} \tag{A1.13d}$$

$$\mathbf{J} = \begin{bmatrix} \dfrac{\partial g_1}{\partial y_1} & \dfrac{\partial g_1}{\partial y_2} & \cdots & \dfrac{\partial g_1}{\partial y_n} \\[2mm] \dfrac{\partial g_2}{\partial y_1} & \dfrac{\partial g_2}{\partial y_2} & \cdots & \dfrac{\partial g_2}{\partial y_n} \\[2mm] \vdots & \vdots & \ddots & \vdots \\[2mm] \dfrac{\partial g_n}{\partial y_1} & \dfrac{\partial g_n}{\partial y_2} & \cdots & \dfrac{\partial g_n}{\partial y_n} \end{bmatrix} = \begin{bmatrix} J_{11} & J_{12} & \cdots & J_{1n} \\ J_{21} & J_{22} & \cdots & J_{2n} \\ \vdots & \vdots & \ddots & \vdots \\ J_{n1} & J_{n2} & \cdots & J_{nn} \end{bmatrix} \tag{A1.13e}$$

$\mathbf{J}$ is the $n \times n$ Jacobian matrix, consisting of all first-order partial derivatives of the functions, $[g_1 \, g_2 \cdots g_i \cdots g_n]^T$ with respect to the dependent variables $[y_1 \, y_2 \cdots y_j \cdots y_n]^T$, that is,

$$J_{ij} = \frac{\partial g_i}{\partial y_j} \tag{A1.13f}$$

$\delta \mathbf{y}$ is the vector of the Newton corrections, which should decrease below a specified tolerance or threshold as the Newton iteration proceeds.

Application of the preceding equations to the 2×2 ODE system of eqs. (A1.2) gives

$$\mathbf{y} = \begin{bmatrix} y_1 \\ y_2 \end{bmatrix}, \quad \delta \mathbf{y} = \begin{bmatrix} \delta y_1 \\ \delta y_2 \end{bmatrix} \tag{A1.14a)(A1.14b}$$

$$\mathbf{g} = \begin{bmatrix} g_1(y_1, y_2, t) \\ g_2(y_1, y_2, t) \end{bmatrix}$$

$$= \begin{bmatrix} h\left[-ay_{i+1,1} + by_{i+1,2} \right] - \left[\alpha_0 y_{i+1,1} + \alpha_1 y_{i,1} + \cdots + \alpha_v y_{i-v+1,1} \right] \\ h\left[+by_{i+1,1} - ay_{i+1,2} \right] - \left[\alpha_0 y_{i+1,2} + \alpha_1 y_{i,2} + \cdots + \alpha_v y_{i-v+1,2} \right] \end{bmatrix}$$
$$\tag{A1.14c}$$

$$
\mathbf{J} = \begin{bmatrix} \dfrac{\partial g_1}{\partial y_1} & \dfrac{\partial g_1}{\partial y_2} \\[2ex] \dfrac{\partial g_2}{\partial y_1} & \dfrac{\partial g_2}{\partial y_2} \end{bmatrix} = \begin{bmatrix} J_{11} & J_{12} \\[1ex] J_{21} & J_{22} \end{bmatrix} = \begin{bmatrix} -ah - \alpha_0 & bh \\[1ex] bh & -ah - \alpha_0 \end{bmatrix}
$$

$$(A1.14d)$$

Thus, eq. (A1.13a) becomes

$$
\begin{bmatrix} -ah - \alpha_0 & bh \\[1ex] bh & -ah - \alpha_0 \end{bmatrix} \begin{bmatrix} \delta y_1 \\[1ex] \delta y_2 \end{bmatrix}
$$
$$
= - \begin{bmatrix} h[-ay_{i+1,1} + by_{i+1,2}] - [\alpha_0 y_{i+1,1} + \alpha_1 y_{i,1} + \cdots + \alpha_v y_{i-v+1,1}] \\[2ex] h[+by_{i+1,1} - ay_{i+1,2}] - [\alpha_0 y_{i+1,2} + \alpha_1 y_{i,2} + \cdots + \alpha_v y_{i-v+1,2}] \end{bmatrix}
$$

$$(A1.14e)$$

Eqs. (A1.14) are programmed in the following R routines. The numerical integration continues until the condition

$$
|\delta y_1| < eps
$$
$$
|\delta y_2| < eps
$$

$$(A1.15)$$

is satisfied, where eps is a tolerance set in the program.

To conclude this section, nonstiff (explicit) and stiff (implicit) integration methods are illustrated by the explicit and implicit Euler methods applied to the single first-order ODE

$$
\frac{dy}{dt} = f(y, t) = \lambda y, \; y(0) = y_0
$$

$$(A1.16a)$$

where we have chosen $Re(\lambda) < 0$ (i.e., λ is in the left half of the complex plane) so that the solution

$$
y(t) = y_0 e^{\lambda t}
$$

$$(A1.16b)$$

is stable (decays exponentially with t).

The explicit Euler method applied to eq. (A1.16a) is

$$y_{i+1} = y_i + f(y_i, t_i)h + O(h) \tag{A1.17a}$$

and the implicit Euler method is

$$y_{i+1} = y_i + f(y_{i+1}, t_{i+1})h + O(h) \tag{A1.17b}$$

where the index for the points along the solution is $i = 0, 1, 2, \ldots$. The important distinction between eqs. (A1.17a) and (A1.17b) is the evaluation of the derivative function at i for the former and $i + 1$ for the latter. This may seem like a minor point, but it has the following important consequences.

- The solution at the advance point, y_{i+1}, appears in only the LHS of eq. (A1.17a) so that it can be calculated directly (explicitly). This makes the calculation of y_{i+1} from the base value y_i straight-forward.
- For the model problem of eq. (A1.16a), application of eq. (A1.17a) gives

$$y_{i+1} = y_i + f(y_i, t_i)h = y_i + \lambda y_i h$$

  or

$$y_{i+1} = (1 + \lambda h)y_i$$

Thus, $(1 + \lambda h)$ is a multiplying factor at each step along the numerical solution, and this stepping will be stable iff $|(1 + \lambda h)| < 1$ or $|\lambda h| < 2$ (recall again that $Re(\lambda) < 0$). The latter result is the stability criterion for the explicit Euler method. We can add two additional points.

- For a system of n linear ODEs, the stability criterion $|\lambda h| < 2$ applies to all n eigenvalues. If h is selected so that this criterion is not satisfied for even one eigenvalue, the numerical explicit Euler integration will be unstable.

— The concept of eigenvalues and the associated eigenfunctions and exponential solutions, for example, eq. (A1.6), originates from linear constant coefficient ODEs. Analogous concepts for nonlinear ODEs are not available, and in this case, we can only infer stiffness indirectly through observed required derivative evaluations and computational times as, for example, with the 7×7 nonlinear ODE system of Chapter 1.

- As eq. (A1.17a) has the stability limit or constraint $|h\lambda| < 2$, for large $|\lambda|$, the integration step h is significantly limited (to maintain stability in the numerical integration of a stiff ODE system with large and small eigenvalues such as eqs. (A1.2) for the stiff case of Table A1.1).

- The solution at the advanced point, y_{i+1}, appears in the LHS and RHS of eq. (A1.17b), so that it can be calculated only indirectly (implicitly). This makes the calculation of y_{i+1} from the base value y_i relatively difficult. In particular, if $f(y,t)$ of eq. (A1.16a) is nonlinear, a nonlinear solver is required, typically a variant of Newton's method.

- For the model problem of eq. (A1.16a), the application of eq. (A1.17b) gives

$$y_{i+1} = y_i + f(y_{i+1}, t_i)h = y_i + \lambda y_{i+1}h$$

or

$$y_{i+1} = \frac{1}{(1 - \lambda h)} y_i$$

$1/(1 - \lambda h)$ is a multiplying factor at each step along the numerical solution that is always less than one in absolute value (for $Re(\lambda) < 0$). In other words, stepping with the implicit Euler method is stable for $|\lambda h| < \infty$ so that h is unlimited with respect to stability (and therefore is limited only by accuracy). In this case, we could solve for y_{i+1} because eq. (A1.16a) is linear in y. More generally, for nonlinear ODEs, this direct algebraic solution for the solution at the advanced point would not be possible.

Rather, the nonlinear equations in y_{i+1} would require a numerical solution.

- Thus, the stability constraint of the explicit Euler method is circumvented because for eq. (A1.17b), the stability criterion is $|h\lambda| < \infty$. That is, the implicit Euler method is unconditionally stable and, therefore, the limitation on the integration step h is from accuracy (it is only first order, $O(h)$) and not stability.

In summary, the additional computation required for y_{i+1} from eq. (A1.17b) is worthwhile if the ODE system is stiff because substantially larger integration steps are possible. The first-order BDF is just the implicit Euler method. To achieve better accuracy as well as stability, higher order BDF methods are available as summarized in Table A1.2 ([2], [5], pp 183–184).

TABLE A1.2   Coefficients for the BDF methods of orders 1–6.

ν	α_0	α_1	α_2	α_3	α_4	α_5	α_6
1	1	−1					
2	3/2	−2	1/2				
3	11/6	−3	3/2	−1/3			
4	25/12	−4	3	−4/3	1/4		
5	137/60	−5	5	−10/3	5/4	−1/5	
6	147/60	−6	15/2	−20/3	15/4	−6/5	1/6

The general BDF formula is

$$\alpha_0 y_{i+1} + \alpha_1 y_i + \cdots + \alpha_\nu y_{i-\nu+1} = hf(y_{i+1} t_{i+1}) \qquad (A1.18)$$

ν is the order of the method. For example, with $\nu = 1$, $\alpha_0 = 1$, $\alpha_1 = -1$ from Table A1.2,

$$y_{i+1} - y_i = hf(y_{i+1} t_{i+1})$$

which is the implicit Euler method of eq. (A1.17b). Eq. (A1.18) was previously applied to the 2×2 ODE system of eqs. (A1.2) as eqs. (A1.12). Note that, in general, y and f in eqs. (A1.18) are n-vectors where n is the number of first-order ODEs to be integrated numerically.

We should also note that the BDF stepping formula, eqs. (A1.18), requires a series of values prior to y_{i+1}, that is, $y_i, y_{i-1}, \ldots, y_{i-\nu+1}$. At the beginning of the solution, when only one value is available, the initial condition y_0, we cannot use eqs. (A1.18) unless we start with the first-order method corresponding to $\nu = 1$. This will permit the calculation of y_1 and now we have two past values to calculate y_2, etc. Thus, we must build up the required past values starting with the $\nu = 1$ method (the implicit Euler method). In other words, the BDFs for $\nu > 1$ are not self-starting (in contrast with Runge–Kutta methods that are self-starting because they require only one past value, y_i, to compute the next solution value y_{i+1}; in fact, implicit Runge–Kutta methods can be used to start the BDF solution from eqs. (A1.18)).

A1.5   R Program for First-Order BDF Method

Eqs. (A1.12) with $\nu = 1$ (first-order BDF or the implicit Euler method) are solved by Newton's method in Listing A1.1.

```
#
# Number of ODEs
  neqn=2;
#
# Convergence tolerance, maximum number of
# iterations to compute Newton corrections
  eps=0.00001;
  maxiter=20;
#
# Initial condition
  y0=rep(2,neqn);
  y0=c(0,2);
  y=rep(0,neqn);
  y=y0;
  t=0;
#
```

```
# Values just for initial output
  dy=rep(0,neqn);
  niter=0;
#
# Integration step, steps/output, number of outputs
  h=0.01;
  nsteps=100;
  nout=11;
#
# Problem parameters
  a=500000.5;
  b=499999.5;
#
# Jacobian matrix
  J=matrix(0,ncol=neqn,nrow=neqn);
  J[1,1]=-a*h-1;
  J[1,2]=b*h;
  J[2,1]=b*h;
  J[2,2]=-a*h-1;
  Jinv=solve(J);
#
# Heading for solution
  cat(sprintf("    t       dy(1)      dy(2)       y(1)        y(2)
     erry(1)    erry(2)   iter\n"));
#
# nout outputs
  for(i in 1:nout){
#
#    Initial output or after nstep integration steps
#    completed; display Newton corrections, numerical and
#    exact solutions for output
     lambda1=-(a-b);
     lambda2=-(a+b);
     exp1=exp(lambda1*t);
     exp2=exp(lambda2*t);
     y1e=exp1-exp2;
     y2e=exp1+exp2;
     erry1=y1e-y[1];
     erry2=y2e-y[2];
     cat(sprintf("%10.1f%10.5f%10.5f%10.5f%10.5f%10.5f%
        10.5f%6d\n",
```

```
      t,dy[1],dy[2],y[1],y[2],erry1,erry2,niter));
#
#   nsteps steps/output
    for(is in 1:nsteps){
#
#     Initialize iteration counter, stopping variable
      niter=1; stop=0;
#
#     Test for the end of the current step
      while(stop==0){
#
#       Functions g1, g2
        g=c(h*(-a*y[1]+b*y[2])-y[1]+y0[1],
            h*( b*y[1]-a*y[2])-y[2]+y0[2]);
#
#       Newton corrections
        dy=-Jinv%*%g;
#
#       Update solution
        y=y+dy;
        stop=1;
#
#       Check if the corrections are within the tolerance
#           eps
        for(ic in 1:neqn){
          if(abs(dy[ic])>eps){
#
#           Convergence not achieved; continue calculation
            niter=niter+1;
            stop=0;
            break;
          }
        }
#
#       If maximum iterations reached, accept current step
        if(niter==maxiter){stop=1;}
      }
#
#     Integration step completed
      y0=y;
      t=t+h;
```

```
#
#    Next integration step
     }
#
# Next output interval
   }
```

Listing A1.1 Solution of eqs. (A1.2) by a first-order BDF.

We can note the following points about Listing A1.1.

- The number of ODEs to be integrated by the BDF method (also, the number of nonlinear algebraic equations, i.e., eqs. (A1.12)) is specified.

```
#
# Number of ODEs
  neqn=2;
```

- The tolerance for the Newton corrections and the maximum number of the Newton iterations are defined numerically.

```
#
# Convergence tolerance, maximum number of
# iterations to compute Newton corrections
  eps=0.00001;
  maxiter=20;
```

- An initial estimate of the solution required by Newton's method is specified, which is taken as the IC for eqs. (A1.2) ($y_1(0) = 0, y_2(0) = 2$ for eqs. (A1.11)). Also, the independent variable, t, in eqs. (A1.2) is initialized.

```
#
# Initial condition
  y0=rep(2,neqn);
  y0=c(0,2);
  y=rep(0,neqn);
  y=y0;
  t=0;
```

- The Newton corrections are zeroed and the counter for the Newton iterations is initialized.

```
#
# Values just for initial output
  dy=rep(0,neqn);
  niter=0;
```

- The variables that control the BDF integration are set, specifically, the integration step in eqs. (A1.12) and (A1.14) (this will be for a fixed step BDF integration), the number of integration steps for each output interval, and the number of outputs.

```
#
# Integration step, steps/output, number of outputs
  h=0.01;
  nsteps=100;
  nout=11;
```

Thus, there will be a total of $100 \times (11 - 1) = 1000$ Newton steps, each of length 0.01 so that the final value of t is $0.01 \times 1000 = 10$.

- The parameters in eqs. (A1.2) (a, b) are defined.

```
#
# Problem parameters
  a=500000.5;
  b=499999.5;
```

These values correspond to the stiff case in Table A1.1 for which the eigenvalues of eq. (A1.5) are $\lambda_1 = -(a - b) = -1, \lambda_2 = -(a + b) = -1{,}000{,}000$.

- The elements of the $n \times n = 2 \times 2$ Jacobian matrix of eq. (A1.14d) are programmed.

```
#
# Jacobian matrix
  J=matrix(0,ncol=neqn,nrow=neqn);
  J[1,1]=-a*h-1;
```

```
J[1,2]=b*h;
J[2,1]=b*h;
J[2,2]=-a*h-1;
Jinv=solve(J);
```

The inverse of the Jacobian matrix, $\mathbf{J}^{-1} = $ Jinv, is also computed by the R inverse matrix operator solve for use in eq. (A1.13a) written as

$$\delta\mathbf{y} = -\mathbf{J}^{-1}\mathbf{g}(\mathbf{y}) \qquad (A1.19)$$

Note that because eqs. (A1.2) are linear constant coefficient ODEs, the Jacobian matrix is constant (the $2 \times 2 = 4$ elements are constant) and therefore has to be evaluated only once. More generally, if the ODEs are nonlinear, the Jacobian matrix would have to be updated at each Newton iteration (which is usually a major portion of the calculation in using Newton's method).

This step (for computing the Newton corrections according to eq. (A1.19)) will fail if the Jacobian matrix is singular or near singular (i.e., ill-conditioned). Thus, the calculation of the condition of J at this point would be a good idea. R has a utility for calculating the condition of a matrix that can then be compared with the machine epsilon that is calculated by the following (separate) coding.

```
eps=1;
while(1+eps >1){
   eps=eps/10;
}
cat(sprintf("\n eps = %12.5e",eps));
```

The output from this program is eps = 1.00000e-16 (the value of eps that produced an exit from the while so that the last value of eps before the exit is 10^{-15}). If the condition number exceeds the reciprocal of the machine epsilon, the linear algebraic system (in this case, eq. (A1.19)) is numerically singular and the Newton solution of the nonlinear system, eq. (A1.12), will not proceed. In other words, the Jacobian matrix condition number should be less than $1/10^{-15} \approx 10^{15}$.

- A heading for the numerical solution is displayed.

```
#
# Heading for solution
  cat(sprintf("   t       dy(1)       dy(2)       y(1)
    y(2)        erry(1)    erry(2)  iter\n"));
```

(this output statement has been put in two lines to fit within the available printed space).

- An outer `for` with index `i` is used to compute and display the solution at the `nout=11` output points.

```
#
# nout outputs
  for(i in 1:nout){
```

- At each of the `nout=11` output points (including $t = 0$), several items are computed and/or displayed: (i) the analytical solution of eq. (A1.11) `y1e,y2e`, (ii) the exact error which is the difference between the numerical and analytical solutions, `erry1,erry2`, and (iii) the Newton corrections, `dy[1],dy[2]`.

```
#
# Initial output or after nstep integration steps
# completed; display Newton corrections, numerical and
# exact solutions for output
  lambda1=-(a-b);
  lambda2=-(a+b);
  exp1=exp(lambda1*t);
  exp2=exp(lambda2*t);
  y1e=exp1-exp2;
  y2e=exp1+exp2;
  erry1=y1e-y[1];
  erry2=y2e-y[2];
  cat(sprintf("%10.1f%10.5f%10.5f%10.5f%10.5f%10.5f%
      10.5f%6d\n",
           t,dy[1],dy[2],y[1],y[2],erry1,erry2,niter));
```

- A second `for` with index `is` performs the calculations through `nsteps` integration steps of length `h`; the iteration counter is initialized for each integration step and a variable is initialized that will indicate when the Newton iterations are stopped.

```
#
#    nsteps steps/output
     for(is in 1:nsteps){
#
#       Initialize iteration counter, stopping variable
        niter=1; stop=0;
```

- A while performs the Newton iterations while nstop=0.

```
#
#       Test for the end of the current step
        while(stop==0){
```

The calculations within the while are explained next.

— The vector of functions to be zeroed is computed according to eq. (A1.12) (with $v = 1$)

```
#
#          Functions g1, g2
           g=c(h*(-a*y[1]+b*y[2])-y[1]+y0[1],
               h*( b*y[1]-a*y[2])-y[2]+y0[2]);
```

This calculation could be moved to a separate function (particularly for larger sets of nonlinear equations to improve the modularity of the coding).

— The linear Newton eq. (A1.19) is then solved for the Newton corrections.

```
#
#          Newton corrections
           dy=-Jinv%*%g;
```

The matrix-vector multiplication between $\mathbf{J}^{-1}$ and g is programmed as %*% (the syntax used with R). Note how easily this calculation is programmed in R; this is due to the facility of R to handle matrices (arrays) without subscripting, plus the definition of basic matrix operations, for example, addition, subtraction, scalar-matrix and vector-matrix multiplications, and matrix inverse.

— The Newton corrections are then applied to the current solution vector to produce (hopefully) an improved solution.

```
#
#         Update solution
          y=y+dy;
          stop=1;
```

If the Newton corrections are small enough (to be tested next), the iterations are terminated by setting stop=1.

— Each Newton correction is tested against the convergence tolerance using a for with index ic. Note the use of abs because the corrections can be either positive or negative.

```
#
#         Check if the corrections are within the
#             tolerance eps
          for(ic in 1:neqn){
            if(abs(dy[ic])>eps){
#
#             Convergence not achieved; continue
#                 calculation
              niter=niter+1;
              stop=0;
              break;
            }
          }
```

If any of the Newton corrections exceed the tolerance, the iteration counter is incremented, the iterations are continued (stop=0), and the testing is ended (break from the for in ic).

— If the maximum number of iterations is reached, the iterations are stopped and the solution at this point is accepted (stop=1). Otherwise, if the iterations are continued (stop=0), the next pass through the while loop (based on stop==0) is initiated.

```
#
#         If maximum iterations reached, accept
```

```
#                current step
        if(niter==maxiter){stop=1;}
    }
```

The final } concludes the while.

- Convergence has been achieved or the maximum number of iterations has been exceeded (stop=1) so the new solution is now used as the old (base) solution in the next step of the ODE integration; the independent variable is incremented for the next step along the solution

```
#
#       Integration step completed
    y0=y;
    t=t+h;
```

- Finally, the nstep integration steps are completed, and the next output interval is covered until all nout output intervals are completed.

```
#
#    Next integration step
    }
#
# Next output interval
  }
```

A1.6   Numerical Output from the BDF Integration

The output from the Listing A1.1 is in Table A1.3.

We can note the following points about this output.

- The numerical solution at $t = 1$ is accurate to

$$(0.00183/0.36971)(100) = 0.5\%$$

This is usually adequate for most applications (e.g., because the original model ODEs may not correspond to the physical system to this accuracy), but improvement in this accuracy by decreasing h is considered subsequently.

TABLE A1.3   Numerical solution from Listing A1.1.

t	dy(1)	dy(2)	y(1)	y(2)	erry(1) erry(2)	iter
0.0	0.00000	0.00000	0.00000	2.00000	0.00000	
					0.00000	0
1.0	0.00000	0.00000	0.36971	0.36971	-0.00183	
					-0.00183	2
2.0	0.00000	0.00000	0.13669	0.13669	-0.00135	
					-0.00135	2
3.0	-0.00000	-0.00000	0.05053	0.05053	-0.00075	
					-0.00075	2
4.0	-0.00000	-0.00000	0.01868	0.01868	-0.00037	
					-0.00037	2
5.0	0.00000	0.00000	0.00691	0.00691	-0.00017	
					-0.00017	2
6.0	0.00000	0.00000	0.00255	0.00255	-0.00007	
					-0.00007	2
7.0	-0.00001	-0.00001	0.00094	0.00094	-0.00003	
					-0.00003	1
8.0	-0.00000	-0.00000	0.00035	0.00035	-0.00001	
					-0.00001	1
9.0	-0.00000	-0.00000	0.00013	0.00013	-0.00001	
					-0.00001	1
10.0	-0.00000	-0.00000	0.00005	0.00005	-0.00000	
					-0.00000	1

- $y_1(t)$ and $y_2(t)$ are identical because for $t = 1$ and beyond to $t = 10$, the exponential $e^{\lambda_2 t} = e^{-10^6 t}$ in eqs. (A1.11) is negligibly small in comparison to $e^{\lambda_1 t} = e^{-t}$ so only the latter remains for both $y_1(t)$ and $y_2(t)$. In other words, $y_1(t = 1)$ and $y_2(t = 1)$ are close to $e^{-1} = 0.3678794$.
- Only 1000 implicit Euler steps were used. This contrasts with the 5×10^6 steps estimated for the explicit Euler method after Table A1.1; thus, there was a reduction of $1/5000$ in the number of steps required by an explicit integrator, which clearly shows the advantage of using an implicit integrator for the stiff ODEs. Again, as discussed after Table A1.1, if this conclusion is not

convincing, using $a = 500{,}000{,}000.5$, $b = 499{,}999{,}999.5$ would result in a reduction of $1/(5 \times 10^6)$ steps!

- The two Newton corrections, δy_1 and $\delta y2$ of eqs. (A1.14b), met the tolerance $eps = 0.00001$ with no more than 2 iterations.

- Accuracy (not stability) was limited by the step size $h = 0.01$; this suggests that a higher order BDF method could be used to good advantage (to increase the accuracy, while maintaining stability). Specifically, the BDF methods are stable along the entire negative real axis and, therefore, would be stable for the 2×2 linear problem of eqs. (A1.2) (because the two eigenvalues are real and negative, e.g., $\lambda_1 = -(a - b) = -1, \lambda_2 = -(a + b) = -1{,}000{,}000$). An extension of Listing A1.1 for BDF methods of order 2 and 3 is discussed subsequently.

As an incidental point, the number of iterations in Table A1.3 corresponds to the last of the nsteps=100 integration steps, that is, after the for in is is completed.

```
#
#    nsteps steps/output
     for(is in 1:nsteps){
```

The number of iterations could vary within this for and displayed during each pass through the for, but we used only the final value (at is=nsteps) to give output of reasonable length (in Table A1.3).

To conclude this section with a brief investigation of h refinement, Listing A1.1 is modified with h=0.001 and nsteps=1000 in place of h=0.01 and nsteps=100. The numerical output from this modification is listed in Table A1.4.

We can note the following details about this output.

- The errors have been reduced by approximately $1/10$ as expected because h was decreased by $1/10$ and the BDF method is first order ($O(h)$). For example,

```
Table A1.3, t = 1, h = 0.01
  1.0 0.00000 0.00000 0.36971 0.36971 -0.00183
                                      -0.00183   2
```

```
Table A1.4, t = 1, h = 0.001
   1.0 0.00000 0.00000 0.36806 0.36806 -0.00018
                                       -0.00018   2
```

so that the error was decreased from -0.00183 to -0.00018 at t = 1 (note also the approach to the exact solution $e^{-1} = 0.3678794$ at t = 1).

- The improvement in accuracy resulted with no increase in the number of iterations.

TABLE A1.4   Numerical solution from Listing A1.1 with h=0.001, nsteps=1000.

t	dy(1)	dy(2)	y(1)	y(2)	erry(1) erry(2)	iter
0.0	0.00000	0.00000	0.00000	2.00000	0.00000 0.00000	0
1.0	0.00000	0.00000	0.36806	0.36806	-0.00018 -0.00018	2
2.0	-0.00000	-0.00000	0.13547	0.13547	-0.00014 -0.00014	2
3.0	0.00000	0.00000	0.04986	0.04986	-0.00007 -0.00007	2
4.0	-0.00000	-0.00000	0.01835	0.01835	-0.00004 -0.00004	2
5.0	-0.00001	-0.00001	0.00675	0.00675	-0.00002 -0.00002	1
6.0	-0.00000	-0.00000	0.00249	0.00249	-0.00001 -0.00001	1
7.0	-0.00000	-0.00000	0.00092	0.00092	-0.00000 -0.00000	1
8.0	-0.00000	-0.00000	0.00034	0.00034	-0.00000 -0.00000	1
9.0	-0.00000	-0.00000	0.00012	0.00012	-0.00000 -0.00000	1
10.0	-0.00000	-0.00000	0.00005	0.00005	-0.00000 -0.00000	1

A1.7   Alternative Programming of the BDF Integration

A variation of the programming in Listing A1.1 follows that includes the evaluation of the Jacobian matrix in a separate routine. As the main program is similar to Listing A1.1, only the differences are considered.

- A routine for the Jacobian matrix of eq. (A1.14d), jacob_1, is accessed by setwd (set working directory) and source statements. Note the use of the forward slash, /, in the setwd.

```
#
# Access jacob_1.R
  setwd("c:/R/bme_ode/app1");
  source("jacob_1.R");
```

This code could be placed any where before jacob_1 is called, but putting it at the beginning of Listing A1.1 follows the usual convention.

- Rather than calculating the Jacobian matrix in-line (see Listing A1.1), it is calculated by a call to jacob_1.

```
#
#         Functions g1, g2
          g=c(h*(-a*y[1]+b*y[2])-y[1]+y0[1],
              h*( b*y[1]-a*y[2])-y[2]+y0[2]);
#
#         Jacobian matrix, inverse
          jacob_1(t,y);
          Jinv=solve(J);
```

Note also that the Jacobian matrix is evaluated in each Newton iteration rather than just once at the beginning. This is not required for eqs. (A1.2) (because they are linear and the Jacobian matrix is constant), but computing the Jacobian matrix during each iteration is more general because it can be used for the numerical solution of nonlinear ODEs (for which the Jacobian matrix changes). This also suggests the possibility of calculating (updating) the Jacobian matrix only when it has changed substantially (to save computations). All that is required is the convergence of the Newton iterations (to give accurate solutions of the nonlinear algebraic equations resulting from the BDF) and this can possibly occur even when the Jacobian matrix is not computed during each iteration.

These are the only changes to Listing A1.1, and as expected, the numerical solutions (for $h = 0.01, 0.001$) remain unchanged (from those in Tables A1.1 and A1.2). Routine jacob_1 is given in Listing A1.2.

```
jacob_1=function(t,y){
#
# Jacobian matrix
  J=matrix(0,ncol=neqn,nrow=neqn);
  J[1,1]=-a*h-1;
  J[1,2]=b*h;
  J[2,1]=b*h;
  J[2,2]=-a*h-1;
#
# Return numerical Jacobian as a matrix
  J <<- J;
#
# End of jacob_1
  }
```

Listing A1.2 Routine jacob_1 for the Jacobian matrix of eqs. (A1.2).

This coding is straightforward (a, b, h are set in Listing A1.1 and are available to jacob_1). The Jacobian matrix is returned to the main program with J <<- J.

Finally, we can note that Listing A1.1 contains a general Newton solver that can be applied to a $n \times n$ system of nonlinear equations; all that is required is to reprogram (i) the Jacobian matrix in jacob_1 of Listing A1.2 and (ii) the vector of functions to be zeroed, g (which could also be placed in a separate function to increase the modularity of the programming). Also, some tuning of the parameters will generally be required (e.g., the tolerance eps and the maximum number of iterations maxiter).

A1.8 Second-Order BDF Integration

The preceding use of the $\nu = 1$ BDF integration can easily be changed to a $\nu = 2$ integration by using the coefficients in Table A1.2. The changes in the preceding routines are straightforward, but the entire main program is in Listing A1.3 to give a complete picture of the coding (routine jacob_1 of Listing A1.2 remains unchanged).

```
#
# Access jacob_1.R
  setwd("c:/R/bme_ode/app1");
  source("jacob_1.R");
#
# Number of ODEs
  neqn=2;
#
# Convergence tolerance, maximum number of
# iterations to compute Newton corrections
  eps=0.00001;
  maxiter=20;
#
# Initial condition
  y0=rep(2,neqn);
  y0=c(0,2);
  y=rep(0,neqn);
  y=y0;
  t=0;
#
# Values just for initial output
  dy=rep(0,neqn);
  niter=0;
#
# Integration step, steps/output, number of outputs
  h=0.01;
  nsteps=100;
  nout=11;
#
```

```
# Problem parameters
  a=500000.5;
  b=499999.5;
#
# BDF coefficients
#
#   First order BDF
    a10=1; a11=-1;
#
#   Second order BDF
    a20=3/2; a21=-2; a22=1/2;
#
# Heading for solution
  cat(sprintf("    t      dy(1)      dy(2)      y(1)
    y(2)      erry(1)   erry(2)  iter\n"));
#
# nout outputs
  for(i in 1:nout){
#
#   Initial output or after nstep integration steps
#   completed; display Newton corrections, numerical and
#   exact solutions for output
    lambda1=-(a-b);
    lambda2=-(a+b);
    exp1=exp(lambda1*t);
    exp2=exp(lambda2*t);
    y1e=exp1-exp2;
    y2e=exp1+exp2;
    erry1=y1e-y[1];
    erry2=y2e-y[2];
    cat(sprintf("%10.1f%10.5f%10.5f%10.5f%10.5f%10.5f
       10.5f%6d\n",
          t,dy[1],dy[2],y[1],y[2],erry1,erry2,niter));
#
#   nsteps steps/output
    for(is in 1:nsteps){
#
#     Initialize iteration counter, stopping variable
      niter=1; stop=0;
#
#     Test for the end of the current step
```

```
        while(stop==0){
#
#         Functions g1, g2
          if(is==1){
             g=c(h*(-a*y[1]+b*y[2])-(a10*y[1]+a11*y0[1]),
                 h*( b*y[1]-a*y[2])-(a10*y[2]+a11*y0[2]));
           }else if(is>=2){
             g=c(h*(-a*y[1]+b*y[2])-(a20*y[1]+a21*y0[1]+
                 a22*y1[1]),
                 h*( b*y[1]-a*y[2])-(a20*y[2]+a21*y0[2]+
                   a22*y1[2]));
           }
#
#         Jacobian matrix, inverse
          jacob_1(t,y);
          Jinv=solve(J);
#
#         Newton corrections
          dy=-Jinv%*%g;
#
#         Update solution
          y=y+dy;
          stop=1;
#
#         Check if the corrections are within the tolerance
#            eps
          for(ic in 1:neqn){
            if(abs(dy[ic])>eps){
#
#               Convergence not achieved; continue calculation
                niter=niter+1;
                stop=0;
                break;
             }
           }
#
#         If maximum iterations reached, accept current step
          if(niter==maxiter){stop=1;}
        }
#
#     Integration step completed
```

```
    if(is>=1){
      y1=rep(0,neqn);
      y1=y0;
    }
      y0=y
      t=t+h;
#
#   Next integration step
    }
#
# Next output interval
  }
```

Listing A1.3 Solution of eqs. (A1.12) by a second-order BDF.

We can note the following details about Listing A1.3 that pertain specifically to the second-order BDF integration.

- The coefficients for the first- and second-order BDFs from Table A1.2 are programmed.

```
#
# BDF coefficients
#
#   First order BDF
    a10=1; a11=-1;
#
#   Second order BDF
    a20=3/2; a21=-2; a22=1/2;
```

- The first- and second-order BDF integrations are programmed according to eqs. (A1.12).

```
#
#      Functions g1, g2
       if(is==1){
         g=c(h*(-a*y[1]+b*y[2])-(a10*y[1]+a11*y0[1]),
             h*( b*y[1]-a*y[2])-(a10*y[2]+a11*y0[2]));
        }else if(is> =2){
          g=c(h*(-a*y[1]+b*y[2])-(a20*y[1]+a21*y0[1]+
            a22*y1[1]),
```

```
                h*( b*y[1]-a*y[2])-(a20*y[2]+a21*y0[2]+
                  a22*y1[2])));
    }
```

Note that for the first (implicit Euler) step (is=1), the first-order BDF coefficients are used. This provides two solutions points at $t = 0$ (the ICs) and $t = h = 0.01$ so that the second-order BDFs can be used subsequently as programmed with if(is>=2).

Thus, the extension of the first-order BDF to second order is straightforward. The numerical output from Listing A1.3 is in Table A1.5.

We can note the following details about this output.

- The errors have been reduced by approximately $1/10$ relative to the first-order BDF. For example,

```
Table A1.3, first order BDF,  t = 1, h = 0.01
  1.0  0.00000  0.00000  0.36971  0.36971 -0.00183
                                          -0.00183  2
```

```
Table A1.5, second order BDF, t = 1, h = 0.01
  1.0  0.00001  0.00001  0.36776  0.36776  0.00012
                                           0.00012  10
```

so that the error was decreased from -0.00183 to -0.00012 at $t = 1$ (note also the approach to the exact solution $e^{-1} = 0.3678794$ at $t = 1$).

- The improvement in accuracy required an increase in the number of Newton iterations (2 to 10). The reason for this increase is not clear and requires some additional analysis for clarification. The increase did not occur because of increased ill-conditioning of the Jacobian matrix because for this application, the Jacobian matrix is constant.

To conclude, the modest increase in the programming and computation for the second-order BDF produced a substantial improvement in the accuracy of the numerical solution of eqs. (A1.2).

TABLE A1.5   Numerical solution from Listing A1.3 with h=0.01, nsteps=100 for the second-order BDF.

t	dy(1)	dy(2)	y(1)	y(2)	erry(1) erry(2)	iter
0.0	0.00000	0.00000	0.00000	2.00000	0.00000	
					0.00000	0
1.0	0.00001	0.00001	0.36776	0.36776	0.00012	
					0.00012	10
2.0	-0.00001	-0.00001	0.13531	0.13531	0.00003	
					0.00003	9
3.0	0.00001	0.00001	0.04989	0.04989	-0.00011	
					-0.00011	8
4.0	0.00001	0.00001	0.01830	0.01830	0.00001	
					0.00001	6
5.0	-0.00001	-0.00001	0.00666	0.00666	0.00008	
					0.00008	5
6.0	-0.00001	-0.00001	0.00257	0.00257	-0.00009	
					-0.00009	3
7.0	0.00001	0.00001	0.00096	0.00096	-0.00005	
					-0.00005	2
8.0	-0.00001	-0.00001	0.00027	0.00027	0.00007	
					0.00007	1
9.0	-0.00000	-0.00000	0.00004	0.00004	0.00009	
					0.00009	1
10.0	-0.00000	-0.00000	0.00000	0.00000	0.00004	
					0.00004	1

A1.9   Third-Order BDF Integration

As a concluding example, we consider the use of a third-order BDF. The programming of Listing A1.3 requires modification in a few places.

- The maximum number of Newton iterations increases from 20 to 50.

```
#
# Convergence tolerance, maximum number of
# iterations to compute Newton corrections
```

```
eps=0.00001;
maxiter=50;
```

The subsequent numerical solution indicates that this is necessary.

• The coefficients from Table A1.2 for the first-, second-, and third-
order BDF integrators are programmed.

```
#
# BDF coefficients
#
#    First order BDF
     a10=1; a11=-1;
#
#    Second order BDF
     a20=3/2; a21=-2; a22=1/2;
#
#    Third order BDF
     a30=11/6; a31=-3; a32=3/2; a33=-1/3;
```

• Eqs. (A1.12) are programmed for the first-, second-, and third-
order BDF integrators.

```
#
# Functions g1, g2
  if(is==1){
      g=c(h*(-a*y[1]+b*y[2])-(a10*y[1]+a11*y0[1]),
          h*( b*y[1]-a*y[2])-(a10*y[2]+a11*y0[2]));
  }else if(is==2){
      g=c(h*(-a*y[1]+b*y[2])-(a20*y[1]+a21*y0[1]+
          a22*y1[1]),
          h*( b*y[1]-a*y[2])-(a20*y[2]+a21*y0[2]+
             a22*y1[2]));
  }else if(is>=3){
      g=c(h*(-a*y[1]+b*y[2])-(a30*y[1]+a31*y0[1]+
          a32*y1[1]+a33*y2[1]),
          h*( b*y[1]-a*y[2])-(a30*y[2]+a31*y0[2]+
             a32*y1[2]+a33*y2[2]));
```

For is=1 corresponding to $t = 0$, the first-order BDF is used. For
is=2 corresponding to $t = h = 0.01$, the second-order BDF is

used, and for `is>=3` corresponding to $t = 2h = 0.02$ and beyond, the third-order BDF is used. In this way, the required initial values of the solution are computed to start the third-order method.

The numerical solution is in Table A1.6.

TABLE A1.6   Numerical solution from Listing A1.3 with `h=0.01`, `nsteps=100` for the third-order BDF.

t	dy(1)	dy(2)	y(1)	y(2)	erry(1) erry(2)	iter
0.0	0.00000	0.00000	0.00000	2.00000	0.00000	
					0.00000	0
1.0	-0.00001	-0.00001	0.36797	0.36797	-0.00009	
					-0.00009	35
2.0	0.00001	0.00001	0.13534	0.13534	-0.00000	
					-0.00000	30
3.0	-0.00001	-0.00001	0.04976	0.04976	0.00003	
					0.00003	25
4.0	0.00001	0.00001	0.01832	0.01832	-0.00000	
					-0.00000	20
5.0	-0.00001	-0.00001	0.00661	0.00661	0.00013	
					0.00013	15
6.0	-0.00001	-0.00001	0.00230	0.00230	0.00018	
					0.00018	9
7.0	0.00001	0.00001	0.00095	0.00095	-0.00004	
					-0.00004	2
8.0	-0.00000	-0.00000	0.00027	0.00027	0.00006	
					0.00006	1
9.0	-0.00000	-0.00000	0.00000	0.00000	0.00012	
					0.00012	1
10.0	-0.00000	-0.00000	0.00000	0.00000	0.00005	
					0.00005	1

We can note the following details about this output.

- The errors have been reduced relative to the first- and second-order BDFs as expected. For example,

```
Table A1.3, first order BDF,  t = 1, h = 0.01
   1.0  0.00000  0.00000  0.36971  0.36971 -0.00183
                                           -0.00183  2

Table A1.5, second order BDF, t = 1, h = 0.01
   1.0  0.00001  0.00001  0.36776  0.36776  0.00012
                                            0.00012  10

Table A1.6, third order BDF,  t = 1, h = 0.01
   1.0 -0.00001 -0.00001  0.36797  0.36797 -0.00009
                                           -0.00009  35
```

so that the error was decreased from -0.00183 to -0.00012 to
-0.00009 at t = 1 (note again the approach to the exact solution
$e^{-1} = 0.3678794$ at t = 1).

- As before, the improvement in accuracy required an increase in
the number of Newton iterations (2 to 10 to 35). The reason
for this continuing increase is not clear and requires some additional analysis for clarification. As noted previously, the increase
did not occur because of increased ill-conditioning of the Jacobian matrix because for this application, the Jacobian matrix is
constant.

We can generally conclude from this numerical output that an
increase in the order of the BDF integrators produced more accurate solutions but at a decreasing rate of improvement and with a
substantial increase in the computational effort (number of Newton iterations). Of course, these conclusions may apply to only the
2×2 system of eqs. (A1.2) and may only offer some guidance about
the expected performance of the BDF integrators. Perhaps the most
important conclusion is that eq. (A1.18) provide a way to integrate a
system of stiff ODEs that can be far more efficient than an explicit
method, depending on the stiffness of the problem system (the spread
or spectrum of the eigenvalues for a linear ODE system).

We should also keep in mind that an analytical (exact) Jacobian
matrix was used in jacob_1 of Listing A1.2. As the number n of
ODEs increases, the Jacobian matrix scales as $n \times n$, which grows

very quickly with n. Thus, using the analytical Jacobian matrix may be infeasible and a numerical approximation of the Jacobian may be a necessary alternative. The details for how this might be done will not be discussed here, but this approach has been widely discussed in the literature ([1], [3], [4], [6]).

Also, because the Jacobian matrix is usually sparse in applications with large n (the Jacobian has mostly zeros), a sparse matrix integrator can be used to good advantage. For example, the ODE BDF integrator lsodes in the R library deSolve takes advantage of the sparsity of the Jacobian matrix, often with substantially reduced computation. lsodes [4] combines the features discussed previously to efficiently compute an ODE solution, that is, variable step (h refinement), variable order (p refinement), and sparse matrix methods (to avoid processing zeros in the Jacobian matrix).

A1.10 Conclusions

In this appendix, we have discussed some basic concepts pertaining to the stiffness of the ODE systems and how large stiffness might be accommodated with a calculation of reasonable length by using an implicit numerical integrator. Specifically, we have tested with the stiff problem of eqs. (A1.2) the BDF integrators that are widely used.

The improved performance of stiff integrators, however, involves greater computational complexity than for explicit methods (generally the solution of linear or nonlinear algebraic or transcendental equations, e.g., eq. (A1.18)), depending on whether the ODE system is linear or nonlinear); therefore implicit methods should be used only if the ODE system is stiff. Also, we should not conclude that a nonlinear ODE system is necessarily stiff, and therefore, an implicit integrator is required.

This final discussion suggests a fundamental question: "How do we know if an ODE system is stiff and therefore an implicit integrator should be used?" In the case of linear ODE systems, we can look at the spectrum (spread) of the eigenvalues, as we did in Table A1.1. However, in the case of nonlinear ODEs, eigenvalues are not defined (and therefore cannot be studied for possible stiffness). For this more general case (of nonlinear ODEs), we suggest the following criterion for determining if an implicit integrator should be used:

maximum stable step $<<$ problem timescale

In other words, observe if the ODE problem timescale is much greater than the largest integration step (h) that can be taken while still maintaining a stable solution, which suggests that stability is the limiting condition on h, and therefore, the ODE system is effectively stiff so that an implicit integrator should be used.

To illustrate the application of this criterion, for the 2×2 ODE system of eqs. (A1.2) with a =5,00,000.5, b = 499999.5, and $\lambda_1 = -(a - b) = -1, \lambda_2 = -(a + b) = -1,000,000$, so that the preceding criterion gives for the explicit Euler method (with $|h\lambda| \le 2$)

$$\frac{2}{1,000,000} << 10$$

which implies that an implicit integrator should be used.

However, we now have two additional questions to answer in applying the preceding criterion for stiffness (involving the maximum integration step and problem timescale):

1. How do we determine the maximum integration step for an explicit integrator that still produces a stable solution? Ans: In general, by trial and error using a computer program with an explicit integrator. Or, if the computer run times for a stable explicit solution are large, or an excessive number of derivative evaluations is required to maintain a stable solution, an implicit integrator may possibly be used to good advantage.

2. How do we determine the timescale for the ODE problem? Ans: Either from some knowledge of the characteristics of the problem such as physical reasoning, or again, by trial and error to observe when a complete solution appears to have been computed.

In other words, some trial and error with an explicit integrator is generally required. If the computational effort required to compute a complete solution appears to be excessive, switch to an implicit integrator.

Admittedly, this procedure is rather vague (to the author's knowledge a general easily applied mathematical test is not available, especially for nonlinear problems), and some trial and error with explicit integrators first, followed possibly by a switch to implicit integrators, may be required (this is the procedure we generally follow for a new ODE problem). Also, lsoda [4] in the R library deSolve switches automatically between nonstiff and stiff options based on an analysis of the apparent largest ODE eigenvalue (the "a" in lsoda stands for "automatic"). Experience has indicated that this quality integrator can be used reliably to avoid having to choose between a nonstiff and a stiff integrator.

References

[1] Brenan, K.E., S.L. Campbell, and L.R. Petzold (1996), *Numerical Solution of Initial-value Problems in Differential-algebraic Equations*, SIAM, Philadelphia, PA.

[2] Gear, C.W. (1971), *Numerical Initial Value Problems in Ordinary Differential Equations*, Prentice-Hall, Englewood Cliffs, NJ.

[3] Hairer, E., and G. Wanner (1991), *Solving Ordinary Differential Equations II: Stiff and Differential-algebraic Problems*, Springer-Verlag, Berlin.

[4] Hindmarsh, A.C. (1983), *ODEPACK, A Systematized Collection of ODE Solvers*, in Scientific Computing, R.S. Stepleman, et al. (eds.), North-Holland, Amsterdam, pp 55–64.

[5] Shampine, L.F. (1994), *Numerical Solution of Ordinary Differential Equations*, Chapman and Hall, New York.

[6] Shampine, L.F., and S. Thompson (2007), Stiff systems, Scholarpedia, vol. 2, no. 3, p 2855; available at: http://www.scholarpedia.org/article/stiff_systems.

■ INDEX

Differential Equation Analysis in Biomedical Science and Engineering: Ordinary Differential Equation
Applications with R, First Edition. William E. Schiesser.
© 2014 John Wiley & Sons, Inc. Published 2014 by John Wiley & Sons, Inc.